Marine Algal Antioxidants

Marine Algal Antioxidants

Editors

Christophe Brunet
Clementina Sansone

MDPI • Basel • Beijing • Wuhan • Barcelona • Belgrade • Manchester • Tokyo • Cluj • Tianjin

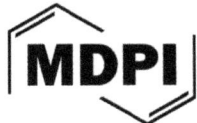

Editors
Christophe Brunet
Stazione Zoologica Anton Dohrn
Italy

Clementina Sansone
Stazione Zoologica Anton Dohrn
Italy

Editorial Office
MDPI
St. Alban-Anlage 66
4052 Basel, Switzerland

This is a reprint of articles from the Special Issue published online in the open access journal *Antioxidants* (ISSN 2076-3921) (available at: https://www.mdpi.com/journal/antioxidants/special_issues/Marine_Algal_Antioxidants).

For citation purposes, cite each article independently as indicated on the article page online and as indicated below:

LastName, A.A.; LastName, B.B.; LastName, C.C. Article Title. *Journal Name* **Year**, *Article Number*, Page Range.

ISBN 978-3-03936-878-5 (Hbk)
ISBN 978-3-03936-879-2 (PDF)

© 2020 by the authors. Articles in this book are Open Access and distributed under the Creative Commons Attribution (CC BY) license, which allows users to download, copy and build upon published articles, as long as the author and publisher are properly credited, which ensures maximum dissemination and a wider impact of our publications.

The book as a whole is distributed by MDPI under the terms and conditions of the Creative Commons license CC BY-NC-ND.

Contents

About the Editors vii

Clementina Sansone and Christophe Brunet
Marine Algal Antioxidants
Reprinted from: *Antioxidants* **2020**, *9*, 206, doi:10.3390/antiox9030206 1

Marie Emilie Wekre, Karoline Kåsin, Jarl Underhaug, Bjarte Holmelid and Monica Jordheim
Quantification of Polyphenols in Seaweeds: A Case Study of *Ulva intestinalis*
Reprinted from: *Antioxidants* **2019**, *8*, 612, doi:10.3390/antiox8120612 5

Mariana Manzoni Maroneze, Leila Queiroz Zepka, Eduardo Jacob Lopes, Antonio Pérez-Gálvez and María Roca
Chlorophyll Oxidative Metabolism During the Phototrophic and Heterotrophic Growth of *Scenedesmus obliquus*
Reprinted from: *Antioxidants* **2019**, *8*, 600, doi:10.3390/antiox8120600 21

Gaurav Rajauria
In-Vitro Antioxidant Properties of Lipophilic Antioxidant Compounds from 3 Brown Seaweed
Reprinted from: *Antioxidants* **2019**, *8*, 596, doi:10.3390/antiox8120596 37

Delphine Nègre, Méziane Aite, Arnaud Belcour, Clémence Frioux, Loraine Brillet-Guéguen, Xi Liu, Philippe Bordron, Olivier Godfroy, Agnieszka P. Lipinska, Catherine Leblanc, Anne Siegel, Simon M. Dittami, Erwan Corre and Gabriel V. Markov
Genome–Scale Metabolic Networks Shed Light on the Carotenoid Biosynthesis Pathway in the Brown Algae *Saccharina japonica* and *Cladosiphon okamuranus*
Reprinted from: *Antioxidants* **2019**, *8*, 564, doi:10.3390/antiox8110564 55

Clementina Sansone and Christophe Brunet
Promises and Challenges of Microalgal Antioxidant Production
Reprinted from: *Antioxidants* **2019**, *8*, 199, doi:10.3390/antiox8070199 79

Ulrike Neumann, Felix Derwenskus, Verena Flaiz Flister, Ulrike Schmid-Staiger, Thomas Hirth and Stephan C. Bischoff
Fucoxanthin, A Carotenoid Derived from *Phaeodactylum tricornutum* Exerts Antiproliferative and Antioxidant Activities In Vitro
Reprinted from: *Antioxidants* **2019**, *8*, 183, doi:10.3390/antiox8060183 89

Arianna Smerilli, Sergio Balzano, Maira Maselli, Martina Blasio, Ida Orefice, Christian Galasso, Clementina Sansone and Christophe Brunet
Antioxidant and Photoprotection Networking in the Coastal Diatom *Skeletonema marinoi*
Reprinted from: *Antioxidants* **2019**, *8*, 154, doi:10.3390/antiox8060154 101

Yanan Xu and Patricia J. Harvey
Red Light Control of β-Carotene Isomerisation to 9-cis β-Carotene and Carotenoid Accumulation in *Dunaliella salina*
Reprinted from: *Antioxidants* **2019**, *8*, 148, doi:10.3390/antiox8050148 121

Bao Le, Kirill S. Golokhvast, Seung Hwan Yang and Sangmi Sun
Optimization of Microwave-Assisted Extraction of Polysaccharides from *Ulva pertusa* and Evaluation of Their Antioxidant Activity
Reprinted from: *Antioxidants* **2019**, *8*, 129, doi:10.3390/antiox8050129 135

Yanan Xu and Patricia J. Harvey
Carotenoid Production by *Dunaliella salina* under Red Light
Reprinted from: *Antioxidants* **2019**, *8*, 123, doi:10.3390/antiox8050123 . . . . **149**

José Joaquín Merino, José María Parmigiani-Izquierdo, Adolfo Toledano Gasca and María Eugenía Cabaña-Muñoz
The Long-Term Algae Extract (*Chlorella and Fucus sp*) and Aminosulphurate Supplementation Modulate SOD-1 Activity and Decrease Heavy Metals (Hg^{++}, Sn) Levels in Patients with Long-Term Dental Titanium Implants and Amalgam Fillings Restorations
Reprinted from: *Antioxidants* **2019**, *8*, 101, doi:10.3390/antiox8040101 . . . . **163**

About the Editors

Christophe Brunet senior researcher, Stazione Zoologica Anton Dohrn, Naples, Italy) obtained his Ph.D. in 1994 in biological oceanography at the University of Paris VI (Pierre et Marie Curie). He became researcher at the Stazione Zoologica di Napoli (SZN, Italy) in 2000. Since 2017, he is senior scientist at the SZN. His research interests deal with and microalgal ecophysiology and biotechnology. C. Brunet is interested in algal growth, production of bioactive compounds from microalgae and technological development for carrying out ecological and biotechnological experiments. He is involved in projects in which he is carrying out fundamental and applied research as well as in technological development for improving the role and importance of microalgae in biotechnological applications. He is author of more than 70 scientific publications and three European or Italian patents. He is involved in the Editorial Board of Antioxidants, Scientific reports and Advances in Oceanography and Limnology journals.

Clementina Sansone is a Researcher since 2012 at Stazione Zoologica Anton Dohrn. Her research activity is focused on Marine Biotechnology for human and ocean health. Her interest lies in drug discovery from marine micro and macro-organisms, for applications as pharmaceuticals, nutraceuticals and cosmetics. She was involved in testing the bioactivity of chemical compounds from marine microalgae and invertebrates on several human cell lines.

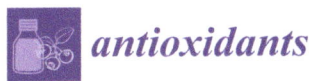

Editorial

Marine Algal Antioxidants

Clementina Sansone * and Christophe Brunet

Stazione Zoologica Anton Dohrn, Villa comunale, 80121 Napoli, Italy; christophe.brunet@szn.it
* Correspondence: clementina.sansone@szn.it

Received: 19 February 2020; Accepted: 28 February 2020; Published: 2 March 2020

Sea and marine biodiversity exploration represents a new frontier for the discovery of new natural products with human health benefits ("the exploitable biology", [1]).

New compounds suitable for nutraceuticals, cosmeceuticals, or pharmaceuticals require (i) eco-friendly production and (ii) bioactivity against illness, thus making microorganisms potential interesting targets. Among them, microalgae provide advantages as they are photosynthetic, high growth rate organisms that are easy to cultivate and require less space than higher plants, together with displaying high chemodiversity—though this has barely been explored—coupled with high biodiversity [2]. Although very attractive compared to higher plants, microalgae biotechnology still requires further research and development to lower its cost and enhance practical and industrial interest [3,4]. One of the main branches of the biotechnological exploration of marine algae concerns bioactive and, especially, antioxidant compounds.

This Special Issue, concerning marine algal antioxidants, contains eleven contributions detailing recent advances in this field; experimental results and technical improvements are presented and discussed.

Antioxidant bioactivity concerns different families of compounds, but this issue is focused on the microalgae richness of such compounds (e.g., [5,6]). Among the huge variety of antioxidant compounds, algae derived carotenoids are the most well known, together with other bioactive compounds, such as polyphenols, sterols, carbohydrates, and vitamins [6]. The synergistic effect of all of these families in unicellular organisms induces the high antioxidant power of microalgae that is comparable, or even higher than, the antioxidant activity of higher plants or fruits [5]. The potentiality of a single microalgae cell compared with that of a multicellular plant presents a biotechnological challenge for developing microalgae as an efficient and ecosustainable "bio factory" of bioactive molecules with antioxidant activity. For this reason, it is very important to invest in research programs aiming to investigate the diversity of bioactive molecules along the microalgal biodiversity scale and its intracellular modulation [2].

In a recent study [7], the coastal diatom *Skeletonema marinoi* was used to investigate the modulation of lipophilic antioxidant compounds and the hydrophilic vitamin c by light manipulation. The results revealed a significant effect of light (intensity and/or distribution) on the production of antioxidants as well as a strong link between carotenoid operating photoprotection and the antioxidant molecules and activity modulation. This study confirms the role of light manipulation as a powerful tool for modulating the synthesis of antioxidant compounds in microalgae.

The most frequently investigated algae compounds are carotenoids due to their well-known bioactivity and human wellness benefits as well as their plasticity which allows them to be enhanced through abiotic factors, for example, light modulation in microalgae [2,8].

Dunaliella salina, a chlorophyte that is mostly used for biotechnological investigations and applications, mainly relies on the production of β-carotene [9], has been used as a model to study the modulation of carotenoids and β-carotene concentration with respect to the light spectrum [10,11]. This study demonstrates that monochromatic red light strongly affects the carotenoid pool, enhancing the β-carotene concentration as well as modifying the ratio between the different forms of β-carotene towards 9-cis β-carotene. These studies confirm the relevant role of light in shaping the carotenoid profile in microalgae, demonstrating that its modulation is of great interest for the biotechnological production of such bioactive compounds.

The enhancement of carotenoid production in algae can use genetic engineering and biomanipulation. In order to reach this goal, it is necessary to increase the knowledge about the biosynthetic pathways of these compounds as well as the modulation factors affecting the gene expression involved. Two brown algae, *Saccharina japonica* and *Cladosiphon okamuranus*, have been investigated thanks to the analysis of Genome–Scale Metabolic Networks (GSMNs, [12]). The authors were able to reconstruct the biosynthetic pathways of the main carotenoids in these two algae, highlighting the interest and scientific richness of such approach for the study of targeted biochemical pathways.

Together with carotenoids, chlorophylls and their derivatives are also of interest for biotechnological applications [13]. Enhancing the production of chlorophylls per biomass unit in microalgae and understanding the biosynthetic and degradation pathways of such molecules is therefore biotechnologically relevant. The study by Maroneze and collaborators [13] reported and discussed the modulation of the chlorophyll and carotenoid contents in the model species *Scenedesmus obliquus* with respect to the growth phase and the presence/absence of light, turning growth from autotrophy to heterotrophy. The authors demonstrated that the content and chemical forms of these compounds are affected by growth conditions, laying the foundation for up-scaling and massive production for industrial application.

On the other hand, i.e., in brown algae, fucoxanthin is now being investigated for its potential activity related to human health protection [14]. This pigment might be extracted from numerous classes of microalgae, including diatoms as well as brown macroalgae [14]. The anti-inflammatory, antioxidant, and antiproliferative effects of fucoxanthin were investigated on blood mononuclear cells and different cell lines [15]. The results clearly displayed the antiproliferative and antioxidant activities of fucoxanthin in vitro, highlighting the great interest in its potential use in nutraceuticals.

Pigments are not the only compounds presenting antioxidant properties; other lipophilic compounds such as phenols and hydrophilic compounds accompany them.

It is therefore of interest to investigate the best solvents for obtaining the best yield from the extraction of bioactive compounds from algal biomass. For this reason, in three brown algae [16], the antioxidant properties and antioxidant compound concentration were compared between seven extraction solvents or mixtures between them. This work defined the best extraction procedure for enhancing the harvesting of phenols, flavonoids, carotenoids, and chlorophylls. In the same framework, a technical approach comparing methodologies for the quantification of polyphenols was undertaken on the macroalga *Ulva intestinalis* [17], highlighting some uncertainties and difficulties in actual methodologies that require further optimization of the extraction, identification, and quantification of polyphenols.

In addition, polysaccharides are also relevant antioxidant compounds, and algae might be a relevant source for their production and use as nutraceuticals [18]. In the contribution by Le et al. [19], the authors compared data from different extraction procedures of the green alga *Ulva pertusa* in terms of antioxidant activity together with polysaccharide and ulvan contents. The differences between the various extracts were compared with regard to operational parameters such as power, time, water-to-raw-material ratio, and pH, in order to optimize the quantity yield of ulvan.

Last, but not least, extracts from *Fucus* spiralis and *Chlorella vulgaris* were tested as enhancers of the removal of heavy metals (Hg^{++}, Ag, Sn, Pb) in patients with long-term dental titanium implants and amalgam filling restoration [20]. The authors demonstrated that long-term effects from nutritional supplementation with these algae result in the enhancement of heavy metal removal.

All of these contributions highlight the great potential of marine algae to provide substances/extracts that are able to protect or increase human wellness, and the need for optimization and technological/technical/scientific improvement to increase the biomass-harvesting efficacy with reduction of the production cost. Marine biotechnology relies on the exploration, discovery, and exploitation of marine algal species and/or products still requires research dealing with biodiversity (searching for new targeted species with peculiar biochemical profiles, for instance), chemodiversity (richness and diversity of bioactive molecule screening), bioactivity (antioxidant ability of the algal extracts), technological cultivation improvement (lowering the costs, co-cultivation, environmental modulation), and optimization of the extraction techniques. These steps are crucial to achieve the challenges offered by the green (blue in case of marine) biotechnological revolution which, in our point of view, cannot exist without deployment of the industrial use of (micro)algae.

Conflicts of Interest: The authors declare no conflict of interest.

References

1. Bull, A.T.; Ward, A.C.; Goodfellow, M. Search and Discovery Strategies for Biotechnology: The Paradigm Shift. *Microbiol. Mol. Biol. Rev.* **2000**, *64*, 573–606. [CrossRef] [PubMed]
2. Barra, L.; Chandrasekaran, R.; Corato, F.; Brunet, C. The challenge of ecophysiological biodiversity for biotechnological applications of marine microalgae. *Mar. Drugs* **2014**, *12*, 1641–1675. [CrossRef] [PubMed]
3. Williams, P.J.B.; Laurens, L.M.L. Microalgae as biodiesel & biomass feedstocks: Review & analysis of the biochemistry, energetics & economics. *Energy Environ. Sci.* **2010**, *3*, 554–590.
4. Kroumov, A.D.; Scheufele, F.B.; Trigueros, D.E.G.; Modenes, A.N.; Zaharieva, M.; Najdenski, H. Modeling and Technoeconomic Analysis of Algae for Bioenergy and Coproducts. *Algal Green Chem.* **2017**, 201–241. [CrossRef]
5. Sansone, C.; Brunet, C. Promises and Challenges of Microalgal Antioxidant Production. *Antioxidants* **2019**, *8*, 199. [CrossRef] [PubMed]
6. Galasso, C.; Gentile, A.; Orefice, I.; Ianora, A.; Bruno, A.; Noonan, D.M.; Sansone, C.; Albini, A.; Brunet, C. Microalgal Derivatives as Potential Nutraceutical and Food Supplements for Human Health: A Focus on Cancer Prevention and Interception. *Nutrients* **2019**, *11*, 1226. [CrossRef] [PubMed]
7. Smerilli, A.; Balzano, S.; Maselli, M.; Blasio, M.; Orefice, I.; Galasso, C.; Sansone, C.; Brunet, C. Antioxidant and Photoprotection Networking in the Coastal Diatom *Skeletonema marinoi*. *Antioxidants* **2019**, *8*, 154. [CrossRef] [PubMed]
8. Brunet, C.; Chandrasekaran, R.; Barra, L.; Giovagnetti, V.; Corato, F.; Ruban, A.V. Spectral radiation dependent photoprotective mechanism in diatom *Pseudo-nitzschia multistriata*. *PLoS ONE* **2014**, *9*, e87015. [CrossRef] [PubMed]
9. Tafreshi, A.H.; Shariati, M. Dunaliella biotechnology: Methods and applications. *J. Appl. Microbiol.* **2009**, *107*, 14–35. [CrossRef] [PubMed]
10. Xu, Y.; Harvey, P. Carotenoid Production by *Dunaliella salina* under Red Light. *Antioxidants* **2019**, *8*, 123. [CrossRef] [PubMed]
11. Xu, Y.; Harvey, P. Red Light Control of β-Carotene Isomerisation to 9-cis β-Carotene and Carotenoid Accumulation in *Dunaliella salina*. *Antioxidants* **2019**, *8*, 148. [CrossRef] [PubMed]
12. Nègre, D.; Aite, M.; Belcour, A.; Frioux, C.; Brillet-Guéguen, L.; Liu, X.; Bordron, P.; Godfroy, O.; Lipinska, A.; Leblanc, C.; et al. Genome–Scale Metabolic Networks Shed Light on the Carotenoid Biosynthesis Pathway in the Brown Algae *Saccharina japonica* and *Cladosiphon okamuranus*. *Antioxidants* **2019**, *8*, 564. [CrossRef]
13. Maroneze, M.; Zepka, L.; Lopes, E.; Pérez-Gálvez, A.; Roca, M. Chlorophyll Oxidative Metabolism During the Phototrophic and Heterotrophic Growth of *Scenedesmus obliquus*. *Antioxidants* **2019**, *8*, 600. [CrossRef] [PubMed]
14. Zhang, H.; Tang, Y.; Zhang, Y.; Zhang, S.; Qu, J.; Wang, X.; Kong, R.; Han, C.; Liu, Z. Fucoxanthin: A Promising Medicinal and Nutritional Ingredient. *Evid. Based Complement. Alternat. Med.* **2015**, *2015*, 723515. [CrossRef] [PubMed]
15. Neumann, U.; Derwenskus, F.; Flaiz Flister, V.; Schmid-Staiger, U.; Hirth, T.; Bischoff, S. Fucoxanthin, A Carotenoid Derived from *Phaeodactylum tricornutum* Exerts Antiproliferative and Antioxidant Activities In Vitro. *Antioxidants* **2019**, *8*, 183. [CrossRef] [PubMed]
16. Rajauria, G. In-Vitro Antioxidant Properties of Lipophilic Antioxidant Compounds from three Brown Seaweed. *Antioxidants* **2019**, *8*, 596. [CrossRef] [PubMed]
17. Wekre, M.; Kåsin, K.; Underhaug, J.; Holmelid, B.; Jordheim, M. Quantification of Polyphenols in Seaweeds: A Case Study of *Ulva intestinalis*. *Antioxidants* **2019**, *8*, 612. [CrossRef] [PubMed]

18. Wells, M.L.; Potin, P.; Craigie, J.S.; Raven, J.A.; Merchant, S.S.; Helliwell, K.E.; Smith, A.G.; Camire, M.E.; Brawley, S.H. Algae as nutritional and functional food sources: Revisiting our understanding. *J. Appl. Phycol.* **2017**, *29*, 949–982. [CrossRef] [PubMed]
19. Le, B.; Golokhvast, K.; Yang, S.; Sun, S. Optimization of Microwave-Assisted Extraction of Polysaccharides from *Ulva pertusa* and Evaluation of Their Antioxidant Activity. *Antioxidants* **2019**, *8*, 129. [CrossRef] [PubMed]
20. Merino, J.; Parmigiani-Izquierdo, J.; Toledano Gasca, A.; Cabaña-Muñoz, M. The Long-Term Algae Extract (*Chlorella* and *Fucus* sp.) and Aminosulphurate Supplementation Modulate SOD-1 Activity and Decrease Heavy Metals (Hg++, Sn) Levels in Patients with Long-Term Dental Titanium Implants and Amalgam Fillings Restorations. *Antioxidants* **2019**, *8*, 101. [CrossRef] [PubMed]

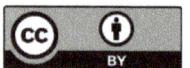

© 2020 by the authors. Licensee MDPI, Basel, Switzerland. This article is an open access article distributed under the terms and conditions of the Creative Commons Attribution (CC BY) license (http://creativecommons.org/licenses/by/4.0/).

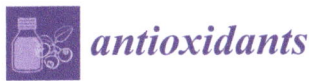

Article

Quantification of Polyphenols in Seaweeds: A Case Study of *Ulva intestinalis*

Marie Emilie Wekre [1,2], Karoline Kåsin [1,3], Jarl Underhaug [1], Bjarte Holmelid [1] and Monica Jordheim [1,*]

1. Department of Chemistry, University of Bergen, Allégt. 41, N-5007 Bergen, Norway; marie.wekre@uib.no (M.E.W.); karoline.kasin@nmbu.no (K.K.); jarl.underhaug@uib.no (J.U.); bjarte.holmelid@uib.no (B.H.)
2. Alginor ASA, Haraldsgata 162, N-5525 Haugesund, Norway
3. Faculty of Chemistry, Biotechnology and Food Science, Norwegian University of Life Science, Universitetstunet 3, N-1433 Ås, Norway
* Correspondence: monica.jordheim@uib.no; Tel.: +47-55-58-35-48

Received: 14 October 2019; Accepted: 30 November 2019; Published: 3 December 2019

Abstract: In this case study, we explored quantitative ^{1}H NMR (qNMR), HPLC-DAD, and the Folin-Ciocalteu assay (TPC) as methods of quantifying the total phenolic content of a green macroalga, *Ulva intestinalis*, after optimized accelerated solvent extraction. Tentative qualitative data was also acquired after multiple steps of purification. The observed polyphenolic profile was complex with low individual concentrations. The qNMR method yielded 5.5% (DW) polyphenols in the crude extract, whereas HPLC-DAD and TPC assay yielded 1.1% (DW) and 0.4% (DW) respectively, using gallic acid as the reference in all methods. Based on the LC-MS observations of extracts and fractions, an average molar mass of 330 g/mol and an average of 4 aromatic hydrogens in each spin system was chosen for optimized qNMR calculations. Compared to the parallel numbers using gallic acid as the standard (170 g/mol, 2 aromatic H), the optimized parameters resulted in a similar qNMR result (5.3%, DW). The different results for the different methods highlight the difficulties with total polyphenolic quantification. All of the methods contain assumptions and uncertainties, and for complex samples with lower concentrations, this will be of special importance. Thus, further optimization of the extraction, identification, and quantification of polyphenols in marine algae must be researched.

Keywords: seaweeds; green algae; marine algae; *Ulva intestinalis*; *Enteromorpha intestinalis*; quantification; polyphenols; flavonoids; apigenin; accelerated solvent extraction; ASE; HPLC-LRMS; HPLC-HRMS; HPLC; TPC; Folin–Ciocalteu; TFC; qNMR

---

1. Introduction

Marine macroalgae, or seaweed, is a large group of macroscopic organisms that are an important component in aquatic ecosystems. The wide diversity of marine organisms is being recognized as a rich source of functional materials and, in 2015, the global seaweed aquaculture production reached 30 million tons [1]. Although marine algae have gained increasing attention over the last years due to the fact of their bioactive natural substances with potential health benefits, they are still identified as an underexploited resource [2–6].

Natural antioxidants with multifunctional potential are of high interest, and numerous studies have focused on natural antioxidants, including polyphenols and flavonoids, from terrestrial plants [7–9]. However, the application potential of polyphenolic analyses of marine sources suffers from several factors, most importantly, the lack of exactness with respect to quantitative and qualitative data at a molecular level. Marine plant material with analytic matrices at very low concentrations and a high and variable dissolved salt concentration makes polyphenol analyses challenging [4,10]. The diversity of phenolic compounds also varies from simple to highly polymerized substances which makes qualitative and quantitative procedures, involving sample preparation and extraction, difficult to standardize. Thus, this makes for a further challenge in the analyses and in furthering the research in this field.

Colorimetric assays, such as Folin-Ciocalteu, have been extensively used to quantify phlorotannins and polyphenolic content in seaweeds. However, since the assay is difficult to standardize and not selective, it has been recommended to use the assay for approximate measurements of an extract's antioxidant potential only [11–15]. Since the colorimetric assays neither separate nor give a correct quantitative measurement of the individual compounds, high-performance liquid chromatography (HPLC) has been the method of choice for separation and quantification of polyphenols in plants. The HPLC with multiple diode array UV-Visible detection (DAD) quantifies according to Lambert-Beer's law ($A = \varepsilon cl$). A compound's ability to absorb UV-Visible light (A) is related to the compound's molar absorptivity value (ε) and molar concentration (c). The diversity of molar absorptivity values of polyphenols is almost as large as the number of polyphenols existing; even within the same polyphenol class, there will be differences [16]. In the lack of commercially available standards, one standard is often chosen when total amounts of polyphenols or phlorotannins are quantified. Gallic acid (GA) seems to be the most used standard for total polyphenolic quantification and phloroglucinol (PG) for the phlorotannin quantification in brow algae [17–20]. In addition to the limitations with commercially available standards, HPLC will also suffer from a lack of separation of complex extract matrices and loss of compound amounts due to the irreversible retention on the HPLC column during elution.

In recent years, quantitative ^{1}H NMR (qNMR) have gained increasing attention as a method for quantitative determination of metabolites in complex biological matrices [21–23]. According to the review by Pauli et al. (2012) [22] and references therein, qNMR methods have proven successful when standard chromatographic methods have been ineffective [22]. In general, qNMR can be considered a primary ratio method of measurement in which the analytes can be correlated directly to a calibration standard, and since the reference compound differs from the analytes, generating a calibration curve becomes unnecessary. However, the quantification needs to be validated with reference compounds. Some work on quantification of phlorotannins in brown algae (*Ascophyllum nodosum*, *Fucus vesiculosus*, and *Cystoseira tamariscifolia*) with qNMR has been done using internal standards [14,23].

In this case study, we examined the polyphenolic content of the green algae *Ulva intestinalis* (syn. *Enteromorpha intestinalis*) collected on the west coast of Norway. An optimized extraction of the polyphenolic content was performed. The extract and semi-purified fractions were further analysed utilizing qNMR with an external reference for quantification of the total phenolic content. For comparison, HPLC-DAD and TPC assay analyses were also performed. To further explore the diverse group of polyphenols in *Ulva intestinalis*, qualitative analyses were performed with HPLC-DAD, HPLC-LR, and HR-MS. We entered this case study with the overarching goal of examining which analytical methods could lead to a more reliable value of polyphenolic content in seaweed and, thus, obtain a better view of the grand potential of seaweed phenolics.

2. Materials and Methods

2.1. Plant Materials

Samples of *Ulva intestinalis* (syn. *Enteromorpha intestinalis*) were collected in June from the western coast of Norway; Rogn, Ormhilleren (60°29'38.8" N 4°55'11.9" E). The voucher specimen of *Ulva intestinalis* was deposited in the Herbarium BG (Voucher no. BG-A-75) at the University Museum of Bergen, Bergen.

2.2. Chemicals

All chemicals used were of analytical grade. Methanol (≥99.9%), acetonitrile (≥99.8%), trifluoroacetic acid (TFA) and Folin-Ciocalteu reagent were all acquired form Sigma-Aldrich (Sigma-Aldrich, St. Louis,

MO, USA). Formic (98–100%) and acetic (99.8%) acids were both acquired from Riedel-de Haën (Honeywell Inc., Charlotte, NC, USA). Luteolin, apigenin, myrcetin, diosmetin, quercetin, caffeic acid, coumaric acid, ferulic acid, sinapic acid, and gallic acid reference standards were all purchased from Sigma–Aldrich (Sigma-Aldrich, St. Louis, MO, USA). The analytical standard of tricin was purchased from PhytoLab (PhytoLab BmbH & Co. KG, Vestenbergsgreuth, Germany), (+)-catechin was purchased from USP (USP, Rockville, MD, USA), and DPPH free radical was purchased from Merck (Merck, Kenilworth, NJ, USA). Deionized water was deionized at the University of Bergen (Bergen, Norway).

2.3. Extraction and Purification

The collected plant material was washed thoroughly in fresh water and air dried. Dried plant material was stored at −20 °C when not used. Dried material was extracted using ASE (Accelerated Solvent Extraction) (Dionex™ ASE™ 350, Thermo Fisher Scientific, Waltham, MA, USA). A dried sample of *Ulva intestinalis* (55.9 g) was mixed with Dionex ASE prep DE sand and added to 66 mL stainless-steel cells with two glass fiber filters placed at the bottom end of the cell, before being extracted using a Dionex ASE 350 Accelerated Solvent Extractor. The extraction procedure consisted of two different methods, one being a pre-soak method, and the other being the primary extraction method. Pre-soaking consisted of extraction at 23 °C under 1500 psi. The static extraction period was 1 min with a flush volume of 50% of cell volume, purged with N_2 for 70 s, and 100% deionized water was used as the solvent in the pre-soak method. The primary extraction method consisted of preheating for 5 min, and samples were then extracted at 70 °C under 1500 psi. Static extraction time was 5 min with a flush volume of 60% of the cell volume, purged with N_2 for 100 sec. The solvent used for the primary extraction was a mixture of deionized water and methanol (40:60, *v/v*). Primary extraction was repeated two times. The volume of the combined extract was reduced using a rotavapor, and the concentrated aqueous extract was partitioned against ethyl acetate (EtOAc) four times. The contents of both the EtOAc phase and the water phase were examined using HPLC-DAD, HPLC-LRMS, HPLC-HRMS, and colorimetric assays including Total Phenolic Content Assay (TPC) and Total Flavonoid Content Assay (TFC). Before analysis, all phases were carefully reduced to dryness using rotavapor, and, finally, the samples were dried under N_2 gas.

The aqueous extract was applied to an Amberlite XAD-7 column and washed with distilled water. Methanol was applied for elution. The pre-eluted washing water was analyzed for polyphenols with HPLC. Collected methanolic fractions (XAD7-A, XAD7-B, XAD7-C) were reduced using a rotavapor and analyzed on analytical HPLC. The XAD-7 fraction A contained the highest number of polyphenols and was chosen to be submitted to preparative HPLC to obtain three purified fractions; prepLC-A1, -A2, and -A3 (Figure 1).

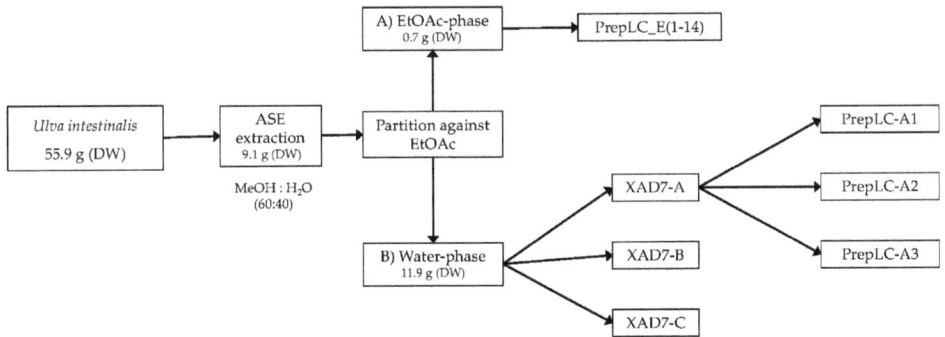

Figure 1. Overview of the extraction and purification steps in the *Ulva intestinalis* analysis.

2.4. General Instrumentation

2.4.1. Preparative HPLC

The preparative HPLC system consisted of a Gilson 321 pump (Gilson Inc., Middleton, WI, USA), an Ultimate 3000 variable wavelength detector (Dionex, Thermo Fisher Scientific, Sunnyvale, CA, USA), and a 25 × 2.12 cm (10 μm) UniverSil C18 column (Fortis Technologies Ltd., Neston, UK). Two solvents were used: (A) super distilled water (0.1% acetic acid) and (B) acetonitrile (0.1% acetic acid) with initial conditions of 90% A and 10% B followed by an isocratic elution for the first 5 minutes, and the subsequent linear gradient conditions, 5–18 min: to 16% B, 18–22 min: to 18% B, 26–31 min: to 28% B, 31–32 min: to 40% B, 32–40 min: isocratic at 40% B, 40–43 min: to 10% B. The flow rate was 15 mL/min, and the aliquots of 750 μL were injected.

2.4.2. Analytical HPLC-DAD

All HPLC-DAD analyses were performed on an Agilent 1260 Infinity HPLC system (Agilent Technologies, Santa Clara, CA, USA) equipped with a 1260 diode array detector (DAD) and a 200× C analysis was performed using two solvents, (A) super distilled water (0.5% TFA) and (B) acetonitrile (0.5% TFA), in a gradient (0–10 min: 95% A + 5% B, 10–20 min: 85% A + 15% B, 20–34 min: 60% A + 40% B. 34–35 min: 95% A + 5% B). The flow rate was 1.0 mL/min, and aliquots of 20 μL were injected with an Agilent 1260 vial sampler. UV-Vis absorption spectra were recorded during the HPLC analysis over the wavelength range of 200–600 nm in steps of 2 nm.

The established HPLC method was validated for linearity, sensitivity, precision, and accuracy. Table 1 presents data for calibration curves, test ranges, limit of detection (LOD), and limit of quantification (LOQ) for gallic acid. The LOD and LOQ were calculated based on the standard deviation of y-intercepts of the regression line (S_y) and the slope (S), using the equations LOD = 3.3 × S_y/S and LOQ = 10 × S_y/S.

Table 1. Calibration curve, limit of detection (LOD), and limit of quantification (LOQ) for gallic acid (GA) (Sigma-Aldrich) at 280 nm and 330 nm.

Standard	Calibration Curve (μg/mL)	R^2	Test Range (μg/mL)	LOD (μg/mL)	LOQ (μg/mL)
Gallic acid (280 nm)	y = 65.536x − 366.51	0.9988	10–500	14.1	42.8
Gallic acid (330 nm)	y = 0.2603x − 0.8339	0.9993	10–500	18.5	56.0

2.4.3. HPLC-LRMS and HPLC-HRMS

Liquid chromatography low-resolution mass spectrometry (HPLC-LRMS) (ESI+/ESI−) was performed using an Agilent Technologies 1260 Infinity Series system and an Agilent Technologies 6420A triple quadrupole mass spectrometry detector. The following conditions were applied: ionization mode: positive/negative, capillary voltage = 3000 V, gas temperature = 300 °C, gas flow rate = 3.0 L/min, acquisition range = 100–800 m/z. The elution profile for HPLC consisted of the following gradient: 0–3 min: 90%A + 10%B, 3–11 min: 86%A + 14%B, 11–15.5 min: 60%A + 40%B, 15.5–17 min: 90%A + 10%B, at a flowrate = 0.3 mL/min, where solvent A was super distilled water (0.5% formic acid), and solvent B was acetonitrile (0.5% formic acid). A 50 × 2.1 mm internal diameter, 1.8 μm Agilent Zorbax SB-C18 column was used for separation. Calibration curve of Apigenin ran on HPLC-LRMS and used for quantification is listed in Table 2.

Table 2. Calibration curve, limit of detection (LOD), and limit of quantification (LOQ) for apigenin (Sigma-Aldrich) acquired using HPLC-LRMS.

Standard	Calibration Curve (mM)	R^2	Test Range (mM)	LOD (mM)	LOQ (mM)
Apigenin	$y = (2.0 \times 10^{-6})x - 2054.6$	0.995	0.00156–0.0125	0.0014	0.0041

Liquid chromatography high-resolution mass spectrometry (HPLC-HRMS) (ESI+/TOF) was performed using an AccuTOF JMS-T100LC (JEOL, Peabody, USA) mass spectrometer in combination with an Agilent Technologies 1200 Series HPLC system. The following instrumental settings/conditions were used: ionization mode: positive, ion source temperature = 220 °C, needle voltage = 2500 V, desolvation gas flow = 4 L/min, nebulizing gas flow = 3 L/min, orifice1 temperature = 125 °C, orifice2 voltage = 10 V, ring lens voltage = 20 V, ion guide RF voltage = 1600 V, detector voltage = 2350 V, acquisition range = 15–1000 m/z, spectral recording interval = 0.50 sec, wait time = 0.033 nsec, and data sampling interval = 2 nsec. The elution profile for HPLC consisted of the same gradient and column as described for HPLC-LRMS, but the flowrate was increased to 0.35 mL/min.

2.4.4. NMR Spectroscopy

Quantification of the extracts of *Ulva intestinalis* was performed using ^{1}H NMR analyses on a Bruker 600 MHz instrument (Bruker BioSpin, Zürich, Switzerland). All spectra were recorded in DMSO-d_6 at 25 °C. The pulse sequence applied was $zg30$ with the following acquisition parameters: sweep width of 19.8 ppm, 64 k data points, 16 scans, and 2 dummy scans. The relaxation delay, d1, was set to 40 sec (equal to $5 \times T_{1,max}$) to ensure complete relaxation between scans. The spectra were processed using a line broadening of 0.3 Hz. The crude extract was used for T_1 measurements, utilizing the *t1ir* pulse sequence with a sweep width of 19.8 ppm, 16 k data points, 8 scans, 2 dummy scans, and 9 different inversion recovery delays between 1 ms and 5 s. Measured T_1 values ranged from 1.0–8.1 s.

Quantification using the ^{1}H NMR spectra was performed using the ERETIC2 function in TopSpin with DMSO$_2$ (10 mM) as an external reference. The DMSO$_2$ signal (~3.0 ppm) was integrated and defined as the ERETIC reference (No. H = 6, Mm = 94.13 g/mol, V(sample) = 0.75 mL, C = 10 mM).

Reference compounds for validation were gallic acid (GA), *p*-coumaric acid, ferulic acid, (+)-catechin, and luteolin (10 mM, DMSO-d_6). An average standard deviation of < 10% was observed. The integrations were repeated three times.

Two-dimensional heteronuclear single quantum coherence (^{1}H-^{13}C HSQC), heteronuclear multiple bond correlation (^{1}H-^{13}C HMBC), and double quantum filtered correlation (^{1}H-^{1}H DQF COSY) spectra were also recorded on the Bruker 600 MHz instrument.

2.5. Total Phenolic Content Assay

For the determination of total phenolic content, the Folin-Ciocalteu total phenolic content assay (TPC) was used. The method used was adapted from Ainsworth and Gillespie (2007) [24]. 200 µL of the sample or standard was added to the cuvettes (10 × 45 mm, 3 mL), followed by 400 µL 10% (*v/v*) Folin–Ciocalteu reagent in super distilled water. Further, 1600 µL 700 mM Na$_2$CO$_3$ in super distilled water was added to the cuvettes. The mixture was incubated for 30 minutes, and the absorbance was measured at 765 nm using a Shimadzu UV-1800 UV spectrophotometer and a Shimadzu CPS-100 cell positioner (Shimadzu, Kyoto, Japan). Data was expressed as gallic acid equivalents (GAE). An incubation time of 2 h was also tested.

2.6. Total Flavonoid Content Assay

For the determination of the total flavonoid content, 2 mL test solution (standard or sample) was added to four cuvettes (10 × 45 mm, 3 mL) and the absorbance measured at 425 nm with solvent in the reference cuvette. An aliquot of AlCl3 solution (0.5 mL, 1%, *w/v*) was added to three of the four cuvettes, and the same volume of solvent was added to the fourth (blank sample). The content of the cuvettes was stirred thoroughly, and the absorbance measured at 1 minute intervals at 425 nm for 10 minutes at 22 °C. For quantitative analysis apigenin was chosen as the reference compound (concentration range of 1–500 µg/mL). Procedure modified from Pękal and Pyrzynska (2014) [25].

3. Results and Discussion

3.1. Quantification of Polyphenols in Ulva Intestinalis

In this work, extraction of polyphenols was performed after optimization of extraction parameters utilizing a Dionex ASE 350 extraction instrument (see Section 2.3). Aliquots (10 mL) of the different phases, ASE (Accelerated Solvent Extractor) Crude, (A) EtOAc and (B) water (see Figure 1) were sampled and dried for weight determination and further quantification with HPLC-DAD, qNMR, TPC, and TFC. The results of the different quantification methods are shown in Tables 3–5.

Table 3. Quantification of polyphenols in the crude extract and liquid–liquid extraction phases of crude with HPLC.

Sample	g DW	%PP GAE	mg (GAE)/g DW
ASE crude	9.1	1.1 ± 0.14	11.3 ± 1.4
(A) EtOAc	0.7	0.7 ± 0.2	6.7 ± 0.2
(B) Water	11.9	0.6 ± 0.1	5.5 ± 0.9
A + B	12.6	1.2 ± 0.1	12.1 ± 0.5

PP = polyphenol; (A) EtOAc = ethyl acetate phase; (B) water phase; GAE = gallic acid equivalents; DW = Dry Weight.

Table 4. Quantification of polyphenols in the crude extract and liquid–liquid extraction phases of crude with qNMR.

Sample	DW	GAE			330 Mw eq.			mg (GAE)/g DW	mg (330 Mw eq.) g DW
	g	%PP			%PP				
		2H	4H	6H	2H	4H	6H	4H	4H
ASE Crude	9.1	5.5 ± 0.5	2.7 ± 0.3	1.8 ± 0.2	10.6 ± 1	5.3 ± 0.5	3.5 ± 0.4	27.3 ± 2.7	52.9 ± 5.2
(A) EtOAc	0.7	0.502 ± 0.002	0.251 ± 0.001	0.167 ± 0.001	1.01 ± 0.07	0.50 ± 0.04	0.30 ± 0.03	2.51 ± 0.01	5.0 ± 0.4
(B) Water	11.9	4.9 ± 0.3	2.5 ± 0.2	1.7 ± 0.1	9.7 ± 0.7	4.8 ± 0.3	3.2 ± 0.1	24.9 ± 1.5	48.5 ± 3.3
A + B	12.6	5.5 ± 0.2	2.7 ± 0.3	1.9 ± 0.1	10.7 ± 0.4	5.3 ± 0.2	3.6 ± 0.1	27.4 ± 1.1	53.5 ± 2.1

PP = polyphenol; (A) EtOAc = ethyl acetate phase; (B) water phase; GAE = gallic acid equivalents; 330 Mw eq. = equivalents of average mass found from MS; 2H, 4H, and 6H = assumptions made related to the number of aromatic ^{1}H in each polyphenolic spin system; DW = Dry Weight.

Table 5. Quantification of polyphenols in the crude extract and liquid–liquid extraction phases of crude with total phenolic content (TPC).

Sample	g DW	GAE %PP	mg (GAE)/g DW
ASE crude	9.1	0.4 ± 0.1	5 ± 1
(A) EtOAc	0.7	0.035 ± 0.001	0.3 ± 0.2
(B) Water	11.9	0.4 ± 0.1	3.6 ± 1.5
A + B	12.6	0.5 ± 0.1	4 ± 1

PP = polyphenol; (A) EtOAc = ethyl acetate phase; (B) water phase; GAE = gallic acid equivalents; DW = Dry Weight.

3.2. Quantification Utilizing High-Performance Liquid Chromatography (HPLC) with Wavelength Detector (DAD)

Quantification of polyphenols in plants and foods has been a topic of discussion and research for years, and among the different methods HPLC-DAD it has been the method of choice due to the possibility of separation of compounds before individual quantification. However, with the use of retention times, absorption spectra, and molar absorptivity, the technique is often limited when it comes to simultaneous determination of polyphenols of different groups [9]. Table 6 illustrates the different area responses observed in HPLC for different standards with the same concentration, reflecting the molar absorptivity differences.

Table 6. Illustration of molar absorptivity differences expressed with HPLC integrated peak areas (280 nm and 330 nm) of selected standards (5 mM) used in polyphenolic quantification.

Standard	Compound Class	λ_{max} (nm)	280 nm	330 nm
p-Coumaric acid	HCA	(230), 310	2754 ± 43	4743 ± 4
Gallic acid (GA)	HBA	272	2884 ± 2	8.7 ± 0.3
(+)-Catechin	Flavan-3-ol	279	5687 ± 6	2.1 ± 0.4
Apigenin	Flavone	(267), 340	801,120 ± 2361	131,812 ± 1525

HCA = hydroxycinnamic acid, HBA = hydroxybenzoic acid

When dealing with complex polyphenolic mixtures with unknown identities, which is the case for seaweeds, one standard is often selected for quantification. Traditionally, gallic acid is chosen for total polyphenolic quantification and phloroglucinol (PGE) for total phlorotannin quantification as seen for brown algae [17–20]. In this work, gallic acid (GA) was chosen as the reference standard, since the nature of the polyphenols in the green algae *U. intestinalis* was unknown, and since we wanted to compare different quantification methods. However, there is no doubt that the estimation of the total polyphenol content will suffer from this.

The HPLC peaks with maximum intensity in the 280 nm (R_t: 1–15 min) were quantified according to the 280 nm GA standard curve (Table 1), while peaks with maximum intensity in the 330 nm (R_t: 15–35 min) window were quantified according to the 330 nm GA standard curve. This resulted in an HPLC-DAD quantification of 1.1% polyphenols in the algae, based on quantification on the ASE crude extract (11.3 ± 1.4 mg GAE/g DW) (Table 3). The recovery of the polyphenols after the liquid-liquid ethyl acetate partition was quantified to be 1.2% (12.1 ± 0.5 mg GAE/g DW), almost evenly distributed into the (A) EtOAc phase (0.7%) and the (B) water phase (0.6%). Thus, the total recovery for A + B was relatively close to the initial amounts found in the crude.

3.3. Quantitative NMR (qNMR)

In order to get closer to a "true" estimation of polyphenol content in seaweeds, quantifications using ^{1}H NMR (qNMR) were performed (Table 4). One of the advantages of qNMR is that there is no need to consider the large variation observed regarding the molar absorptivity of different phenolic compounds (Table 6) nor the loss of sample during chromatography as with HPLC analyses. When quantifying polyphenols from NMR, one can consider two regions for quantification: the –OH spectral region, as shown by Nerantzakie et al. [23], or the aromatic 1H region [14,26]. Nerantzaki et al. presented a method for total phenolic content determination of crude plant extracts based on phenol type –OH resonances in the region between 14–8 ppm. Signals were selected after observation of elimination, or reduction, of the signal intensities after irradiation of the residual water resonance. In our marine *U. intestinalis* samples, the phenol –OH type resonances were observed at low intensities and were too broad to perform reliable integration. The broad signals may be attributed to the nature of the marine extract, containing many different types of phenol –OH resonances. Additionally, the ASE crude and the water phase contained some water, even after careful drying, which increases the phenol –OH exchange with the water peak. The 10–8.5 ppm region of the EtOAc phase (Figure 2) showed several sharp signals; however, these signals were found to not represent phenol –OH resonances due to the fact of their observed $^1J_{CH}$ correlations in the HSQC spectrum.

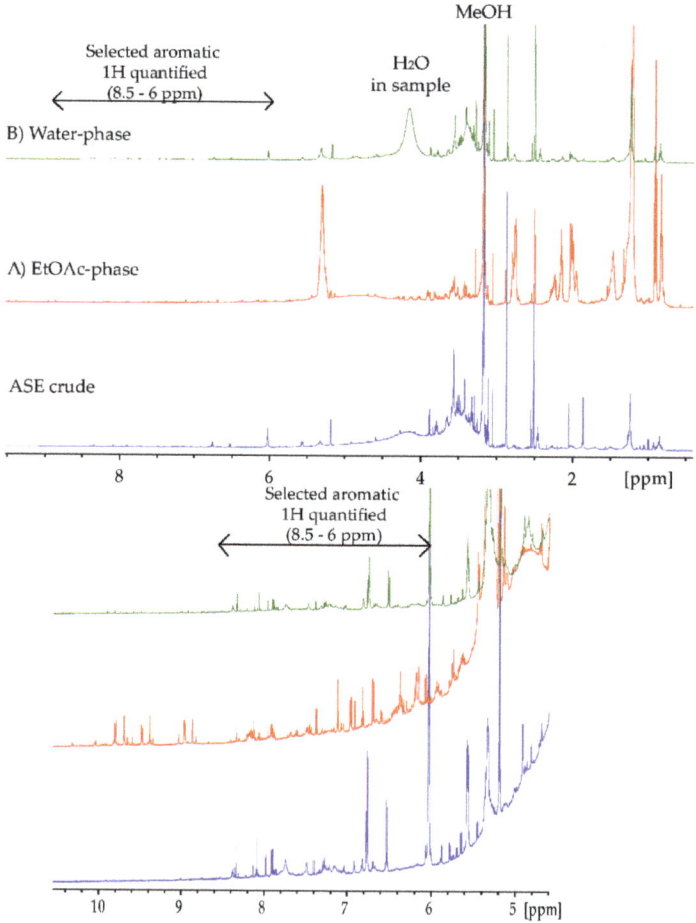

Figure 2. ^{1}H-NMR spectrum (600 MHz) for ASE crude (blue), (**A**) EtOAc phase (red), and (**B**) water phase (green) recorded in DMSO-d_6 at 25 °C. 2D spectra were used to deselect peaks in the 8.5–6 ppm region belonging to the same spin system, avoiding multiple quantification.

For qNMR calculations, characteristic aromatic signals in the 8.5–6 ppm region of the ^{1}H NMR spectra were integrated individually, and quantifications were added together to yield the total phenolic content (Section 2.4.4, Figure 2) [21,25]. Additionally, two-dimensional NMR spectra, such as COSY, HSQC and HMBC, were recorded to deselect signals belonging to the same molecule as far as possible in order to avoid multiple quantifications. The qNMR calculations were validated with quantification of standards (Section 2.4.4). Quantifications were calculated using the ERETIC2 function in TopSpin (Bruker) with DMSO$_2$ as an external reference (C = 10 mM). However, to quantify the signals, a molar mass is needed. The molar mass of gallic acid was chosen in order to obtain comparable results. Quantifications were also calculated using an average molar mass of 330 g/mol based on observed masses from the MS analyses (Table 4). Additionally, an average value of aromatic protons found in each polyphenolic spin system must be chosen. This assumption will also introduce uncertainty. Nerantzakie et al. [23] made their quantification on phenol –OH and used an average of 2 OH for each spin system related to their standard, caffeic acid. In Table 4, the polyphenolic content calculation utilizing different average aromatic protons are shown, resulting in a 33% difference between the maximum (2 aromatic H) and minimum (6 aromatic H) values calculated. Based on our tentatively identified compounds in Table 7 it seemed like 4 aromatic protons (H) was a reasonable assumption. The qNMR method thus yielded a polyphenolic content of 5.3% in the crude (52.9 ± 5.2 mg 330 Mw eq./g DW). Due to the parallel numbers, using gallic acid (170 g/mol) and 2 aromatic protons yielded similar results (Table 4).

Table 7. Overview of tentatively identified low-mass polyphenols/simple phenolics at different stages of purification with HPLC-LRMS.

Observed R_t (min)	$(M+H)^+$	Tentative identification	LC-MS R_t Confirmed with Standard	Compound Class	Phase
1.56	171	Gallic acid	+	HBA	XAD7-A
4.74	127	Phloroglucinol *	−	benzentriol	EtOAc
6.93	291	Catechin	+	flavan-3-ol	EtOAc
8.11	181	Caffeic acid	+	HCA	EtOAc, XAD7-C
8.67	169	Vanilic acid *	−	HBA	EtOAc
9.02	165	Coumaric acid	+	HCA	EtOAc
10.10	475	Chicoric acid *	−	HCA	XAD7-B
10.27	195	Ferulic acid	+	HCA	EtOAc
10.27	183	Veratric acid *	−	HBA	EtOAc
10.51	225	Sinapic acid	+	HCA	XAD7-B
10.65	321	Luteic acid *	−	HBA	XAD7-A
12.31	475	Valoneic acid *	−	HBA	Crude, H$_2$O, XAD7-A
12.50	319	Myricetin *	−	flavone	XAD7-A, prepLC-A3
12.90	287	Luteolin *, HR	+	flavone	EtOAc, prepLC-A3
12.98	303	Quercetin	+	flavonol	EtOAc, PrepLC-A3
13.16	273	Naringenin *	−	flavanone	PrepLC-A3
13.69	271	Apigenin (2.62 ng/g)	+	flavone	PrepLC-A3
14.43	303	Hesperetin *	−	flavanone	PrepLC-A3
14.76	289	Aromadendrin/eriodictyol *	−	flavanonol/flavanone	EtOAc
14.93	301	Diosmetin	+	flavone	XAD7-A, PrepLC-A2
14.95	303	Ellagic acid *	−	HT	XAD7-A
15.61	331	Rhamnazin *, HR	−	flavone	EtOAc, prepLC-A3
16.12	579	Procyanidin B1 *	−	PAC	PrepLC-A2, EtOAc
16.76	256	Chrysin *	−	flavone	Crude
16.80	317	Isorhamnetin *	−	flavonol	PreLC-A3

HCA = hydroxycinnamic acid, HBA = hydroxybenzoic acid, HT = hydrolysable tannins, PAC = proanthocyanidin. * Several possible isomers; HR HR-LC-MS mass; + = identity confirmed with standard on LR-LC-MS, - = identity not confirmed with standard on LR-LC-MS.

3.4. Colorimetric Assays: Total Phenolic Content (TPC) and Total Flavonoid Content (TFC)

The Folin–Ciocalteu assay is the most common assay used to quantify phenolic content (TPC) in both terrestrial plants and seaweeds. However, the assay is debatable due to the lack of standardization and lack of specificity in the reaction mechanism resulting in the colorimetric quantification [11–15,27]. This is of importance for all colorimetric assays, including the total flavonoid content (TFC) assay [25,28]. With increasing purity of the samples, direct quantitative measurements seem to be more reliable. However, the difficulty of standardizing this assay does not seem to be without importance.

The TPC assay (Table 5) resulted in a total of 0.4% in the ASE crude (5 ± 1 mg GAE/g DW), with a recovery of 0.04% in the (A) EtOAc phase (0.035 ± 0.001 mg GAE/g DW) and 0.4% in the (B) water phase (0.4 ± 0.1 mg GAE/g DW). Relatively high standard deviations were observed for the aqueous phases, potentially reflecting the lack of reliability of the method and difficulties with standardization.

The relative partition of polyphenols found between the two phases (A:B) in the TPC assay seem to follow the pattern observed from the qNMR quantification (10:90) (Table 4), rather than the partition ratio found in the HPLC-DAD analyses (50:50) (Table 3). The different ratio observed from the HPLC analyses is most likely due to the impact of molar absorptivity difference between the standard used and the compounds present.

The occurrence of flavonoids in algae is a central topic [29–32], and we chose to run a TFC assay in parallel with our attempts to identify flavonoids in our extracts (Table 8). The TFC assay gave a total of 0.03% flavonoids in the ASE Crude (0.2 ± 0.4 mg apigenin eq./g DW) and 0.13% in the (A) EtOAc phase (0.2 ± 0.4 mg apigenin eq./g DW). No flavonoids were detected in the (B) water phase with the TFC method.

Table 8. Quantification of flavonoids in the crude extract and liquid–liquid extraction phases of crude with total flavonoid content (TFC).

Sample	g DW	mg Apigenin Equivalents	mg (Apigenin eq.)/g DW
ASE crude extract	9.1	0.03 ± 0.04 [a]	0.3 ± 0.4 [a]
(A) EtOAc phase	0.7	0.13 ± 0.01	1.3 ± 0.1
(B) Water phase	11.9	n.d.	n.d.
A + B	12.6	0.13 ± 0.01	1.3 ± 0.1

[a] Three parallels measured from (0–34 mg); n.d.= not detected; PP = polyphenol; FL = flavonoid; (A) EtOAc = ethyl acetate phase; (B) water phase; TFC = total flavonoid content; DW = Dry Weight.

3.5. Qualitative Analysis of Polyphenols in Ulva intestinalis

After ASE extraction of the polyphenols (Figure 3; HPLC profile and selected UV-Vis spectra) and partition of the aqueous crude extract against ethyl acetate, the concentrated water phase (B) was applied to a XAD-7 column, washed with distilled water, and then eluted with methanol (Figure 1). The pre-eluted washing water was analyzed for polyphenols with HPLC-DAD. Collected methanolic fractions (XAD7 A–C) were reduced using a rotavapor and analyzed using analytical HPLC. The XAD-7 fraction A showed the highest polyphenol content and was chosen to be submitted to preparative HPLC to obtain three major fractions (prepLC A1–A3, Figure 1). The EtOAc phase was also submitted to preparative HPLC. The liquid–liquid partition with ethyl acetate gave some selectivity with respect to separation of compounds as seen in Figure 4. The compounds found in the EtOAc phase were most likely less polar and seemed to have a shorter chromophore compared to compounds observed in the water phase. The compounds in the water phase also showed an additional absorption band around 412–414 nm.

The preparative HPLC gave some separation of compounds; however, the samples were still complex. All the phases and fractions underwent extensive analyses with HPLC-DAD, HPLC-LRMS, HPLC-HRMS, and NMR. The results of the HPLC-LRMS analyses are shown in Table 7, giving an overview of the tentatively identified compounds.

Fragmentation patterns were difficult to obtain due to low concentrations. The ESI-MS spectra were recorded in both positive and negative modes. The masses of a luteolin-isomer ($(M+H)^+$, calculated: 287.05556, exact: 287.05599, $C_{15}H_{10}O_6$, Δppm 1.5) and a rhamnazin-isomer ($(M+H)^+$, calculated: 331.08178, exact: 331.08178, $C_{17}H_{14}O_7$, Δppm 1.24) were confirmed with HPLC-HRMS. The rhamnazin-isomer (m/z 331.08178) did not overlap with the commercial standard tricin (330 Mw) in the HPLC-LRMS SIM scan.

The most conclusive evidence of the presence of flavonoids in the green algae U. intestinalis was found in the late preparative fraction: prepLC-A3 (Figure 5). This fraction contained many of the peaks observed between 15 and 35 min in the HPLC profile of the crude (330 nm) (Figure 3). Several of the flavonoid masses found were tentatively identified from this fraction (Table 7) which has its origin from the water phase (B). The TFC assay did not detect any flavonoids in the water phase (Table 8) which illustrates the problem with relaying on these colorimetric assays. One flavonoid in the prepLC-A3 fraction was identified to be apigenin, using overlaid an HPLC-LRMS SIM scan at m/z 271 $(M+H)^+$ with an apigenin standard (Figure 5). The amount of the apigenin in the algae was found to be 2.617 ng/g (DW) using an apigenin calibration curve (Table 2).

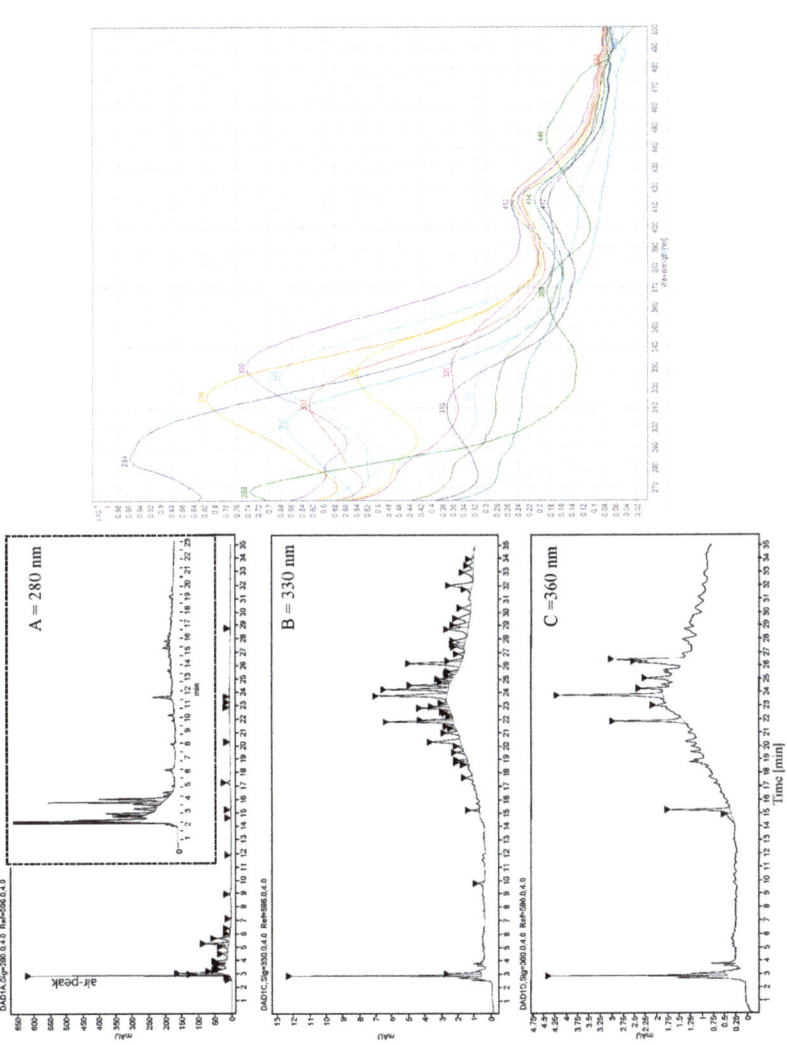

Figure 3. (**Left**) HPLC profile of ASE crude extract of *U. intestinalis* shown at three different wavelengths (A: 280 nm, B: 330 nm, and C: 360 nm). (**Right**) UV-Visible spectrum of selected HPLC-peaks from 15 to 35 min in the (B) 330 nm window.

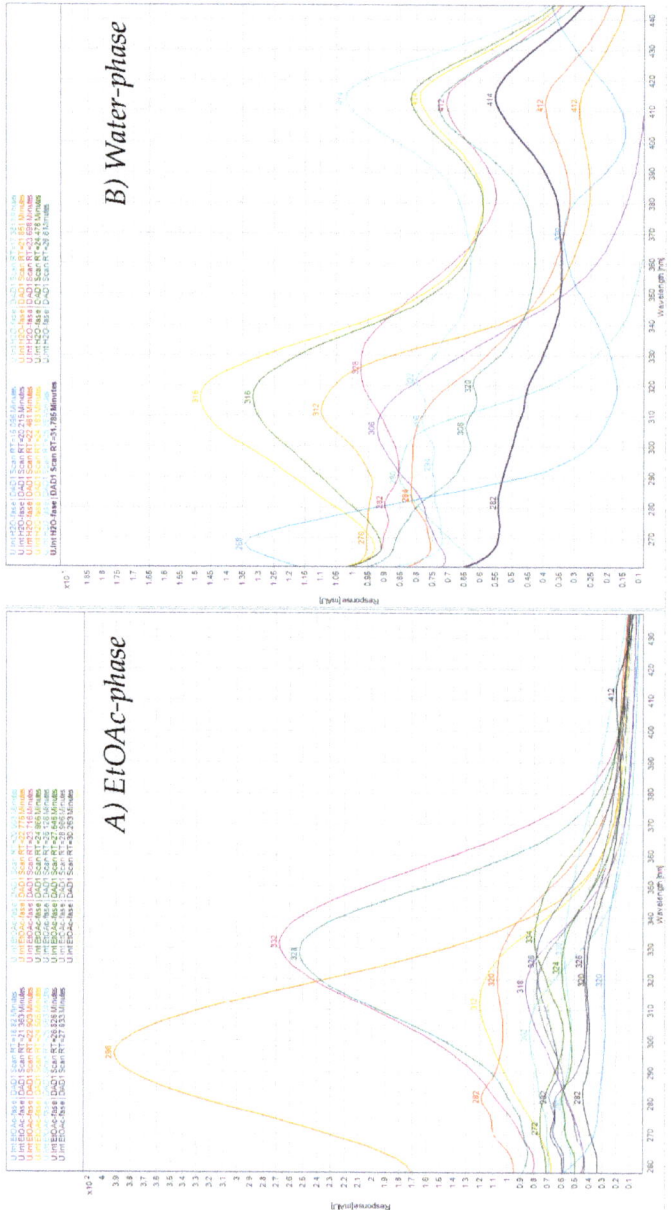

Figure 4. UV-Visible spectra of HPLC peaks found in the (A) EtOAc phase (**left**) and the (B) water phase (**right**) recorded at 330 nm from 15 to 35 min in the chromatograms.

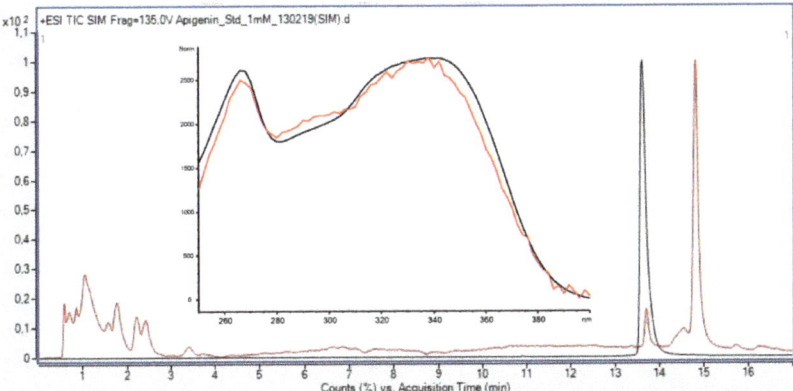

Figure 5. Overlaid HPLC-LRMS (+ESI) SIM Scan at *m/z* 271 of prepLC-A3 fraction (red line, C (Api, HPLC-LRMS) = 2.62 ng/g DW) and apigenin standard (C = 1.00 mM) (black line).

4. Conclusion

This case study provides an optimized extraction process for polyphenolic extraction of algae. The total polyphenolic content was quantified with qNMR (5.3%), HPLC-DAD (1.1%), and TPC (0.4%). Flavonoids and polyphenolic acids were tentatively identified in *Ulva intestinalis* samples. Apigenin was confirmed in one of the semi-purified fractions.

The same samples yielded different total phenolic contents when utilizing the different analytical methods, highlighting the difficulties related to polyphenolic quantification in extracts. All methods utilized in this study depend on assumptions and, thus, also uncertainty. This will be of special importance when analyzing complex samples at low concentrations as is the case for the polyphenolic content in marine algae. Further standardization and optimization of total phenolic quantifications of marine algae samples should be researched.

Author Contributions: M.J. and M.E.W. conceived and designed the experiments; M.J. collected the algae materials; J.U. contributed with support and discussions concerning the qNMR experiments; B.H. contributed with support and discussions concerning the HPLC-LRMS methods and instrumentation; B.H. recorded the HPLC-HRMS data; M.E.W. performed all the laboratory work, the HPLC-DAD, TPC, qNMR, and HPLC-LR and HRMS experiments; K.K. developed the ASE-350 extraction method and the HPLC-LRMS method, and modified and performed the TFC assay. M.E.W. and M.J. analyzed the data. M.J. and M.E.W. wrote the paper. All authors read and approved the final manuscript.

Funding: The authors are grateful to the University of Bergen, Norway, for Open Access funding (710029/884). This work was partly supported by the Bergen Research Foundation (BFS-NMR-1), Sparebankstiftinga Sogn og Fjordane (509-42/16), and the Research Council of Norway through the Norwegian NMR Platform, NNP (226244/F50).

Acknowledgments: M.E.W. gratefully acknowledges the Norwegian Research Council, NFR, and Alginor ASA (Haugesund) for her fellowship

Conflicts of Interest: The authors declare no conflict of interest.

References

1. Food and Agriculture Organization of the United Nations (FAO). *The State of World Fisheries and Aquaculture 2018—Meeting the Sustainable Development Goals*; License: Rome, Italy, 2018; CC BY-NC-SA 3.0 IGO.
2. Hu, J.; Yang, B.; Lin, X.; Zhou, X.-F.; Yang, X.-W.; Liu, Y. Bioactive metabolites from seaweeds. In *Handbook of Marine Macroalgae: Biotechnology and Applied Phycology*, 1st ed.; Kim, S.-K., Ed.; John Wiley & Sons: Hobroken, NJ, USA, 2012; Volume 1, pp. 262–284.
3. Pangestuti, R.; Kim, S.-K. Biological activities and health benefit effects of natural pigments derived from marine algae. *J. Funct. Foods.* **2011**, *3*, 255–266. [CrossRef]

4. Rajauria, G. Optimization and validation of reverse phase HPLC method of qualitative and quantitative assessment of polyphenol in seaweed. *J. Pharm. Biomed. Anal.* **2018**, *148*, 230–237. [CrossRef]
5. Gómez-Guzmán, M.; Rodríguez-Nogales, A.; Algieri, F.; Gálvez, J. Potential role of seaweed polyphenols in cardiovascular-associated disorders. *Mar. Drugs* **2018**, *16*, 250. [CrossRef] [PubMed]
6. Ganesan, A.R.; Tiwari, U.; Rajauria, G. Seaweed nutraceuticals and their therapeutic role in disease prevention. *Food Sci. Hum. Wellness* **2019**, *8*, 256–263. [CrossRef]
7. Pietta, P.-G. Flavonoids as antioxidants. *J. Nat. Prod.* **2000**, *63*, 1035–1042. [CrossRef]
8. Crozier, A.; Jaganath, I.B.; Clifford, M.N. Dietary phenolics: Chemistry, bioavailability and effects on health. *Nat. Prod. Rep.* **2009**, *26*, 1001–1043. [CrossRef]
9. Ignat, I.; Volf, I.; Popa, V.I. A critical review of methods for characterisation of polyphenolic compounds in fruit and vegetables. *Food Chem.* **2011**, *126*, 1821–1835. [CrossRef]
10. Monbet, P.; Worsfold, P.; McKelvie, I. Advances in marine analytical chemistry. *Talanta* **2019**, *202*, 610. [CrossRef]
11. van Alstyne, K.L. Comparison of three methods for quantifying brown algal polyphenolic compounds. *J. Chem. Ecol.* **1995**, *21*, 45–58. [CrossRef]
12. Singleton, V.L.; Orthofer, R.; Lamuela-Raventós, R.M. Analysis of total phenols and other oxidation substrates and antioxidants by means of Folin-Ciocalteu reagent. *Methods Enzymol.* **1999**, *299*, 152–178.
13. Ikawa, M.; Schaper, T.D.; Dollard, C.A.; Sasner, J.J. Utilization of Folin–Ciocalteu phenol reagent for the detection of certain nitrogen compounds. *J. Agric. Food Chem.* **2003**, *51*, 1811–1815. [CrossRef] [PubMed]
14. Parys, S.; Rosenbaum, A.; Kehraus, S.; Reher, G.; Glombitza, K.-W.; König, G.M. Evaluation of quantitative methods for the determination of polyphenols in algal extracts. *J. Nat. Prod.* **2007**, *70*, 1865–1870. [CrossRef] [PubMed]
15. Jackobsen, C.; Sørensen, A.-D.; Holdt, S.L.; Akoh, C.C.; Hermund, D.B. Source, extraction, characterization, and applications of novel antioxidants from seaweed. *Annu. Rev. Food Sci. Technol.* **2019**, *10*, 541–568. [CrossRef] [PubMed]
16. Jordheim, M.; Aaby, K.; Fossen, T.; Skrede, G.; Andersen, Ø.M. Molar absorptivities and reducing capacity of pyranoanthocyanins and other anthocyanins. *J. Agric. Food Chem.* **2007**, *55*, 10591–10598. [CrossRef]
17. Li, X.; Fu, X.; Duan, D.; Liu, X.; Xu, J.; Gao, X. Etraction and identification of phlorotannins from the brown alga, *Sargassum fusiforme* (Harvey) Setchell. *Mar. Drugs* **2017**, *15*, 49. [CrossRef]
18. Barbosa, M.; Lopes, G.; Ferreres, F.; Andrade, P.B.; Pereira, D.M.; Gil-Izquierdo, Á.; Velntãno, P. Phlorotannin extracts from Fucales: Marine polyphenols as bioregulators engaged in inflammation-related mediators and enzymes. *Algal Res.* **2017**, *28*, 1–8. [CrossRef]
19. Machu, L.; Misurcova, L.; Ambrozova, J.V.; Orsavova, J.; Mlcek, J.; Sochor, J.; Jurikova, T. Phenolic content and antioxidant capacity in algal food products. *Molecules* **2015**, *20*, 1118–1133. [CrossRef]
20. Duan, X.-J.; Zhang, W.-W.; Li, X.-M.; Wang, B.-G. Evaluation of antioxidant property of extract and fractions obtained from a red alga, *Polysiphonia urceolata*. *Food Chem.* **2006**, *95*, 37–43. [CrossRef]
21. Pauli, G.F.; Jaki, B.U.; Lankin, D.C. Quantitative ^{1}H NMR: Development and potential of a method for natural products analysis. *J. Nat. Prod.* **2005**, *68*, 133–149. [CrossRef]
22. Pauli, G.F.; Gödecke, T.; Jaki, B.U.; Lankin, D.C. Quantitative ^{1}H NMR: Development and potential of an analytical method: An update. *J. Nat. Prod.* **2012**, *75*, 834–851. [CrossRef]
23. Nerantzaki, A.A.; Tsiafoulis, C.G.; Charisiadis, P.; Kontogianni, V.G.; Gerothanassis, I.P. Novel determination of the total phenolic content in crude plant extracts by the use of 1H NMR of the–OH spectral region. *Anal. Chim. Acta* **2011**, *688*, 54–60. [CrossRef] [PubMed]
24. Ainsworth, E.A.; Gillespie, K.M. Estimation of total phenolic content and other oxidation substrates in plant tissues using Folin-Ciocalteu reagent. *Nat. Protoc.* **2007**, *2*, 875–877. [CrossRef]
25. Pękal, A.; Pyrzynska, K. Evaluation of aluminium complexation reaction for flavonoid content assay. *Food Anal. Methods* **2014**, *7*, 1776–1782. [CrossRef]
26. Jégou, C.; Kervarec, N.; Cérantola, S.; Bihannic, I.; Stiger-Pouvreau, V. NMR use to quantify phlorotannins: The case of *Cystoseira tamariscifolia*, a phloroglucinol producing brown macroalga in Brittany (France). *Talanta* **2015**, *135*, 1–6. [CrossRef] [PubMed]
27. Ford, L.; Theodoridou, K.; Sheldrake, G.N.; Walsh, P.J. A critical review of analytical methods used for the chemical characterisation and quantification of phlorotannin compounds in brown seaweeds. *Phytochem. Anal.* **2019**, 1–13. [CrossRef] [PubMed]

28. Chang, C.-C.; Yang, M.-H.; Wen, H.-M.; Chern, J.-C. Estimation of total flavonoid content in propolis by two complementary colorimetric methods. *J. Food Drug Anal.* **2002**, *10*, 178–182.
29. Markham, K.R. Distribution of flavonoids in the lower plants and its evolutionary significance. In *The Flavonoids, Advances in Research since 1980*, 1st ed.; Harborne, J.B., Ed.; Academic Press: Boston, MA, USA, 1988; Volume 3, pp. 427–468.
30. Stafford, H.A. Flavonoid evolution: An enzymic approach. *Plant Physiol.* **1991**, *96*, 680–685. [CrossRef]
31. Goiris, K.; Muylaert, K.; Voorspoels, S.; Noten, B.; de Paepe, D.; Baart, G.J.E.; de Cooman, L. Detection of flavonoids in microalgae from different evolutionary lineages. *J. Phycol.* **2014**, *50*, 483–492. [CrossRef]
32. de Vries, J.; de Vries, S.; Slamovits, C.H.; Rose, L.E.; Archibald, J.M. How embryophytic is the biosynthesis of phenylpropanoids and their derivatives in streptophyte algae? *Plant Cell Physiol.* **2017**, *58*, 934–945. [CrossRef]

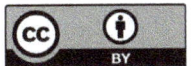

© 2019 by the authors. Licensee MDPI, Basel, Switzerland. This article is an open access article distributed under the terms and conditions of the Creative Commons Attribution (CC BY) license (http://creativecommons.org/licenses/by/4.0/).

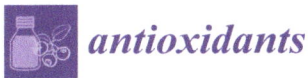

Article

Chlorophyll Oxidative Metabolism During the Phototrophic and Heterotrophic Growth of *Scenedesmus obliquus*

Mariana Manzoni Maroneze [1], Leila Queiroz Zepka [1], Eduardo Jacob Lopes [1], Antonio Pérez-Gálvez [2] and María Roca [2,*]

1. Department of Food Science and Technology, Federal University of Santa Maria (UFSM), 97105-900 Santa Maria, Brazil; mariana_maroneze@hotmail.com (M.M.M.); lqz@pq.cnpq.br (L.Q.Z.); jacoblopes@pq.cnpq.br (E.J.L.)
2. Food Phytochemistry Department, Instituto de la Grasa, Consejo Superior de Investigaciones Científicas (CSIC), University Campus, Building 46, Carretera de Utrera km. 1, 41013 Sevilla, Spain; aperez@ig.csic.es
* Correspondence: mroca@ig.csic.es; Tel.: +34-954-611550

Received: 21 October 2019; Accepted: 27 November 2019; Published: 29 November 2019

Abstract: Different cultivation strategies have been developed with the aim of increasing the production rate of microalgal pigments. Specifically, biotechnological approaches are designed to increase antioxidant metabolites as chlorophyll and carotenoids. However, although significant advances have been built up, available information regarding both the chlorophyll metabolism and their oxidative reactions in photobioreactors is scarce. To unravel such processes, the detailed chlorophyll and carotenoid fraction of *Scenedesmus obliquus* has been studied by HPLC-ESI/APCI-hrTOF-MS from phototrophic and heterotrophic cultures. *Scenedesmus* is provided with a controlled strategy of interconversion between chlorophyll *a* and *b* to avoid the formation of reactive oxygen species (ROS) at high irradiances in addition to the photoacclimation of carotenoids. Indeed, precise kinetics of 13^2-hydroxy- and 15^1-hydroxy-lactone chlorophyll metabolites shows the existence of a chlorophyll oxidative metabolism as a tool to manage the excess of energy at high light conditions. Unexpectedly, the oxidation under phototrophy favored chlorophyll *b* metabolites over the chlorophyll *a* series, while the heterotrophic conditions exclusively induced the formation of 13^2-hydroxy-chlorophyll *a*. In parallel, during the first 48 h of growth in the dark, the chlorophyll fraction maintained a promising steady state. Although future studies are required to resolve the biochemical reactions implied in the chlorophyll oxidative metabolism, the present results agree with phytoplankton metabolism.

Keywords: phototrophic; heterotrophic; *Scenedesmus*; chlorophylls; carotenoids; hydroxy-chlorophyll; oxidative metabolism; ROS; lactone-chlorophyll; photoacclimation

1. Introduction

Chlorophyll and carotenoids are challenging compounds in microbial biotechnology that find several applications in the food industry. The present food market trend is towards more natural ingredients, and colorants are not an exception [1]. Hence, artificial food colorants have been associated with health problems and consequently new sources of natural colorants are under investigation. Although natural food colorants have been traditionally extracted from fruits and vegetables sources, microalgae are currently a promising natural resource. Several advantages as the fast growth, the high pigment concentration, and the physiologically plasticity, make microalgae the new objective of biotechnological companies for pigment production. Among them, *Scenedesmus obliquus* stands out as source of pigments in food and cosmetics as well as is considered for human consumption [2,3].

In addition, chlorophyll and carotenoids exert beneficial health properties for human beings that increase their value as functional ingredients [4]. Specifically, both groups of pigments have shown to develop antioxidant activities. The antioxidant behavior of chlorophylls is highly dependent of the type of chlorophyll derivative, with significant antioxidative performances among metabolites [5]. The porphyrin structure, the central magnesium, and the functional group at C7 seem to be determinants for the antioxidant activity [6–9]. In the same line, carotenoids are highly appreciated by their antioxidant properties [10]. Consequently, the production of chlorophyll and carotenoids is one of the most successful applications of microalgal biotechnology [11], although the improvement of the feasibility of their commercial production through better cultivation strategies is still the main goal.

Photo-autotrophy is the classical culture system to grow microalgae, where the energy source comes from the sunlight and the carbon source from the atmospheric CO_2. Different light regimes (intensity, photoperiod, and wavelengths) generate different chlorophyll and carotenoid patterns. It is generally assumed that sub saturating light intensities induce higher chlorophyll synthesis, while high light irradiation reduces the chlorophyll content [12]. On the contrary, specific microalgae (*Haematococcus pluviales*, *C. zofingiensis*) enhance the production of secondary carotenoids when grown with high light intensities [13].

Open and closed photobioreactors present several disadvantages, such as the presence of contaminants, the need of robust species, or the requirement of vigorous mixing [13]. Consequently, growing microalgae in heterotrophic conditions in conventional bioreactors is at present an attractive and economical option. An additional advantage is that green algae can synthesize chlorophylls in dark conditions unlike angiosperms. This is possible thanks to the presence of a light-independent POR (protochlorophyllide *a* oxidoreductase) enzymatic process, one of the key enzymes in the chlorophyll biosynthetic pathway [14]. However, only a few microalgal species have been shown to grow in the dark so far, because the capacity of sugar utilization is not a universal strategy. In this sense, a constitutive glucose transport and utilization system has been reported for *Scenedesmus obliquus* growth [15]. In fact, different new strategies are continuously developing. Cyclic autotrophic/heterotrophic cultivation, where organic carbon is added during light or during the dark phase has been studied to optimize the production of chlorophylls and carotenoids [16]. The strategy of cultivation in two stages has been explored as an alternative to avoid the division between cell growth and the production of secondary metabolites [17]. The first phase is dedicated to obtaining the maximum biomass production, followed by a stressed second phase to increase the accumulation of lipid-derived compounds. In fact, such strategy (two-stage heterotrophy/photoinduction) has been successfully applied in *Scenedesmus* reaching values of lutein productivity 1.6 times higher than in autotrophic conditions [18]. With the same aim, that is, to enhance the lutein productivity, the conditions during mixotrophic cultures of *S. obliquus* have been optimized, determining the best operating parameters for photoperiod, source of light, nutrients and batch system [11]. Different conditions have been established to modulate, improve, or control the chlorophyll content in different *Scenedesmus* sp. [19,20]. Light conditions, stirring, depletion of nutrients, open fields or bioreactors, and carbon source are among the most explored variables [12]. *Scenedesmus* seems to have a lower sensitivity to photoinhibition and a higher capacity to adapt to high irradiance conditions by increasing its photosynthetic capacity, in comparison with other species such as *Chlorella* [21]. However, the following step is to analyze the chlorophyll profile in detail, to decipher the responsible mechanism(s) for the synthesis and degradation of chlorophylls in response to modifying parameters.

The biochemical reactions implied during the chlorophyll degradation pathway have been unraveled in higher plants [22], but in green microalgae only a few steps have been discovered [23,24]. Thus, the initial catabolic steps of chlorophyll *a* are the de-esterification of phytol (Figure 1) and the loss of the central magnesium to finally yield pheophorbide *a*. For these consecutive reactions, two plausible alternative routes have been proposed [22], which are potentially catalyzed by different enzymes. The last proposal has been to postulate that both enzymatic systems can operate simultaneously, although at different functional levels [25]. Next, the macrocycle of the pheophorbide *a* intermediate is oxygenolytically open, yielding a sequence of linear chlorophyll catabolites denominated phyllobilins (Figure 1). Regardless, it has been established that knowledge level of chlorophyll degradation in microalgae is at present in a preliminary stage. Specifically, as it was regarding that of the higher plants 30 years ago. A very close relationship has been always suggested between the chlorophyll catabolic pathway in chlorophytes and in higher plants [26], which is not unlikely assuming the phylogenetic relationship between both taxonomic groups. In fact, open chlorophyll catabolites with similar structures to those of phyllobilins have been identified in *Chlorella* [26,27] or in *Desmodesmus subpicatus* [28]. In parallel, chlorophylls are subjected to an oxidative metabolism [29,30]. At present, two reactions have been identified. Hence, the chlorophyll skeleton can be oxidized at $C13^2$ to form 13^2-hydroxy-compounds and secondly, while the isocyclic ring can further react to form a lactone group, that is, the 15^2-hydroxy-lactone chlorophyll derivatives [31] (Figure 2). Their formation could arise from different pathways, enzymatic [30] or by an increase in oxygen reactive species, and even they can also be produced in dark anoxic conditions [32]. Regardless, the presence of hydroxy-chlorophylls has been related with conditions of high environmental presence of peroxide species, as the former are the main products of chlorophyll *a* in presence of the latter [33]. Therefore, hydroxy-chlorophylls are related to the response to oxidative stress. Physiologically, they have been associated with senescence [34], virus infection [35], and even cell death [36]. In any case, hydroxy-chlorophylls are common chlorophyll metabolites found in phytoplankton species in their natural environments [36,37]. For some authors, oxidative chlorophylls are the origin of "petrochlorophylls", as they have been identified in numerous phytoplankton sediments [38]. However, to the best of our knowledge, chlorophyll oxidation has not been analyzed in relation to microalgae cell culture.

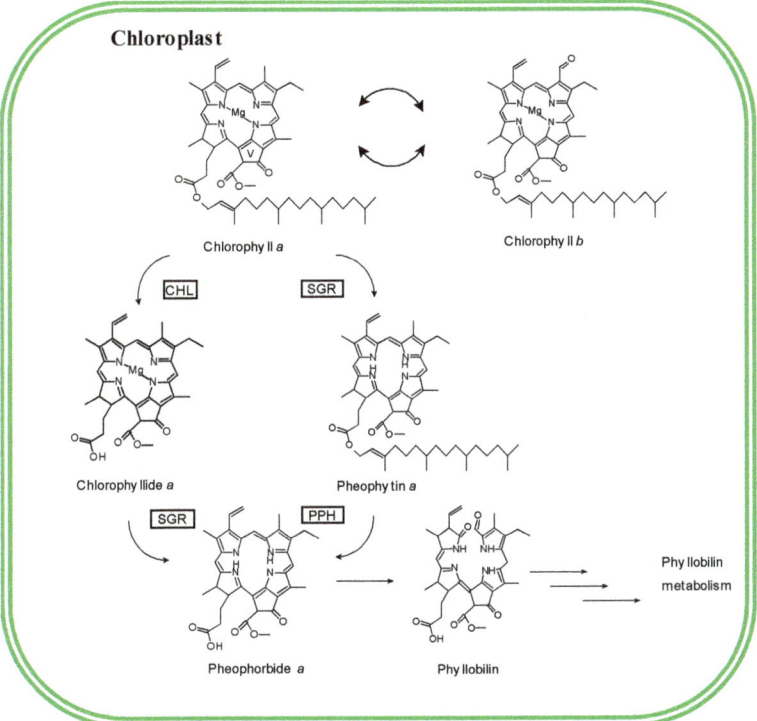

Figure 1. Chlorophyll degradation pathway. CHL: chlorophyllase, SGR: stay-green, PPH: pheophytinase.

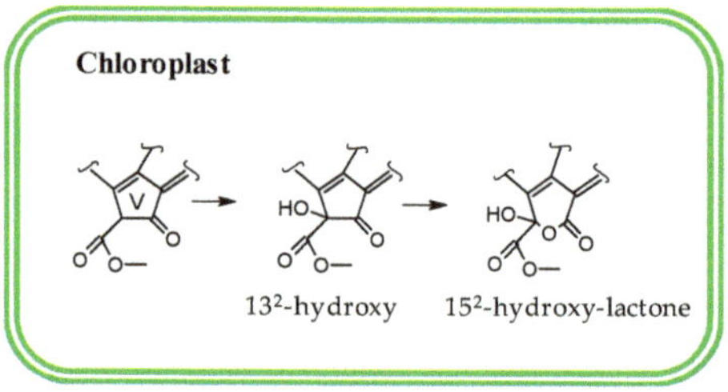

Figure 2. Oxidative chlorophyll reactions, following previous proposal [31]. The structures correspond only with the V ring (or isocyclic ring) of the chlorophyll molecule. The wavy line means the rest of the chlorophyll structure (see Figure 1). The oxidative reactions can be performed over diverse chlorophyll compounds (see the tables).

As stated before [39], a deep knowledge of their metabolic pathways is necessary to select the best cultivation conditions to improve the microalgal pigment production. Although significant advances have been developed to maximize the total chlorophyll and carotenoid content in some microalgae species, it is necessary to understand the individual behavior within the heterogenous pigment profile. It is necessary not only to consider the total pigment content, but also to determine which metabolites are producing or degrading. The aim of this study was to analyze in detail the chlorophyll and carotenoid metabolism during the phototrophic and heterotrophic cultivation of *Scenedesmus* with special emphasis in the oxidative reactions occurring at the chlorophyll fraction.

2. Materials and Methods

2.1. Microorganisms and Culture Media

The axenic culture of *Scenedesmus obliquus* (CPCC05) was supplied by the Canadian Phycological Culture Centre (Waterloo, Canada). We applied the following incubation conditions, 26 °C, photon flux density of 30 µmol m^{-2} s^{-1} and a photoperiod of 12 h to obtain the stock cultures, which were propagated and maintained in synthetic BG11 medium [40].

2.2. Cultivation Conditions

The phototrophic experiments were carried out in a 2 L bubble column photobioreactor (Tecnal, Piracicaba-SP, Brazil) operated in batch mode [41]. We applied the following experimental conditions: 100 mg/L for the initial cell concentration, and 26 °C for the isothermal reactor, which was fed with 2 L of B11 medium, pH set to 7.6, 150 µmol m^{-2} s^{-1} for the photon flux density and a light cycle of 24:0 h (light:dark). Continuous aeration of 1 VVM (volume of air per volume of culture per minute) was applied with the injection of air enriched with 15% carbon dioxide. The conditions for the heterotrophic cultivations were set up in a 2 L bubble column bioreactor operating under a batch regime [42]. It was operated at 26 °C in the absence of light, with a carbon/nitrogen ratio of 20, pH adjusted to 7.6, aeration of 1 VVM, and initial cell concentration of 100 mg/L. The culture medium consisted of BG11 synthetic medium supplemented with 12.5 g/L of D-glucose.

2.3. Kinetic Parameters

We used the biomass data to calculate the biomass productivity [$P_X = (X_i - X_{i-1}) \times (t_i - t_{i-1})^{-1}$, mg/L h], the maximum specific growth rate [$\ln(X_i/X_0) = \mu_{max} \times t$, 1/h], and generation time [$tg = 0.693/\mu_{max}$, h]. Hence the X_i is the biomass concentration at time t_i (mg/L), while X_{i-1} is the biomass concentration at time t_{i-1} (mg/L) and X_0 is the biomass concentration at time 0. μ_{max}: maximum specific growth rate (h−1). Residence time (t, in h) is defined as the time required for cells to reach the end of the stationary phase.

2.4. Extraction of Photosynthetic Pigments

Aliquots of microalgae or cyanobacteria biomass (5 mL) were filtered with a Whatman grade GF/F glass microfiber filter (47-mm diameter, Merck, Darmstadt, Germany), and immediately frozen at −80 °C [43]. The filter was grinded with liquid nitrogen into powder and mixed with 10 mL of DMF:water (9:1) under stirring at 4 °C for 15 min and spinning (10,000 rpm, 5 min). Subsequently, the solvent phase was collected in a separation funnel whereas the solid residue was re-extracted with 10 mL hexane, ultrasonicated (5 min, 720 W), and vortexed (5 min). Then, 10 mL NaCl solution (10% *w/v*) was added to the mixture, centrifuged (10,000 rpm, 5 min) and the supernatant was added to the first extract in the funnel. Finally, the pellet was dissolved with 10 mL diethyl ether in an ultrasonic bath (5 min, 720 W) and finally vortexed for 5 min. Then, the solution was mixed with 10 mL NaCl solution (10% *w/v*) and the mixture was centrifuged (10,000 rpm, 5 min) and added to the previous extracts in the funnel. There, the mixed solvent layers were extracted with diethyl ether and NaCl solution (10% *w/v*). The water layer was discarded, and the organic phase was concentrated to dryness in a rotary evaporator. The residue was dissolved in acetone. Samples were stored at −20 °C until analysis within 1 week.

2.5. Identification of Photosynthetic Pigments by HPLC-ESI/APCI-HRTOF-MS^n

The chromatographic separation of the individual chlorophyll derivatives and carotenoids was achieved in a Dionex Ultimate 3000RS U-HPLC equipment (Thermo Fisher Scientific, Waltham, MA, USA). The column applied for chlorophyll pigments was a reversed-phase C18 column (200 × 4.6 mm i.d., Teknokroma, Barcelona, Spain), 3 µm particle size, while the elution gradient was the one described previously [44]. The separation of the carotenoid profile required different chromatographic conditions. A reversed-phase C30 column (250 × 4.6 mm i.d., YMC, Schermbeck, Germany), with 3 µm particle size, was applied with the elution gradient described earlier [45,46]. For chlorophyll and carotenoids, the injection volume was 30 µL and the flow rate utilized was 1 mL/min. The UV-visible spectra of the chromatographic peaks were recorded in the 300–700 nm range with a PDA detector. Subsequently, a split post-column of 0.4 mL/min was introduced directly on the mass spectrometer ion source (micrOTOF-QII™ High Resolution Time-of-Flight mass spectrometer with Qq-TOF geometry, Bruker Daltonics, Bremen, Germany). The analysis was developed with an ESI interface (for chlorophyll compounds) or an APCI source (for carotenoid compounds). The instrument was operated in positive ion mode and scanning the *m/z* values in the 50–1200 Da range. We operated the acquisition of the mass spectra in broad-band Collision Induced Dissociation mode (bbCID), so that MS and MS/MS spectra were recorded simultaneously. The instrument control was performed with Bruker Compass HyStar software (Bruker Daltonics version 3.2, Bremen, Germany), whereas the processing of MS data was made with the Bruker Compass DataAnalysis software (Bruker Daltonics version 4.1, Bremen, Germany). For the automated screening of signals corresponding to identified chlorophyll derivatives and carotenoids on the EICs, we applied the TargetAnalysis™ software (Bruker Daltonics version 1.2, Bremen, Germany). The validation of the automated identifications was carried out according to different filtering rules, including mass accuracy (tolerance limit set at 5 ppm) and isotopic pattern comparison calculated with the SigmaFit™ (Bremen, Germany) algorithm (tolerance limit set at 50) [44]. The interpretation of the MS/MS spectra and the consistency of the product ions, which have to fulfil the previous filtering rules for mass accuracy and isotopic pattern, was developed with the SmartFormula3D™ (Bremen, Germany) module [44]. The software MassFrontier™ software (Thermo Scientific™ version 4.0, Waltham, MA, USA) allowed the acquisition of the in silico tandem MS spectra of the filtered analytes to compare the theoretical product ions with the corresponding experimental ones. This software allows the evaluation of different product ions when different isomers show the same bbCID spectrum.

2.6. Quantification of Photosynthetic Pigments by HPLC-UV-Visible Detection

The identified pigments were quantified by reversed-phase HPLC using a Hewlett-Packard HP 1100 liquid chromatograph with the same columns and eluent gradients as for the MS analyses. The on-line UV-visible spectra were recorded in the 350–800 nm wavelength range. Sequential detection was performed at 410, 430, 450, and 666 nm with a photodiode-array detector. Data were collected and processed with the HP ChemStation (Rev.A.05.04) software (Agilent Technologies, Waldbronn, Germany). Calibration curves (amount versus integrated peak area) were obtained by the least-squares linear regression analysis for quantification of pigments. The concentration range considered to build the calibration equations was ascertained from the observed levels of the pigments in the samples. Triplicate injections were made for five different volumes of each standard solution.

2.7. Statistical Analysis

Normality of data (mean values of three independent measurements) was checked with the Shapiro-Wilk test, and one-way analysis of the variance was performed using the Statistica software (version 6, StatSoft, Inc., 2001, Palo Alto, Santa Clara, CA, USA). Post-hoc comparison for detecting statistic significant differences was made with the Tukey test, setting the significance value a $p < 0.05$.

3. Results

3.1. Microalgae Growth/Kinetic Parameters

Knowledge regarding the growth pattern of microalgae and its parameters is not only interesting for the quantitative production of both biomass and metabolites, but also for increasing our comprehension of both the synthesis regulation and degradation dynamics of photosynthetic products. In this sense, Figure 3 depicts representative growth curves for the microalgae *Scenedesmus obliquus* through phototrophic and heterotrophic metabolic pathways, whereas the growth parameters are presented in Table 1. Hence, both culture conditions followed an exponential growth from the beginning without lag phase, at the specific growth rates of 0.023 and 0.024 h^{-1}, generation intervals of 30.13 and 28.8 h, and finally reaching a stationary phase at 144 h and at 96 h in photosynthetic and heterotrophic cultures, respectively. The highest biomass accumulation was achieved under the photosynthetic cultivation (2650 mg/L) which was only 2% higher than the high biomass concentration of heterotrophic condition (2600 mg/L). The greatest impact of the type of cultivation was on the biomass productivity, where the highest value was obtained under heterotrophy (19.75 mg/L h), which is a consequence of the low residence time (120 h) reached in this condition, when compared with the phototrophic culture (216 h) that resulted in a productivity of 10.87 mg/L h. Regardless, at very long incubation times during the phototrophic growth, it is impossible to ensure that no nutrient deprivation occurs. However, assuming this possibility, we extended the study to analyze the effects of excess of light on pigment composition.

Table 1. Kinects parameters of *Scenedesmus obliquus* in phototrophic and heterotrophic growth conditions (mean ± SD).

Parameter	Phototrophic	Heterotrophic
X_{max} (mg/L)	2650 ± 111.8	2600 ± 97.5
μ_{max} (h^{-1})	0.023 ± 0.00	0.024 ± 0.00
RT (h)	216 ± 0.00	120 ± 0.00
GT (h)	30.13 ± 0.60	28.8 ± 0.49
P_X (mg/L h)	10.87 ± 0.43	19.75 ± 0.29

X_{max}: maximum cell biomass; μ_{max}: maximum specific growth rate (h^{-1}); RT: residence time (h); GT: generation time (h); P_X: average biomass productivity (mg/L h).

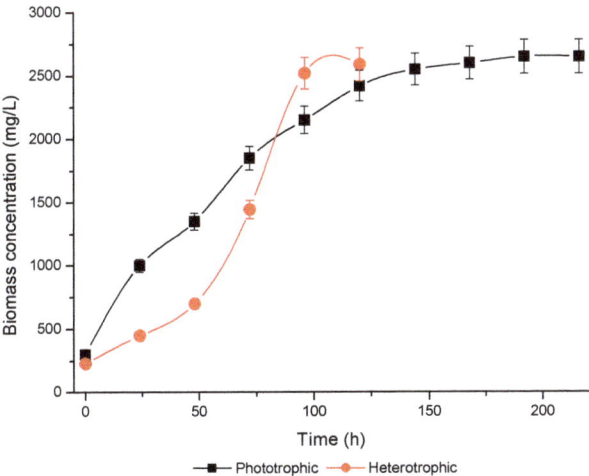

Figure 3. Growth curves in phototrophic and heterotrophic culture regimes of *Scenedesmus obliquus*.

3.2. Pigment Profile During Phototrophic Growth

The characteristics of the chromatographic and mass spectrometric data for the different pigments analyzed in the present study are shown in Table S1. *Scenedesmus* exhibits the typical carotenoid profile of the Chlorophyta taxon, which mainly contains lutein, β-carotene, and relative amounts of minor xanthophylls, such as violaxanthin and neoxanthin [47]. The chlorophyll fraction has been generally described as comprised by chlorophyll *a* and chlorophyll *b*, a feature of this taxonomic group of green algae. However, our detailed analysis reveals the presence of intermediary chlorophyll metabolites within the chlorophyll profile. Figure 4 displays the structures of the chlorophyll derivatives present in the profile of *Scenedesmus obliquus*.

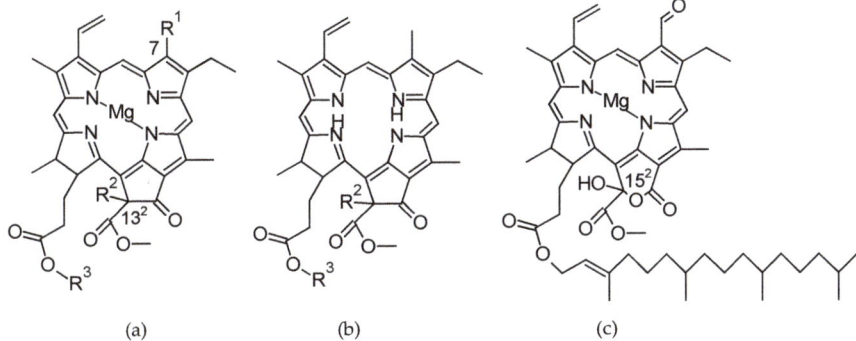

Figure 4. Chlorophyll structures identified in *Scenedesmus obliquus*: (**a**) chlorophyll (R^3 is phytol, $C_{20}H_{40}$) and chlorophyllide (R^3 is H) structure, R^1 is CH_3 for chlorophyll *a*, and CHO for chlorophyll *b*, R^2 is H for chlorophyll (*a* and *b*) and OH for 13^2-hydroxy-chlorophyll (*a* and *b*); (**b**) pheophytin (R^3 is phytol, $C_{20}H_{40}$) and pheophorbide (R^3 is H) structure, R^2 is H for pheophorbide, and OH for 13^2-hydroxy-pheophorbide; (**c**) 15^2-hydroxy-lactone chlorophyll *b* structure.

It was observed that the total amount of carotenoids (Table 2) increased with the radiation time until the microalgae reached the stationary phase (144 h), to subsequently present a steady state until the end of the phase. In *Scenedesmus*, this behavior is due to the response of the main carotenoids, lutein and β-carotene, to the continuous illumination. As it has been stated [39], the same carotenoid kind may develop different roles in the cell depending on its location. According to the observed data (Table 2), lutein and β-carotene behave as primary photosynthetic pigments in *Scenedesmus*, although β-carotene could perform secondary activities in other chlorophytes, and even transported into oil droplets where they accumulate under stress conditions [17]. Regardless, lutein and β-carotene are photoprotective pigments, minimizing the photoinhibition through additional roles as quenchers or scavengers [39]. However, the minor xanthophylls display a different behavior under continuous radiation in *Scenedesmus* cells. Neoxanthin, violaxanthin, luteoxanthin, and antheraxanthin increased their concentrations in the microalgae culture even after the stationary growth phase. Specifically, violaxanthin and antheraxanthin are involved in the so-called xanthophyll cycle, intimately related with the ability to dissipate the excess of absorbed light. During high light irradiance conditions, the de-epoxidation reaction of violaxanthin to produce antheraxanthin reduces the light-harvesting efficiency in the antenna [48]. Finally, although neoxanthin could be considered as a light harvesting pigment, it also develops a role as photoprotective compound, reacting towards reactive oxygen species and preventing cell damage [49].

Table 2. Evolution of the carotenoid profile during the phototrophic growth of *Scenedesmus obliquus* (mg/kg dw).

Time (h)	Neox	Violax	Luteox	Antherax	Lutein	β-Carotene	Total
0	+	+	+	0.0	703.3	30.0	703.3
24	127.0	11.0	20.0	0.0	689.5	30.1	877.2
48	142.0	10.4	26.3	0.0	860.7	38.9	1174.3
72	130.3	28.1	37.0	7.0	795.4	45.9	1044.0
96	83.7	25.8	40.7	15.6	931.2	53.2	1150.1
120	146.7	28.5	36.7	20.4	1238.3	176.4	1647.0
144	147.0	40.0	45.1	32.0	1443.9	224.7	1952.4
168	122.3	19.8	51.3	26.2	1125.0	220.0	1679.6
192	156.2	38.9	67.0	30.0	1313.2	227.1	1832.4
216	321.9	108.9	44.0	49.2	1408.7	212.6	2145.3

Neox: neoxanthin, Violax: violaxanthin, Luteox: luteoxanthin, Anterax: anteraxanthin, Total: total carotenoids. +, means presence but under the LOQ. (coefficient of variance < 10% in all cases).

In relation to the response of the chlorophyll fraction to the continuous irradiance (Table 3), it was observed that light exposure initially induces chlorophyll synthesis. Although this result was anticipated, prolonged irradiance times (which means an excess of light) result in a net degradation of the chlorophyll fraction. The detailed analysis of the chlorophyll profile during the phototrophic growth of *Scenedesmus* shows chlorophyll *a* and *b* as the main pigments, but the accumulation of the intermediary metabolites pheophytin and pheophorbide *a* was also concomitant. Pheophytin *a* (Figure 4b) is produced by the substitution of the central Mg^{2+} ion by hydrogens, while pheophorbide *a* (Figure 4a) involves an additional dephytylation step at the $C17^3$ position. However, the outstanding results are the production of a heterogeneous profile of oxidized chlorophylls. Among them, the 13^2-hydroxy-compounds stand out, which result from the oxidation at the $C13^2$ carbon atom (R^2 is OH in Figure 4) in chlorophyll of the *a* and *b* series, and in pheophorbide *a*. Furthermore, the formation of a lactone functional group is considered a further step in the oxidative level of the original chlorophyll structure [31]. In this sense, it was very surprising to find 15^1-hydroxy-lactone chlorophyll *b* (Figure 4c) in the chlorophyll profile of *Scenedesmus* under radiation conditions.

Table 3. Evolution of the chlorophyll profile from series *a* during the phototrophic growth of *Scenedesmus obliquus* (mg/kg dw).

Time (h)	Pheo *a*	OH-Pheo *a*	OH-Chl *a*	Chl *a*	Phy *a*
0	0.0	0.0	0.0	2438.3	2787.7
24	0.0	0.0	85.0	2420.0	3350.0
48	20.4	0.0	111.1	3955.2	2950.7
72	33.0	0.0	148.6	3718.6	2375.9
96	155.6	0.0	114.0	4079.3	2413.7
120	210.0	22.9	133.3	3981.3	2590.0
144	262.7	13.7	127.5	7417.5	897.8
168	86.7	8.3	134.6	5935.8	878.5
192	31.7	11.3	0.0	6170.0	708.7
216	8.5	0.0	0.0	6878.1	192.1

Pheo: pheophorbide, OH-Pheo *a*: 13^2-hydroxy-chlorophyll *a*, Chl: chlorophyll, OH-Chl *a*: 13^2-hydroxy-chlorophyll *a*, Phy: pheophytin. (CV < 10% in all cases).

It is noteworthy to highlight the different behavior of chlorophyll derivatives from *a* series (Figure 4a, CH_3 at C7) from that observed for the *b* series (Figure 4a, CHO at C7). The chlorophyll compounds from *a* series, except pheophytin *a*, were biosynthesized until the maximum growth stage was reached (144 h), and subsequently a progressive degradation initiated. However, metabolites from chlorophyll *b* series (chlorophyll *b*, 13^2-hydroxy-chlorophyll *b* and 15^1-hydroxy-lactone chlorophyll *b*) showed their maximum concentrations between 48 and 72 h of illumination, around half of the period required to reach the residence time. After the apex peak, the metabolites of the chlorophyll *b* initiated a net degradation. The interconversion of chlorophyll *a* and *b*, through the denominated chlorophyll cycle (Figure 1 [50]), is an essential mechanism in photosynthetic organisms, as they can adapt their photosynthetic apparatus to the irradiance level. At high levels of illumination, the organism reduces the antenna complexes to avoid excess of photons, so that the production of reactive oxygen species (ROS) is minimized. As antenna complexes are rich in chlorophyll b compounds, at high irradiances the relative amounts of chlorophyll *b* decreased. On the contrary, at low irradiance (shadow) conditions, the organism rises the antenna complexes to capture as many photons as possible, which results in an increase of the chlorophyll compounds of the *b* series. Consequently, microalgae modify the ratio of chlorophyll *a/b* according to the irradiance levels [51]. As it can be observed in Table 4, at the initial 72 h of growth the ratio of *a/b* series decreased in *Scenedesmus*, as the biosynthesis rate of chlorophyll *b* was higher than that for the chlorophyll *a*. However, when the quantity of light was excessive for the culture (after 72 h of continuous illumination), the antenna complexes decreased, the concentration of chlorophyll *b* diminished and, consequently, the *a/b* ratio increased. Similar changes in the *a/b* ratio have been observed for *Chlorella* and *Dunalliela* [52]. At high irradiances, the energy received by chlorophyll *a* molecule is higher than its capacity to transfer it towards the photosynthetic electron transport chain, and chlorophyll *a* switches to the triplet excited stage [39]. Next, overexcited chlorophyll *a* molecule is quenched by molecular oxygen yielding ROS. As we can observe in Tables 3 and 4, the interconversion between chlorophyll *a* and *b* contents is the preferred mechanism of *Scenedesmus* cells to avoid the formation of ROS at high irradiances.

Nevertheless, once the maximum concentrations for chlorophyll *a* (144 h, Table 3) and *b* (72 h in Table 4) were reached, the net degradation of chlorophyll compounds was not exhaustive. Otherwise, *Scenedesmus* cells reached a steady state for the chlorophyll content (around 6200 mg/kg dw. for chlorophyll *a*, 1900 mg/kg dw. for chlorophyll *b*) until the end of the controlled period. It seems that once the top biosynthetic capabilities were accomplished, the microalgae found an 'ideal' chlorophyll content, which allows an equilibrated photosynthetic performance, that is, a productive one but not harmful, at least at the irradiance assayed for *Scenedesmus*. As it has been previously stated, photoacclimation is complete only when a balanced growth condition is achieved [53]. However, this is accurate when the chlorophyll content is determined as a whole value. As we have shown, a detailed study of the complete chlorophyll profile allows to observe different biosynthetic capabilities with some chlorophyll metabolites reaching steady state earlier, precisely to fit with the photoacclimation at 144 h.

Table 4. Evolution of the chlorophyll profile from series *b* during the phototrophic growth of *Scenedesmus obliquus* (mg/kg dw).

Time (h)	OH-Lact.-Chl *b*	OH-Chl *b*	Chl *b*	Series *a/b*
0	100.0	116.7	1408.3	3.22
24	175.0	124.5	1472.5	3.30
48	179.3	418.1	2023.0	2.71
72	275.1	437.6	5557.0	1.02
96	122.6	308.6	1757.2	3.02
120	116.7	310.4	1724.0	3.13
144	132.0	231.8	2016.7	3.55
168	90.0	286.3	1802.7	3.19
192	56.8	31.1	1878.3	3.50
216	40.9	50.6	1747.2	3.85
240	51.0	63.5	2038.6	3.14

OH-Lact.-Chl *b*: 15^1-hydroxy-chlorophyll *b*; OH-Chl *b*: 13^2-hydroxy-chlorophyll *b*; Chl *b*: chlorophyll *b*. (CV < 10% in all cases).

Pheophorbide *a* and pheophytin *a* are currently considered the metabolites of the chlorophyll degradation pathway (Figure 1). In fact, pheophorbide, pheophytin, and pyropheophorbide have been associated with the chlorophyll degradation in cyanobacteria in sedimentary surfaces [54] and chlorophyll senescence in marine environments [34]. Recently, the gene responsible of the formation of pheophytin (SGR) a has been identified in *Chlamidomonas reinharditii* [24]. However, while the kinetics of production and degradation of pheophorbide *a* is parallel to the chlorophyll *a*, the profile of metabolism of pheophytin *a* seems to progress in a different fashion and not correlated with the metabolism of chlorophyll *a*. The maximum concentration of pheophytin *a* was observed at 24 h, while its progressive decay through the continuous illumination period made the interpretation of the results in base to its implication in the chlorophyll degradation pathway challenging.

In addition, the HPLC-ESI/APCI-hrTOF-MS analyses of the chlorophyll fraction revealed the existence of a specific chlorophyll oxidative metabolism (Tables 2 and 3) during the *Scenedesmus* phototrophic cultivation. As stated before (Figure 2), hydroxylation at $C13^2$ is the first step in the oxidative pathway of chlorophylls. Hence, 13^2-hydroxy-chlorophyll *a* and *b* increased their concentrations in the cell with the continuous illumination for the initial 72 h period, and afterwards a progressive degradation was observed. In any case, it is important to highlight that the maximum of 13^2-hydroxy-chlorophyll *a* cellular content was not concurrent with the maximum concentration of chlorophyll *a*, which pointed towards a specific linking reaction between both compounds instead of an unspecific process. Noteworthy, 13^2-hydroxy-pheophorbide *a* was also produced around 3 days of illumination, once pheophorbide *a* is biosynthesized in the microalgae. A further oxidative process is the generation of the lactone rearrangement at the $C15^1$ position (Figure 4). During the phototrophic growth of *Scenedesmus* a progressive accumulation of 15^1-hydroxy-lactone chlorophyll *b* is observed, reaching the maximum value after 72 h (Table 3). In our experimental conditions it seems 72 h is the timeframe for *Scenedesmus* to reach the 'buffer capacity' (from the point of view of chlorophylls) and manage both the excess of energy and, consequently, the potential accumulation of ROS. Afterwards, profound physiological changes are required to avoid oxidative stress, as the commented restructuration of antenna complexes.

Moreover, no 15^1-hydroxy-lactone chlorophyll *a* formation was detected in any moment of the phototrophic growth, although chlorophyll *a* is the main chlorophyll pigment in the chlorophyll profile of *Scenedesmus*. In fact, although a chlorophyll metabolite with this functional group is not easy to distinguish [1], it is the 15^1-hydroxy-lactone chlorophyll *a* catabolite observed (if any) in photosynthetic organisms, but not the 15^1-hydroxy-lactone chlorophyll *b* catabolic product [30]. Indeed, both proportionally and in absolute concentration, the total biosynthesized chlorophyll oxidative compounds of the *b* series overcame those of the *a* series. To the best of our knowledge, this is the first time to describe such phenomenon. The biochemical origin of the oxidized chlorophyll metabolites is still under discussion. In higher plants, different enzymatic systems have been assumed as responsible for such oxidation (lipoxygenase and/or peroxidase) [29–31]. However, although different oxidative mechanisms have been observed in microalgae (peroxidase, superoxide dismutase, polyphenol oxidase, glutathione peroxidase, etc.) [55,56], none of them have been correlated with the chlorophyll metabolism so far. Two possible hypotheses can explain the higher rate of oxidation of chlorophyll *b* catabolism. Thus, the preferential accumulation of chlorophyll *b* catabolites could be due to an unknown chlorophyll *b* affinity by the pool of oxidative enzymes pool, or this singularity could be caused by the different localization of both chlorophyll series in the photosynthetic apparatus. Further research is required to unravel the exact mechanism.

3.3. Pigment Evolution During Heterotrophic Growth

As it can be seen in Table 5, heterotrophy means carotenoid degradation for *Scenedesmus obliquus* in our experimental conditions, although at very different rates depending on the carotenoid sort. The initial 24 h in darkness produces a significant carotenoid degradation except for neoxanthin, while the concentration of β-carotene and violaxanthin decreased by half. This decrease was extended in a lower degree for lutein. From 24 to 48 h of growth in the darkness, carotenoids were highly stable, the next 24 h interlude (72 h) only being a significant stage for the stability of neoxanthin and violaxanthin. Extending the heterotrophic culture of *Scenedesmus obliquus* far from 96 h implied a carotenoid degradation of at least 85%. In fact, carotenoid production in heterotrophic cultivation requires additional oxidative stress: high salt concentration, high light, etc. [13]. In any case, it is important to highlight the different stability of carotenoids in heterotrophic conditions, to face the future biotechnological strategies aimed to enhance the production of carotenoids.

Table 5. Evolution of the chlorophyll and carotenoid profile during the heterotrophic growth of *Scenedesmus obliquus* (mg/kg dw).

Pigment	Residence Time (h)					
	0	24	48	72	96	120
Neoxanthin	86.4	76.9	80.0	43.5	36.5	13.3
Violaxanthin	42.2	18.7	18.4	10.4	8.5	1.8
Lutein	429.3	323.2	318.3	319.2	284.3	63.2
β-carotene	241.5	144.3	151.2	131.8	128.8	6.6
Chld *a*	3.4	3.5	3.5	3.5	8.5	108.0
Pheo *a*	78.3	157.7	145.0	67.2	37.2	299.9
Chl *b*	2284.0	2644.4	2778.2	1992.9	1164.0	895.4
OH-chl *a*	15.1	111.6	187.5	3.5	3.5	202.5
Chl *a*	4407.1	4343.0	4190.2	4636.3	2841.9	825.4
Phy *a*	1063.5	1102.6	766.1	326.4	262.0	207.0
Tot. carot	799.4	563.2	568.0	505.1	458.2	85.0
Tot. chls	7851.6	8362.9	8070.7	7030.1	4317.4	2538.3

Chld *a*: chlorophyllide *a*; Pheo *a*: pheophorbide *a*; Chl *a*, Chl *b*: chlorophyll *a*, chlorophyll *b*; OH-chl *a*: 13^2-hydroxy-chlorophyll *a*; Phy *a*: pheophytin *a*; carot: carotenoids. (CV < 10% in all cases).

On the contrary, it was remarkable to observe the behavior of the chlorophyll fraction at heterotrophic culture conditions. During the initial 48 h of growth, the total amount of chlorophylls was constant and after that time interval, the chlorophyll profile initiated a phase of net degradation with increased rate at the end of the controlled period. Such modification in the chlorophyll metabolism is coincident with an increase of biomass. The initial steady state of the chlorophyll content means that the biosynthetic and the degradative reactions are evolving at the same rate. Although the exact quantity is unknown, the half-life of a chlorophyll molecule is estimated around several hours [57]. This fact implies that during the steady state of chlorophylls in the initial 48 h of heterotrophic culture, biosynthetic and degradative reactions are running in *Scenedesmus* cells. Regarding the biosynthetic metabolism, as stated before green algae can synthesize chlorophylls in dark conditions. Consequently, during 48 h of heterotrophic cultivation of *Scenedesmus*, a continuous synthesis of chlorophylls took place, although at the same rate as the degradative reactions. The first assumption to consider is that under heterotrophic conditions, the cell does not invest energy in chlorophyll synthesis but focuses on the cell division and growth process with the available resources. In fact, it has been argued that glucose can inhibit the chlorophyll biosynthesis, by means of an inhibitory activity towards the precursor coprophorphyrin III [58]. On the contrary, some reports have shown a certain degree of chlorophyll retention during heterotrophic growth [59], as we have found for *Scenedesmus*. The exact physiological meaning of such energetic investment is unknown to date, although our results are an important starting point for future biotechnological applications aimed to enhance the chlorophyll production.

In addition, the detailed analysis of the chlorophyll profile during the heterotrophic growth of *Scenedesmus* shows accumulation of chlorophyll metabolites produced during the chlorophyll degradation, that mirror the masked reactions that were under progress. Pheophorbide, chlorophyllide, and pheophytin are intermediary catabolites during the chlorophyll degradation pathway. Table 5 shows a significant increment of pheophorbide and chlorophyllide *a* at the end of the controlled period, concomitant with the main degradation of chlorophylls. However, pheophytin levels continuously decreased through the cycle, showing no parallelism with the chlorophyll breakdown. The results suggest that the operating pathways during the heterotrophic cultivation of *Scenedesmus* are better related with the chlorophyllase (CHL) pathway (Figure 1) than with pheophytinase one (PPH). Homologous PPH proteins have been found through BLASTP (Basic Local Alignment Search Tool for Proteins) searches in green algae but not in cyanobacteria, and it has been proposed that PPHs are also likely to be operative in the green algae [60], although no functional analysis has been developed so far. Although such data are not available, PPH seems to not be responsible for the chlorophyll degradation during heterotrophic conditions, at least during the culture conditions assayed in *Scenedesmus*.

To the best of our knowledge, accumulation of 13^2-hydroxy-chlorophylls is described for the first time in this study during the heterotrophic culture of green microalga, although no 15^1-hydroxy-lactone derivatives were detected. Interestingly, the heterotrophic strategy only induced oxidation in chlorophyll *a* molecules and no oxidized chlorophyll *b* compounds were detected in any moment of the cycle. 13^2-hydroxy-chlorophyll *a* production, observed during the initial 48 h of growth in the darkness could involve a role during the chlorophyll turnover, although the main synthesis is accomplished with the net degradation of chlorophylls at the end of the cultivation period. As stated before, the exact role of oxidized chlorophylls in phytoplankton is unclear, but associated with defense, grazing, senescence, or even death cell [33–38]. Our results show both production and degradation kinetics during the heterotrophic culture of *Scenedesmus*, with more than a plausible role during the chlorophyll degradation. Consequently, the results obtained in Table 5 open a door for future research, with a focus on the biochemical mechanisms involved in the chlorophyll oxidative metabolism during the heterotrophic cultivation of green microalgae.

4. Conclusions

As stated in the introduction, the improvement of pigment production with biotechnological parameters requires a deep understanding of the reactions that take place during the different culture approaches. In this sense, it is essential to know the physiological strategies that green microalgae develop to become acclimatized to the environmental conditions. In addition to the technological data, our study introduces a specific and different chlorophyll oxidative metabolism during phototrophic and heterotrophic cultivation, which agrees with the measurement of oxidized chlorophyll metabolites in natural phytoplankton environment [35,36]. Future assays in controlled bioreactors are required to unravel the precise implication of such oxidative metabolism.

Supplementary Materials: The following are available online at http://www.mdpi.com/2076-3921/8/12/600/s1, Table S1: Photosynthetic pigments identified by HPLC-PDA-ESI/APCI(+)-Q-TOF in the study.

Author Contributions: Conceptualization, L.Q.Z., E.J.L. and M.R.; methodology, M.M.M. and M.R.; software, A.P.-G.; validation, M.M.M.; formal analysis, M.M.M. and M.R.; investigation, M.M.M.; resources, L.Q.Z. and E.J.L.; data curation, A.P.-G. and M.R.; writing—original draft preparation, M.R.; writing—review and editing, L.Q.Z., E.J.L., A.P.-G. and M.R.; supervision and funding acquisition, M.R.

Funding: This work was supported by the Ministerio de Ciencia, Investigación y Universidades, Agencia Estatal de Investigación y Fondo Europeo de Desarrollo Regional (FEDER), grant number RTI2018-095415-B-I00. MM was supported with a fellowship from the Coordenação de Aperfeiçoamento de Pessoal de Nível Superior - Brasil (CAPES) - Finance Code 001 and the Brazilian Funding Agency FAPERGS (Fundação de Amparo a pesquisa do estado do Rio Grande do Sul). The APC was partially funded by CSIC.

Acknowledgments: The authors would like to thank to Sergio Alcañiz for his technical assistance.

Conflicts of Interest: The authors declare no conflict of interest.

References

1. Viera, I.; Roca, M.; Perez-Galvez, A. Mass Spectrometry of Non-allomerized Chlorophylls *a* and *b* Derivatives from Plants. *Curr. Org. Chem.* **2018**, *22*, 842–876. [CrossRef]
2. Catarina, M.M.; Duarte, F.; Malcata, X. Supercritical fluid extraction of carotenoids and chlorophylls *a*, *b* and *c*, from a wild strain of *Scenedesmus obliquus* for use in food processing. *J. Food Eng.* **2013**, *116*, 478–482.
3. Chacon-Lee, T.L.; González-Marino, G.E. Microalgae for "Healthy" Foods—Possibilities and Challenges. *Compr. Rev. Food Sci. Food Saf.* **2010**, *9*, 655–675. [CrossRef]
4. Viera, I.; Pérez-Gálvez, A.; Roca, M. Green Natural Colorants. *Molecules* **2019**, *24*, 154. [CrossRef]
5. Queiroz Zepka, L.; Jacob-Lopes, E.; Roca, M. Catabolism and bioactive properties of chlorophylls. *Curr. Opin. Food Sci.* **2019**, *26*, 94–100. [CrossRef]
6. Ferruzzi, M.G.; Böhm, V.; Courtney, P.D.; Schwartz, S.J. Antioxidant and antimutagenic activity of dietary chlorophyll derivatives determined by radical scavenging and bacterial reverse mutagenesis assays. *Food Chem. Toxicol.* **2002**, *67*, 2589–2595. [CrossRef]
7. Kang, Y.R.; Park, J.; Jung, S.K.; Chang, Y.H. Synthesis, characterization, and functional properties of chlorophylls, pheophytins, and Zn-pheophytins. *Food Chem.* **2018**, *245*, 943–950. [CrossRef]
8. Hoshina, C.; Tomita, K.; Shioi, Y. Antioxidant Activity of Chlorophylls: Its Structure-Activity Relationship. In *Photosynthesis: Mechanisms and Effects*; Garab, G., Ed.; Springer: Berlin, Germany, 1998; pp. 3281–3284.
9. Lanfer-Marquez, U.M.; Barros, R.M.C.; Sinnecker, P. Antioxidant activity of chlorophylls and their derivatives. *Food Res. Int.* **2005**, *38*, 885–891. [CrossRef]
10. Xavier, A.A.; Pérez-Gálvez, A. Carotenoids as a Source of Antioxidants in the Diet. *Subcell. Biochem.* **2016**, *79*, 359–375. [CrossRef]
11. Chen, W.; Hsu, Y.; Chang, J.; Ho, S.; Wang, L.; We, Y. Enhancing production of lutein by a mixotrophic cultivation system using microalga *Scenedesmus obliquus* CWL-1. *Bioresour. Technol.* **2019**, *291*, 121891. [CrossRef]
12. Ferreira, V.S.; Sant'Anna, C. Impact of culture conditions on the chlorophyll content of microalgae for biotechnological applications. *World J. Microbiol. Biotechnol.* **2017**, *33*, 20. [CrossRef] [PubMed]
13. Hu, J.; Nagarajan, D.; Zhanga, Q.; Chang, J.; Lee, D. Heterotrophic cultivation of microalgae for pigment production: A review. *Biotechnol. Adv.* **2018**, *36*, 54–67. [CrossRef] [PubMed]
14. Armstrong, G.A. Greening in the dark: Light-independent chlorophyll biosynthesis from anoxygenic photosynthetic bacteria to gymnosperms. *J. Photochem. Photobiol. B Biol.* **1998**, *43*, 87–100. [CrossRef]
15. Abeliovich, A.; Weisman, D. Role of heterotrophic nutrition in growth of the alga *Scenedesmus obliquus* in high-rate oxidation ponds. *Appl. Environ. Microbiol.* **1978**, *35*, 32–37. [PubMed]
16. Van Wagenen, J.; De Francisci, D.; Angelidaki, I. Comparison of mixotrophic to cyclic autotrophic/heterotrophic growth strategies to optimize productivity of *Chlorella sorokiniana*. *J. Appl. Phycol.* **2015**, *27*, 1775–1782. [CrossRef]
17. Sun, X.; Ren, L.; Zhao, Q.; Ji, X.; Huang, H. Microalgae for the production of lipid and carotenoids: A review with focus on stress regulation and adaptation. *Biotechnol. Biofuels* **2018**, *11*, 272. [CrossRef] [PubMed]
18. Flórez-Miranda, L.; Cañizares-Villanueva, O.; Melchy-Antonio, O.; Martínez-Jerónimo, F.; Mateo Flores-Ortíz, C. Two stage heterotrophy/photoinduction culture of *Scenedesmus incrassatulus*: Potential for lutein production. *J. Biotechnol.* **2017**, *262*, 67–74. [CrossRef]

19. Ferreira, V.S.; Pinto, R.F.; Sant'Anna, C. Low light intensity and nitrogen starvation modulate the chlorophyll content of *Scenedesmus dimorphus*. *J. Appl. Microbiol.* **2015**, *120*, 661–670. [CrossRef]
20. Chen, D.M.; Li, J.; Dai, X.; Sun, Y.; Chen, F. Effect of phosphorus and temperature on chlorophyll a contents and cell sizes of *Scenedesmus obliquus* and *Microcystis aeruginosa*. *Limnology* **2011**, *12*, 187–192. [CrossRef]
21. Masojídek, J.; Torzillo, G.; Koblízek, M.; Kopecký, J.; Bernardini, P.; Sacchi, A.; Komenda, J. Photoadaptation of two members of the Chlorophyta (*Scenedesmus* and *Chlorella*) in laboratory and outdoor cultures: Changes in chlorophyll fluorescence quenching and the xanthophyll cycle. *Planta* **1999**, *209*, 126–135. [CrossRef]
22. Kuai, B.; Chen, J.; Hörtensteiner, S. The biochemistry and molecular biology of chlorophyll breakdown. *J. Exp. Bot.* **2018**, *69*, 751–767. [CrossRef] [PubMed]
23. Gao, C.; Wang, Y.; Shen, Y.; Yan, D.; He, X.; Dai, J.; Wu, Q. Oil accumulation mechanisms of the oleaginous microalga Chlorella protothecoides revealed through its genome, transcriptomes, and proteomes. *BMC Genom.* **2014**, *10*, 582. [CrossRef] [PubMed]
24. Matsuda, K.; Shimoda, Y.; Tanaka, A.; Ito, H. Chlorophyll a is a favorable substrate for Chlamydomonas Mg-dechelatase encoded by STAY-GREEN. *Plant Physiol. Biochem.* **2016**, *109*, 365–373. [CrossRef] [PubMed]
25. Guyer, L.; Schelbert Hofstetter, S.; Christ, B.; Silvestre Lira, B.; Rossi, M.; Hörtensteiner, S. Different Mechanisms Are Responsible for Chlorophyll Dephytylation during Fruit Ripening and Leaf Senescence in Tomato. *Plant Physiol.* **2014**, *166*, 44–56. [CrossRef]
26. Engel, N.; Curty, C.; Gossauer, A. Chlorophyll catabolism in *Chorella protothecoides*. Part 8: Facts and artefacts. *Plant Physiol. Biochem.* **1996**, *34*, 77–83.
27. Bale, N.J.; Llewellyn, C.A.; Airs, R.L. Atmospheric pressure chemical ionisation liquid chromatography/mass spectrometry of type II chlorophyll—A transformation products: Diagnostic fragmentation patterns. *Org. Geochem.* **2010**, *41*, 473–481. [CrossRef]
28. Grabski, K.; Baranowski, N.; Skórko-Glonek, J.; Tukaj, Z. Chlorophyll catabolites in conditioned media of green microalga Desmodesmus subspicatus. *J. Appl. Phycol.* **2016**, *28*, 889–896. [CrossRef]
29. Hynninen, P.H.; Hyvärinen, K. Tracing the Allomerization Pathways of Chlorophylls by 18O-Labeling and Mass Spectrometry. *J. Org. Chem.* **2002**, *6712*, 4055–4061. [CrossRef]
30. Vergara-Domínguez, H.; Gandul-Rojas, B.; Roca, M. Formation of oxidised chlorophyll catabolites in olives. *J. Food Compos. Anal.* **2011**, *24*, 851–857. [CrossRef]
31. Hynninen, P.H. Chemistry of chlorophylls: Modifications. In *Chlorophylls*; Scheer, H., Tsuchiya, T., Ohta, H., Okawa, K., Iwamatsu, A., Shimada, H., Masuda, T., Eds.; CRC Press: Boca Raton, FL, USA, 1991; pp. 145–209.
32. Louda, W.; Mongkhonsri, P.; Baker, E.W. Chlorophyll degradation during senescence and death-III: 3–10 yr experiments, implications for ETIO series generation. *Org. Geochem.* **2011**, *42*, 688–699. [CrossRef]
33. Walker, J.S.; Squier, A.H.; Hodgson, D.A.; Keely, B.J. Origin and significance of 132-hydroxychlorophyll derivatives in sediments. *Org. Chem.* **2002**, *33*, 1667–1674.
34. Bale, N.J.; Airs, R.L.; Martin, P.; Lampitt, R.S.; Llewellyn, C.A. Chlorophyll-a transformations associated with sinking diatoms during termination of a North Atlantic spring bloom. *Mar. Chem.* **2015**, *172*, 23–33. [CrossRef]
35. Steele, D.J.; Kimmance, S.A.; Franklin, D.J.; Airs, R.L. Occurrence of chlorophyll allomers during virus-induced mortality and population decline in the ubiquitous picoeukaryote *Ostreococcus tauri*. *Environ. Microbiol.* **2018**, *20*, 588–601. [CrossRef] [PubMed]
36. Steele, D.J.; Tarran, G.A.; Widdicombe, C.E.; Woodward, E.M.S.; Kimmance, S.A.; Franklin, D.J.; Airs, R.L. Abundance of a chlorophyll *a* precursor and the oxidation product hydroxychlorophyll a during seasonal phytoplankton community progression in the Western English Channel. *Prog. Oceanogr.* **2015**, *137*, 434–445. [CrossRef]
37. Walker, J.S.; Keely, B.J. Distribution and significance of chlorophyll derivatives and oxidation products during the spring phytoplankton bloom in the Celtic Sea April 2002. *Org. Geochem.* **2004**, *35*, 1289–1298. [CrossRef]
38. Naylor, C.C.; Keely, B.J. Sedimentary purpurins: Oxidative transformation products of chlorophylls. *Org. Geochem.* **1998**, *28*, 417–422. [CrossRef]
39. Mulders, K.J.M.; Lamers, P.P.; Martens, D.E.; Wijffels, R.H. Phototrophic pigment production with microalgae: Biological constraints and opportunities. *J. Phycol.* **2014**, *50*, 229–242. [CrossRef]
40. Rippka, R.; Stanier, R.Y.; Deruelles, J.; Herdman, M.; Waterbury, J.B. Generic Assignments, Strain Histories and Properties of Pure Cultures of Cyanobacteria. *Microbiology* **1979**, *111*, 1–61. [CrossRef]

41. Maroneze, M.M.; Siqueira, S.F.; Vendruscolo, R.G.; Wagner, R.; de Menezes, C.R.; Zepka, L.Q.; Jacob-Lopes, E. The role of photoperiods on photobioreactors—A potential strategy to reduce costs. *Bioresour. Technol.* **2016**, *219*, 493–499. [CrossRef]
42. Francisco, É.C.; Franco, T.T.; Wagner, R.; Jacob-Lopes, E. Assessment of different carbohydrates as exogenous carbon source in cultivation of cyanobacteria. *Bioprocess Biosyst. Eng.* **2014**, *37*, 1497–1505. [CrossRef]
43. Jeffrey, S.W.; Wright, S.W.; Zapata, M. Microalgal Classes and their Signature Pigments. In *Phytoplankton pigments*; Roy, S., Llewellyn, C.A., Egeland, E.S., Johnsen, G., Eds.; Cambridge University Press: Cambridge, UK, 2011; pp. 3–77.
44. Chen, K.; Ríos, J.J.; Pérez, A.; Roca, M. Development of an accurate and high-throughput methodology for structural comprehension of chlorophylls derivatives. (I) Phytylated derivatives. *J. Chromatogr. A* **2015**, *1406*, 99–108. [CrossRef] [PubMed]
45. Breithaupt, D.E.; Wirt, U.; Bamedi, A. Differentiation between lutein monoester regioisomers and detection of lutein diesters from marigold flowers (*Tagetes erecta*, L.) and several fruits by liquid chromatography-mass spectrometry. *J. Agric. Food Chem.* **2002**, *50*, 66–70. [CrossRef] [PubMed]
46. Ríos, J.J.; Xavier, A.A.O.; Díaz-Salido, E.; Arenilla-Vélez, I.; Jarén-Galán, M.; Garrido-Fernández, J.; Pérez-Gálvez, A. Xanthophyll esters are found in human colostrum. *Mol. Nutr. Food Res.* **2017**, *61*, 1700296. [CrossRef] [PubMed]
47. Paliwal, C.; Ghosh, T.; George, B.; Pancha, Y.; Maurya, R.; Chokshi, K.; Ghosh, A.; Mishra, S. Microalgal carotenoids: Potential nutraceutical compounds with chemotaxonomic importance. *Algal Res.* **2016**, *15*, 24–31. [CrossRef]
48. Jahns, P.; Latowski, D.; Strzalka, K. Mechanism and regulation of the violaxanthin cycle: The role of antenna proteins and membrane lipids. *Biochim. Biophys. Acta* **2009**, *1787*, 3–14. [CrossRef]
49. Telfer, A.; Pascal, A.; Gall, A. Natural functions. In *Carotenoids*; Britton, G., Liaanen-Jensen, S., Pfander, H., Eds.; Birkhauser: Basel, Switzerland, 2008; Volume 4, pp. 189–211.
50. Tanaka, R.; Tanaka, A. Chlorophyll cycle regulates the construction and destruction of the light-harvesting complexes. *Biochim. Biophys. Acta* **2011**, *1807*, 968–976. [CrossRef]
51. Richardson, K.; Beardall, J.; Raven, J.A. Adaptation of Unicellular Algae to Irradiance: An Analysis of Strategies. *New Phytol.* **1983**, *93*, 157–191. [CrossRef]
52. Falkowski, P.G.; Owens, T.G. Light-Shade Adaptation. Two strategies in marine phytoplankton. *Plant Physiol.* **1980**, *66*, 592–595. [CrossRef]
53. MacIntyre, H.L.; Kana, T.M.; Anning, T.; Geider, R.J. Photoacclimation of photosynthesis irradiance response curves and photosynthetic pigments in microalgae and cyanobacteria. *J. Phycol.* **2002**, *38*, 17–38. [CrossRef]
54. Airs, R.L.; Keely, B.J. A high resolution study of the chlorophyll and bacteriochlorophyll pigment distributions in a calcite/gypsum microbial mat. *Org. Geochem.* **2003**, *34*, 539–551. [CrossRef]
55. Cirulis, J.T.; Ashley Scott, J.; Ross, G.M. Management of oxidative stress by microalgae. *Can. J. Physiol. Pharmacol.* **2013**, *91*, 15–21. [CrossRef] [PubMed]
56. Kumar, R.R.; Hanumantha Rao, P.; Subramanian, V.V.; Sivasubramanian, V. Enzymatic and non-enzymatic antioxidant potentials of *Chlorella vulgaris* grown in effluent of a confectionery industry. *J. Food Sci. Technol.* **2014**, *51*, 322–328. [CrossRef] [PubMed]
57. Beisel, K.G.; Jahnke, S.; Hofmann, D.; Köppchen, S.; Schurr, U.; Matsubara, S. Continuous Turnover of Carotenes and Chlorophyll *a* in Mature Leaves of Arabidopsis Revealed by $^{14}CO_2$ Pulse-Chase Labeling. *Plant Physiol.* **2010**, *152*, 2188–2199. [CrossRef] [PubMed]
58. Stadnichuk, I.N.; Rakhimberdieva, M.G.; Bolychevtseva, Y.V.; Yurina, N.P.; Karapetyan, N.V.; Selyakh, I.O. Inhibition by glucose of chlorophyll *a* and phycocyanobilin biosynthesis in the unicellular red alga *Galdieria partita* at the stage of coproporphyrinogen III formation. *Plant Sci.* **1998**, *136*, 11–23. [CrossRef]
59. Kamalanathan, M.; Dao, T.L.; Panjhaphol, C.; Gleadow, R.; Beardall, J. Photosynthetic physiology of Scenedesmus sp. under photoautotrophic, and molasses-based heterotrophic and mixotrophic conditions. *Phycologia* **2017**, *56*, 666–674. [CrossRef]
60. Guyer, L.; Salinger, K.; Krügel, U.; Hörtensteiner, S. Catalytic and structural properties of pheophytinase, the phytol esterase involved in chlorophyll breakdown. *J. Exp. Bot.* **2018**, *69*, 879–889. [CrossRef]

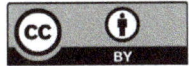

© 2019 by the authors. Licensee MDPI, Basel, Switzerland. This article is an open access article distributed under the terms and conditions of the Creative Commons Attribution (CC BY) license (http://creativecommons.org/licenses/by/4.0/).

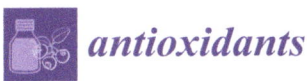

Article

In-Vitro Antioxidant Properties of Lipophilic Antioxidant Compounds from 3 Brown Seaweed

Gaurav Rajauria

School of Agriculture and Food Science, University College Dublin, Lyons Research Farm, Celbridge, Co. Kildare W23 ENY2, Ireland; gaurav.rajauria@ucd.ie; Tel.: +353-1-601-2167

Received: 21 October 2019; Accepted: 26 November 2019; Published: 28 November 2019

Abstract: Lipophilic compounds of seaweed have been linked to their potential bioactivity. Low polarity solvents such as chloroform, diethyl ether, *n*-hexane and their various combinations were used to extract the lipophilic antioxidants from brown seaweed namely *Himanthalia elongata*, *Laminaria saccharina* and *Laminaria digitata*. An equal-volume mixture of chloroform, diethyl ether and *n*-hexane (Mix 4) gave the highest total phenol (52.7 ± 1.93 to 180.2 ± 1.84 mg gallic acid equivalents/g), flavonoid (31.9 ± 2.65 to 131.3 ± 4.51 mg quercetin equivalents/g), carotenoid (2.19 ± 1.37 to 3.15 ± 0.91 µg/g) and chlorophyll content (2.88 ± 1.08 to 3.86 ± 1.22 µg/g) in the tested seaweeds. The extracts were screened for their potential antioxidant capacity and the extracts obtained from the selected solvents system exhibited the highest radical scavenging capacity against 2,2′-diphenly-1-picrylhydrazyl radical (EC_{50} 98.3 ± 2.78 to 298.8 ± 5.81 mg/L) and metal ions (EC_{50} 228.6 ± 3.51 to 532.4 ± 6.03 mg/L). Similarly, the same extract showed the highest ferric reducing antioxidant power (8.3 ± 0.23 to 26.3 ± 0.30 mg trolox equivalents/g) in all the seaweeds. Rapid characterization of the active extracts by liquid chromatography coupled with photodiode array detector and electrospray ionization tandem mass spectrometry (LC-PDA–ESI-MS/MS) identified cyanidin-3-*O*-glucoside, fucoxanthin, violaxanthin, β-carotene, chlorophyll *a* derivatives and chlorophyll *b* derivatives in the tested seaweed. The study demonstrated the use of tested brown seaweed as potential species to be considered for future applications in medicine, cosmetics and as nutritional food supplement.

Keywords: lipophilic antioxidant; solvent blending; macroalgae; LC-ESI-MS/MS; carotenoid pigment; anthocyanin; chlorophyll derivative

1. Introduction

The concepts of nutrition are changing rapidly as consumers all over the world have become more cautious regarding nutritionally healthier food and its ingredients. Recently, a great interest in using natural plant-derived bioactive compounds in foods, cosmetics and pharmaceuticals has arisen, due to their nutritional and therapeutic effects [1,2]. The epidemiological and observational literatures suggest that free radicals play an important role in affecting human health by causing cancers or age associated neurodegenerative diseases. However, antioxidant-rich foods have shown their relevance in the prevention of these diseases by mitigating the harmful free radicals or reactive oxygen species (ROS) [3]. Chemical compounds such as butylated hydroxytoluene (BHT; E-321), butylhydroxyanisole (BHA; E-320) and ascorbic acid (E-300) are commonly used as synthetic antioxidants in food products to improve the product quality and shelf life. However, due to possible toxicity of synthetic antioxidants as well as consumer preference towards natural substances, natural antioxidants are considered safe and more acceptable for use as ingredients in functional foods, nutraceuticals and cosmetics [4,5]. Among the most studied classes of natural antioxidants, phenolic compounds and carotenoid pigments are widely distributed in the plant kingdom and have received much attention for their high antioxidant activity [6]. Although these functional ingredients are not restricted to terrestrial resources, plants in general and seaweeds (marine plants) in particular, are good sources of natural antioxidants. Seaweed grows in extreme environmental conditions thus producing a variety of antioxidant compounds to counteract environmental stresses [7]. The most important naturally occurring seaweed substances showing antioxidant properties are polyphenols, phlorotannins, flavonoids, carotenoids, fatty acids, polysaccharides and amino acids, which in varying proportion and quantities, are reported in different seaweed species [8–10]. A variety of in vitro studies have shown that lipophilic compounds such as carotenoid pigments and some polyphenols and flavonoids exhibit strong antioxidant activity [11–14]. These compounds are capable of acting as primary antioxidants by reacting with free radical species or could act as secondary antioxidants (metal chelator) by blocking the generation of hypervalent metal forms [15]. Such antioxidant activities of carotenoids and polyphenols may protect cells from ROS-induced cellular damage, thereby reducing the risk of diseases associated with oxidative stress [16].

Multiple compounds from hundreds of algal species have been studied up until now and a range of compounds possessing antioxidant properties have been discovered. Among these compounds, some compounds are of polar or hydrophilic nature (e.g., phlorotannins), some are semi-polar (e.g., phenolic acids and simple flavonoids), some and others are non-polar or lipophilic in nature (e.g., carotenoids, fatty acids). They may also exist as complexes with sugar, proteins and other cell membrane components; which make them quite insoluble and a selective solvent system is required to solubilize and extract them [17]. Extractability of bioactive compounds is associated with the polarity of solvents (polar/semi-non-polar) used, as well as their complexity with other constituents. Finding a solvent system suitable for the extraction of all classes or a specific class of antioxidant is restricted by the chemical nature of these bioactive compounds. These bioactives are present in matrices as a complex mixture of compounds that provide a cocktail of many active components present in the free, esterified, glycosylated and bound states as conjugates with other components that lead to the formation of insoluble complexes. The solubility of these compounds is administered by the nature of raw material, degree of polymerization and the polarity of solvent used [1]. Therefore, the extraction of these active ingredients from seaweed matrices is the key step to utilizing them for pharmaceutical, cosmeceutical, and foods as well as nutraceutical preparations. Thus, to obtain extracts enriched in lipophilic compounds, it is of critical importance to select efficient extraction solvent systems to improve their extractability and to maintain stability. Additionally, extraction solvent can have a significant effect on the performance of antioxidant reaction mechanisms which can change the chemical behavior of antioxidant compounds [18]. Therefore, there is no uniform or completely satisfactory procedure that is suitable for extraction of all compounds or a specific class of compounds from plant materials [17]. Thus, the objective of the present study was to select the appropriate solvent system that is capable of extracting lipophilic compounds from Irish brown seaweeds and to evaluate the antioxidant capacity and phytochemical constituents of those extracts. Seaweeds were extracted with semi/non-polar solvents and their mixtures, in order to get the lipophilic antioxidant compounds. The crude extracts were screened for total polyphenol, flavonoid, chlorophyll and carotenoid content along with antioxidant reducing power and potential radical scavenging capacity against 2,2'-diphenyl-1-picrylhydrazyl (DPPH) radicals and metal-ions. The identification and characterization of antioxidant compounds were carried out by using liquid chromatography coupled with electrospray ionization tandem mass spectrometry (LC-ESI-MS/MS) and UV-visible spectroscopy.

2. Materials and Methods

2.1. Chemicals, Solvents and Standards

Folin-Ciocalteu's phenol reagent, 2,2'-diphenyl-1-picrylhydrazyl (DPPH), 3-(2-pyridyl)-5,6-diphenyl-1,2,4-triazine-4',4''-disulphonic acid monosodium salt (ferrozine), 2,4,6-tripyridyl-s-triazine (TPTZ) and 6-hydroxy-2,5,7,8-tetramethylchroman-2-carboxylic acid (Trolox) were purchased from Sigma-Aldrich Chemical Co. (Steinheim, Germany). For LC-MS analysis, solvents such as water, methanol and acetonitrile were chromatography grade which was purchased from Fisher Chemicals

(Thermo Fisher Scientific Inc., Dublin, Ireland). Authentic standards including L-ascorbic acid, gallic acid, quercetin, cyanidin 3-glucoside, fucoxanthin and violaxanthin were purchased from Sigma-Aldrich Chemical Co. (Arklow, Co. Wicklow, Ireland). All other chemicals used in the study were analytical grade and purchased from Sigma-Aldrich Chemical Co. (Ireland).

2.2. Seaweed Materials and Extraction Procedure

Irish brown seaweeds (Figure 1) used in this study namely, *Laminaria digitata*, *Laminaria saccharina* and *Himanthalia elongata* (*Phaeophyta*) were purchased from Quality Sea Veg., Co Donegal, Ireland. Among the tested seaweeds, *L. digitata* and *L. saccharina* (also known as *Saccharina latissima*) are large conspicuous dark brown and yellow brown kelp, commonly found down to a maximum depth of 20 m and 30 m in clear waters respectively. The stipes of *L. digitata* are smooth, flexible and oval in cross section while *L. saccharina* has a long undivided frond with a distinct bullations and a distinctive frilly undulating margin. Both are usually found attached to bedrock or other suitable hard substrata in the low water in Intertidal pools and occasionally in the shallow subtidal zones. *H. elongata* is a light yellow-brown fucoid species which has long, narrow, strap-like branched fronds with basal mushroom-like buttons. It is found attached to rocks or hard substrata on moderately semi-wave-exposed shore. Seaweed species were harvested and collected in winter (January/February), washed thoroughly with fresh water to remove epiphytes, eliminate salt, sand or shells and stored at −20 °C until analysis.

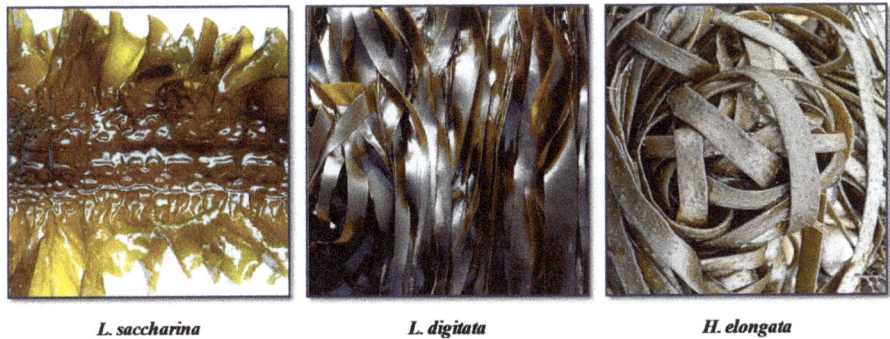

Figure 1. Images of brown Irish seaweeds studied.

Extraction of lipophilic components from seaweed was carried out by crushing the fresh sample with liquid nitrogen followed by extraction with semi/non-polar organic solvents such as chloroform, diethyl ether, *n*-hexane and thereof mixtures according to the method described earlier [19,20]. The mixtures of solvents used were; Mix 1 (*n*-hexane and diethyl ether), Mix 2 (*n*-hexane and chloroform), Mix 3 (diethyl ether and chloroform) and Mix 4 (*n*-hexane, diethyl ether and chloroform). All the solvents were mixed either 1:1 (*v/v*) or 1:1:1 ratio (*v/v/v*) depending upon the mixtures, and dielectric constant (ε) of individual solvent as well as their mixture were taken into account. The extracted samples were filtered with Whatman #1 filter paper and centrifuged at 9168× *g* (Sigma 2–16PK, Sartorius AG, Gottingen, Germany) for 15 min. The resulting supernatant was evaporated to dryness, and the dried lipophilic extract was dissolved in HPLC (high performance liquid chromatography) grade methanol for further analysis. The whole extraction procedure was carried out under dark conditions to minimize the possibility of oxidation/degradation of antioxidant compounds by light.

2.3. Phytochemical Constituent Analysis

Crude lipophilic extracts of seaweed were screened for total phenolic content (TPC), total flavonoid content (TFC), total chlorophyll content (TChC) and total carotenoid content (TCC). TPC was determined according to Ganesan et al. [9]. Samples were read at 720 nm and the results were expressed as mg gallic acid equivalents (GAE)/g dry weight (dw) extract. TFC and TTC were determined according to Liu et al. [21]. Samples were read at 510 nm and 500 nm, and the results were expressed as mg quercetin equivalents (QE)/g extract (dw) and mg (+)-catechin equivalents (ChE)/g extract (dw), respectively. TChC and TCC were determined according to Arnon (1949) and Kirk and Allen (1965) respectively. For chlorophyll, the samples were read at 645 nm and 663 nm, and total content was calculated by using Equation (1), while for total carotenoids, the absorbance of the same chlorophyll samples was recorded at 480 nm and content was calculated by using Equation (2).

$$\text{TChC (µg/g; dw)} = 20.2 \times (A_{645}) + 8.02 \times (A_{663}) \quad (1)$$

where A = Absorbance at respective wavelength

$$\text{TCC (µg/g; dw)} = A_{480} + (0.114 \times A_{663}) - (0.638 \times A_{645}) \quad (2)$$

where, A = Absorbance at respective wavelength

2.4. Antioxidant Capacity Analysis

2.4.1. DPPH Radical Scavenging Capacity Assay

This assay was carried out according to the method reported earlier [22]. Ascorbic acid was used as a standard and the absorbance of the standard or samples was recorded at 517 nm using a 96-well plate reader. The ability of samples to scavenge the DPPH radical was calculated using Equation (3):

$$\text{DPPH radical scavenging capacity (\%)} = [1 - (A_{\text{sample}} - A_{\text{sample blank}})/A_{\text{control}}] \times 100 \quad (3)$$

where, A = Absorbance of sample/sample blank or control

2.4.2. Ferric Reducing Antioxidant Power (FRAP) Assay

Total antioxidant reducing power of various extracts of seaweed was measured using modified FRAP assay [23]. Trolox was used as a standard and the absorbance of the standard or samples was recorded at 593 nm, and the results were expressed as mg trolox equivalents (TE)/g extract (dw).

2.4.3. Metal Ion-Chelating Ability Assay

The chelating ability of metal ion (ferrous ion) by seaweed extracts was estimated using the original method of Decker and Welch [24] with minor modifications. This assay is based upon the formation of blue colored ferrous ion-ferrozine complex which has a maximum absorbance at 562 nm. EDTA (ethylenediaminetetraacetic acid) was used as a standard compound. The percentage of inhibition of ferrozine-Fe^{2+} complex formation was calculated using Equation (3).

2.5. Characterization of Lipophilic Compounds using Liquid Chromatography Mass Spectrometry (LC–MS)

Antioxidant compounds in the lipophilic extracts were analyzed on 6410 Triple Quadrupole LC/MS, fitted with Agilent 1200 series LC, G1315B variable-wavelength photodiode array (PDA) detector and MassHunter Workstation software (version B.04.00, Agilent Technologies, Santa Clara, CA, USA). The separation was performed at 25 °C using an Atlantis C-18 (250 × 4.6 mm, 5 µm particle size) column fitted with a suitable C-18 (4.0 × 3.0 mm) guard cartridge (Waters, Dublin, Ireland). The mobile phase consisting of ternary solvents of acetonitrile/methanol/water (75:15:10, *v/v/v*) containing 1.0 g/L ammonium acetate, eluted at 1.0 mL/min for 25 min, was adopted from Sugawara [25]. The injection volume of 10 µL was kept constant for samples and standard compounds. UV-vis absorption of the selected extracts was recorded from 190 to 600 nm using LC-PDA detector and the $\lambda_{\max}$ (absorption maxima) of each peak was noted. Peaks assignments were made by comparing the UV/visible spectra of analytes to standard compounds, and available literature. Mass spectral data were recorded on positive ionization mode using electrospray ionization (ESI) interface with 3.5 kV capillary voltage, 120 V fragmentor voltage and 10 eV collision energy in the mass range of m/z 100–1000. Nitrogen gas was used as the nebulizer and drying gas with 50 psi pressure, 10 L/min flow rate, 350 °C drying temperature and 35 nA capillary current. The identification of the peaks was carried out using mass spectral data of standard compounds where possible. Identification of remaining peaks was based on UV-visible spectral (λ_{max}) characteristics and the results were compared with the literature when no standards were available.

2.6. Statistical Analysis

Statistical analyses were carried out using STATGRAPHICS Centurion XV software (version XV, Statgraphics Technologies, Inc., The Plains, VA, USA). All the experiments were carried out in triplicate and repeated twice. Results are expressed as mean ± standard deviation. Statistical differences between antioxidant activities or phytochemical content of extracts were determined using Analysis of Variance (ANOVA) followed by Least Significant Difference (LSD) testing. Differences were considered statistically significant when $p < 0.05$.

3. Results and Discussion

3.1. Phytochemical Content in Lipophilic Extracts

It is widely accepted that bioactive compounds can be classified by their solubility into hydrophilic and lipophilic compounds. Similar to hydrophilic compounds, lipophilic compounds also play an important role in a wide spectrum of biochemical and physiological processes [11]. These lipophilic compounds can be extracted with semi/non-polar solvents in plants wherein polarity of the solvents play a significant role in the resulting yield, extractability and biological activity of bioactive compounds. In this study, various organic solvents and their combinations with varying dielectric constant were used to extract lipophilic compounds from 3 brown seaweed.

Results from Table 1 have shown a considerable variation in the extraction yield among the extracts recovered from various low polarity solvents and their mixtures. The extraction yield varied from 0.05% to 0.20% among all the tested seaweeds. The extracts recovered from n-hexane and Mix 1 solvents exhibited significantly ($p > 0.05$) the highest and the lowest extraction yield respectively. It is reported that low polarity (semi/non-polar) solvents generally give less extraction yield as compared to polar solvents [26] which is in agreement with the results obtained in this study.

Table 1. Extraction yield and phytochemical content of lipophilic extracts of brown seaweed obtained from various organic solvents and their mixtures (semi/non-polar solvents).

Organic Solvents	Dielectric Constant (ε)	Yield %	TPC mg GAE/g	TFC mg QE/g	TCC (µg/g)	TChC (µg/g)
H. elongata						
n-hexane	2.0	0.20 ± 0.02 [a,p]	14.1 ± 0.79 [a]	11.3 ± 2.50 [a]	1.55 ± 0.12 [a]	3.23 ± 1.01 [a]
Diethyl ether	4.3	0.17 ± 0.01 [b]	165.2 ± 1.46 [b]	92.1 ± 5.64 [b]	2.18 ± 0.93 [b]	2.41 ± 1.00 [b]
Chloroform	5.0	0.11 ± 0.01 [c]	71.2 ± 2.33 [c]	37.5 ± 3.75 [c]	2.81 ± 1.03 [c]	6.62 ± 1.34 [c]
Mix 1	3.2	0.05 ± 0.02 [e]	121.5 ± 3.67 [d]	60.4 ± 4.02 [d]	1.79 ± 0.22 [d]	1.70 ± 0.91 [d]
Mix 2	3.5	0.16 ± 0.03 [b,d]	152.3 ± 1.98 [e]	55.8 ± 2.60 [d]	1.93 ± 0.31 [d]	1.56 ± 0.61 [d]
Mix 3	4.7	0.16 ± 0.02 [b]	88.9 ± 2.96 [f]	85.8 ± 3.82 [b]	2.66 ± 1.04 [e]	3.68 ± 1.12 [e]
Mix 4 *	3.8	0.14 ± 0.01 [d]	180.2 ± 1.84 [g,p]	131.3 ± 4.51 [e,p]	3.15 ± 0.91 [f,p]	3.86 ± 1.22 [e,p]
L. saccharina						
n-hexane	2.0	0.19 ± 0.03 [a,q]	9.5 ± 1.93 [a]	6.9 ± 0.88 [a]	1.45 ± 0.42 [a]	4.66 ± 1.03 [a]
Diethyl ether	4.3	0.12 ± 0.01 [b]	53.4 ± 0.96 [b]	33.1 ± 2.65 [b]	2.14 ± 0.83 [b]	3.48 ± 0.93 [b]
Chloroform	5.0	0.08 ± 0.02 [c,d]	12.5 ± 0.32 [c]	7.5 ± 0.00 [a]	2.59 ± 0.91 [c]	7.82 ± 1.54 [c]
Mix 1	3.2	0.06 ± 0.01 [d]	29.1 ± 0.64 [d]	17.5 ± 1.77 [c]	1.86 ± 0.63 [d]	2.75 ± 1.08 [d]
Mix 2	3.5	0.11 ± 0.04 [b]	25.2 ± 1.61 [e]	15.0 ± 3.54 [c]	2.08 ± 0.39 [b]	2.46 ± 1.17 [e]
Mix 3	4.7	0.09 ± 0.01 [c]	39.8 ± 1.61 [f]	22.5 ± 1.77 [d]	2.73 ± 0.84 [e]	3.48 ± 1.32 [b]
Mix 4 *	3.8	0.07 ± 0.01 [c,d]	73.4 ± 0.32 [g,q]	56.3 ± 1.77 [e,q]	2.75 ± 0.88 [e,q]	3.62 ± 1.22 [f,p]

Table 1. Cont.

Organic Solvents	Dielectric Constant (ε)	Yield %	TPC mg GAE/g	TFC mg QE/g	TCC (μg/g)	TChC (μg/g)
L. digitata						
n-hexane	2.0	0.17 ± 0.02 [a,r]	7.7 ± 0.64 [a]	4.4 ± 0.88 [a]	1.20 ± 1.24 [a]	6.19 ± 1.42 [a]
Diethyl ether	4.3	0.14 ± 0.02 [a,d]	48.9 ± 2.25 [b]	29.4 ± 2.65 [b]	1.35 ± 1.64 [b]	5.65 ± 1.64 [b]
Chloroform	5.0	0.09 ± 0.01 [b,c]	15.2 ± 2.25 [c]	8.1 ± 0.88 [c]	1.93 ± 1.17 [c]	8.86 ± 1.93 [c]
Mix 1	3.2	0.08 ± 0.02 [c]	29.1 ± 2.57 [d]	18.1 ± 0.88 [d]	1.39 ± 1.28 [b]	4.62 ± 1.76 [d]
Mix 2	3.5	0.11 ± 0.04 [b]	29.5 ± 2.57 [e]	18.1 ± 2.65 [d]	1.44 ± 0.68 [d]	2.47 ± 1.48 [e]
Mix 3	4.7	0.12 ± 0.00 [b,d]	46.8 ± 2.57 [f]	26.3 ± 1.77 [b,e]	1.43 ± 1.29 [d]	2.71 ± 1.39 [f]
Mix 4 *	3.8	0.11 ± 0.02 [b]	52.7 ± 1.93 [g,r]	31.9 ± 2.65 [e,r]	2.19 ± 1.37 [e,r]	2.88 ± 1.08 [f,q]

Values are expressed as mean ± standard deviation (SD). Values within a species with different letters (a–g) in columns are significantly different ($p < 0.05$), n = 6. * Values among the three species with different letters (p–r) in columns, are significantly different ($p < 0.05$). Yield (%) is calculated in terms of g of dry extracts/100 g of fresh weight. TPC (total phenolic content) and TFC (total flavonoid content) are expressed as mg gallic acid equivalents/g (dw) and mg quercetin equivalents/g (dw), respectively. TCC (total carotenoid content) and TChC (total chlorophyll content) are reported in μg/g (dw). Mix 1: *n*-hexane and diethyl ether; Mix 2: *n*-hexane and chloroform; Mix 3: diethyl ether and chloroform; Mix 4: *n*-hexane, diethyl ether and chloroform. All the solvents were mixed in 1:1 or 1:1:1 (v/v/v) ratio.

Phytochemical content was majorly affected by the polarity of the extraction solvents as depicted in Table 1. In each of the tested seaweed, TPC from all the extracts was significantly different ($p > 0.05$) among the tested solvent systems. The extracts obtained from *n*-hexane exhibited the lowest TPC (varied from 7.7 ± 0.64 to 14.1 ± 0.79 mg GAE/g) while the extracts recovered from Mix 4 (*n*-hexane, diethyl ether and chloroform) solvents showed the highest TPC (ranging from 52.7 ± 1.93 to 180.2 ± 1.84 mg GAE/g), in all the species studied. The highest and significantly different ($p < 0.05$) amount of TPC was obtained in *H. elongata* followed by *L. saccharina* and *L. digitata* with the Mix 4 solvent system.

In the case of total flavonoid, the results showed that TFC in seaweeds varied considerably with the solvent polarity. The TFC of extracts obtained from different low polarity solvents and their mixtures ranged from 11.3 ± 2.5 to 131.3 ± 4.51 mg QE/g in *H. elongata*, 6.9 ± 0.88 to 56.3 ± 1.77 mg QE/g in *L. saccharina* and 4.4 ± 0.88 to 31.9 ± 2.65 mg QE/g in *L. digitata*. The extract from Mix 4 solvents exhibited the highest and significantly different ($p < 0.05$) TFC in *H. elongata* followed by *L. saccharina* and *L. digitata*. However, the extract obtained from *n*-hexane showed the lowest TFC in all the seaweed species (Table 1). There was no significant difference observed in TFC between the extract of Mix 1 (*n*-hexane: diethyl ether) and Mix 2 (*n*-hexane: chloroform) solvents within an individual seaweed species.

Pigments such as carotenoids play an important role in seaweed reproduction and are responsible for different colors. Fucoxanthin, a major pigment of brown seaweeds, is one of the most abundant carotenoids in nature and constitute 10% to total carotenoid production [27]. It is an orange-colored pigment, found along with chlorophyll pigment (a and c) and β-carotene, to give a brown or olive-green color to brown seaweed [28–30]. Numerous studies have shown that brown seaweed pigments such as fucoxanthin, violaxanthin and β-carotene have substantial applications in human health. These pigments have been explored for its potential bioactivities including antioxidant, anti-inflammatory, anticancer, anti-obese and antidiabetic property [14,31,32]. Table 1 shows that the spectrophotometric measurement of total carotenoids and total chlorophyll content in various extracts of 3 brown seaweed studied. The results revealed that the Mix 4 solvent system produced significantly higher TCC in *H. elongata* followed by *L. digitata* and *L. saccharina* whereas *n*-hexane extracts presented the lowest values among the tested seaweed. In the case of chlorophyll content, extracts from chloroform (instead of Mix 4 solvents) exhibited the highest TChC while extracts recovered from Mix 2 solvents showed the lowest TChC ($p < 0.05$), among the tested seaweeds and their extracts (Table 1). It was observed that the chloroform extract of *L. digitata* exhibited the highest TChC ($p < 0.05$) whereas *H. elongata* extract presented the lowest TChC.

Furthermore, upon analyzing TPC, TFC, TChC and TCC results against the polarity or dielectric constant of extraction solvents and their mixtures, an interesting relationship was observed. The results interpreted that the phytochemical content was primarily affected by the semi/non-polar extraction solvents. The dielectric constant of solvents and their mixtures was in the range of 5.0 to 2.0 with the following decreasing order: chloroform (5.0) > Mix 2 (4.7) > diethyl ether (4.3) > Mix 4 (3.8) > Mix 3 (3.5) > Mix 1 (3.2) > n-hexane (2.0). The dielectric constant of the mixed solvents is calculated on the basis of percentage (v/v) of each solvent used for the combinations. The dielectric constant of a solvent is an index of its polarity, and an increase in polarity shows a similar increase in the dielectric constant [10]. Mixing of solvents with different polarities is an approach to form a solvent system of optimum polarity to extract the various bioactive compounds. This approach is referred to as "solvent blending" or "co-solvency" and uses the dielectric constant as a guide to develop the co-solvent system [33]. The results indicated that the polarity/dielectric constant of Mix 4 solvent system (n-hexane, diethyl ether and chloroform) was more selective to the lipophilic phenolic compounds present in selected seaweeds than the other tested solvents and their mixtures. These findings are also in agreement with the report of Sahreen [34] wherein a range of polarity solvents gave different values of TPC, TFC and extraction yield. Furthermore, these findings also suggest that yield may not be a good indicator of phytochemical content of extracts based on the fact that phytochemical content was the lowest in the n-hexane extract, but had the highest extraction yield in all the studied seaweeds, which agrees with the previous reported results [35].

This study, as well as other previously reported publications [1,17,36], clearly illustrates that it is essential to systematically evaluate and optimize the extraction solvent composition for accurate and reproducible estimation of structurally diverse antioxidant compounds from different plants. In the present study, the highest recoveries of lipophilic antioxidants from seaweeds samples were obtained from Mix 4 solvents mixture using a solvent extraction technique.

3.2. Antioxidant Capacity of Lipophilic Extracts

The lipophilic extracts of all the three tested seaweed, obtained from various solvents and their mixtures, were screened for their potential antioxidant capacity using the stable DPPH radicals, FRAP reagent and by metal ion-chelating ability assay. The results of antioxidant capacity are illustrated in Figures 2 and 3. It was observed that all the seaweed exhibited a treatment effect and the scavenging of DPPH radicals by the seaweed extracts was dose-dependent. Results interpreted that EC_{50} values of all the extracts obtained from different solvents were significantly different ($p < 0.05$) in each seaweed species. The extracts from Mix 4 solvent exhibited the highest scavenging (lowest EC_{50} values) while the extracts from n-hexane depicted the lowest scavenging capacity (highest EC_{50} values) against DPPH radicals (Figure 2a). Among the tested seaweed, H. elongata showed the highest scavenging capacity (EC_{50} 98.3 ± 2.78 μg/mL) followed by L. saccharina (EC_{50} 222.4 ± 0.84 μg/mL) and L. digitata (EC_{50} 298.8 ± 5.81 μg/mL). The scavenging capacity of the standard ascorbic acid (EC_{50} 50.6 ± 0.79 μg/mL) was recorded higher than the seaweed extracts.

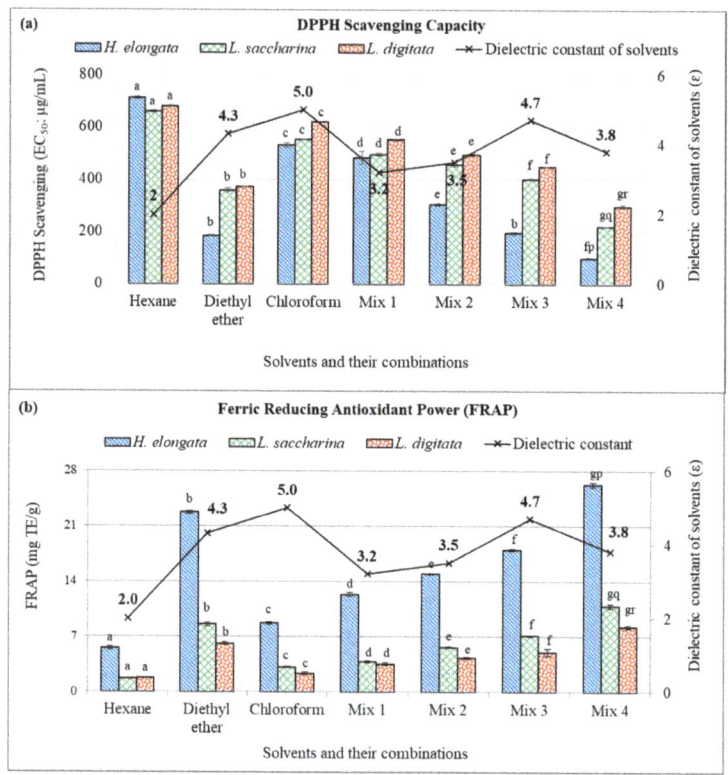

Figure 2. 2,2′-diphenyl-1-picrylhydrazyl (DPPH) radical scavenging capacity (**a**) and ferric reducing antioxidant power (**b**) of the Irish brown seaweeds extracts obtained from semi/non-polar organic solvents and thereof mixtures (1:1 or 1:1:1, $v/v/v$). [Mix 1: *n*-hexane and diethyl ether; Mix 2: *n*-hexane and chloroform; Mix 3: diethyl ether and chloroform; Mix 4: *n*-hexane, diethyl ether and chloroform]. [▨: *H. elongata*; ▨: *L. saccharina*; ▨: *L. digitata*]. Data are expressed as mean ± SD (n = 6). Ferric Reducing Antioxidant Power (FRAP) values are expressed as mg Trolox equivalent (TE)/g extract (dry weight). Letters (a–g) on each bar are significantly different ($p < 0.05$) for various solvents, for each individual species. Letters (p–r) on bars at a specific solvent (Mix 4) are significantly different ($p < 0.05$) among the three species. Mix 1: *n*-hexane and diethyl ether; Mix 2: *n*-hexane and chloroform; Mix 3: diethyl ether and chloroform; Mix 4; *n*-hexane, diethyl ether and chloroform. All the solvents were mixed either 1:1 or 1:1:1 ratio (v/v).

Reducing power appears to be related to the degree of hydroxylation and the extent of conjugation in polyphenols. The ferric reducing antioxidant power in the various extracts of brown seaweeds was studied and the results are presented in Figure 2b. The reducing ability of all the extracts were significantly different within each species and ranged from 5.5 ± 0.20 to 26.3 ± 0.30 mg TE/g dw extract in *H. elongata*, 1.6 ± 0.06 to 10.9 ± 0.29 mg TE/g dw extract in *L. saccharina* and 1.7 ± 0.06 to 8.3 ± 0.23 mg TE/g dw extract in *L. digitata*. Of the tested extracts, Mix 4 solvent extracts (*n*-hexane, diethyl ether and chloroform) exhibited the highest and statistically different ($p < 0.05$) FRAP value in *H. elongata* followed by *L. saccharina* and *L. digitata*, while the extract obtained from the *n*-hexane showed the lowest reducing power in the tested seaweed. Jiménez-Escrig [37] reported that *Fucoid* species contained more reducing power than *Laminaria* species which is in agreement with the present results.

Ferrous ions are the most powerful pro-oxidants among various species of transition metals present in food systems. Dietary antioxidants (nutrients) having the metal chelating ability, form σ-bonds with metal ions and reduce the redox potential thereby stabilizing the oxidized form of the metal ions [38]. As seen in Figure 3, the formation of Fe^{2+}-ferrozine complex is disrupted in the presence of various extracts from brown seaweeds. The absorption of this complex decreased linearly in a dose-dependent manner. All the extracts had a high level of metal ion chelating ability but were significantly lower as compared to the EDTA. Among all the tested solvents, the extract from Mix 4 solvents showed the highest chelating ability ($p < 0.05$) while extracts from n-hexane showed the lowest metal chelating ability at any tested concentration. In contrast to FRAP and DPPH scavenging activity, the metal chelating ability was recorded higher in *Laminaria* species compared to *H. elongata*. The percentage of the metal chelating ability of all the extracts at 1000 µg/mL concentration was found to be 22.7 to 57.8% in *H. elongata*, 48.9 to 81.9% in *L. digitata* and 52.8 to 82.3% in *L. saccharina*, while standard EDTA exhibited almost 100% chelating ability even at very low (125 µg/mL) concentration (Figure 3).

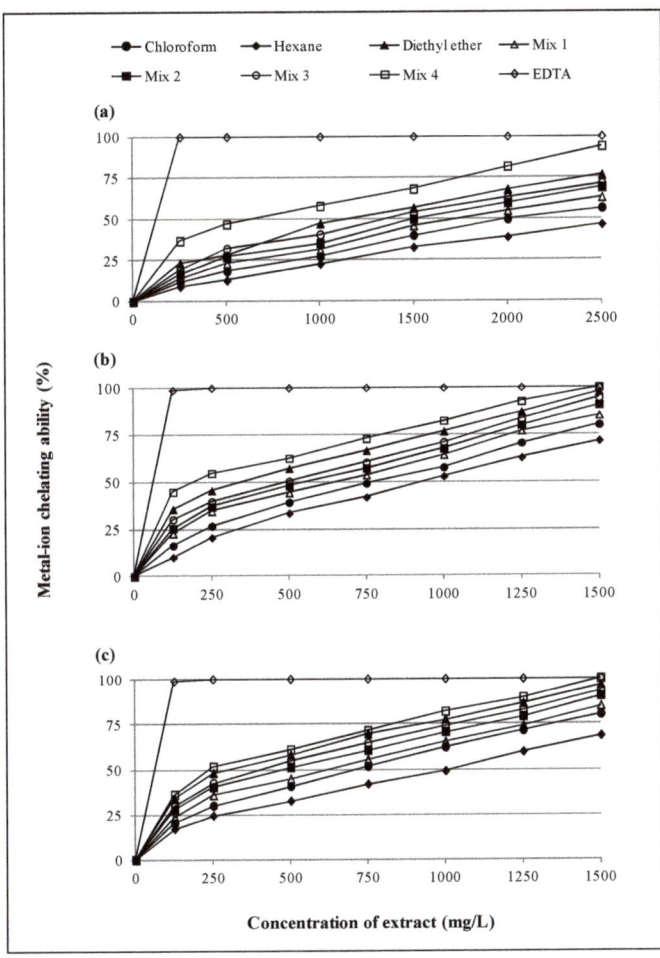

Figure 3. Metal-ion chelating ability of ethylenediaminetetraacetic acid (EDTA) standard and the Irish brown seaweeds extracts obtained from semi/non-polar solvents and mixtures (1:1 or 1:1:1, *v/v/v*) thereof (**a**) *H. elongata*; (**b**) *L. saccharina*; (**c**) *L. digitata*. [Mix 1: *n*-hexane and diethyl ether; Mix 2: *n*-hexane and chloroform; Mix 3: diethyl ether and chloroform; Mix 4: *n*-hexane, diethyl ether and chloroform].

Results also concluded that dielectric constant of extraction solvent has a significant role in antioxidant properties of extracted compounds. In this study, the results interpreted that the *n*-hexane (ε = 2.0) extracts exhibited the lowest while Mix 4 (ε = 3.8) extracts demonstrated the highest DPPH scavenging capacity, reducing power and metal ion chelating ability among the tested seaweed. The pattern of DPPH radical scavenging capacity shown by different solvent extracts were in the order of Mix 4 > diethyl ether > Mix 3 > Mix 1 > Mix 2 > chloroform > *n*-hexane (Figure 2a). While the arrangement of reducing power (FRAP) and metal chelating ability shown by different solvent extracts was as follows: Mix 4 > diethyl ether > Mix 3 > Mix 2 > Mix 1 > chloroform > *n*-hexane (Figures 2b and 3). The recovery of lowest antioxidant activity by *n*-hexane extracts is in agreement with the previous findings wherein, *Carissa opaca* fruit extract obtained from *n*-hexane showed the lowest antioxidant capacity as compared to other higher polarity solvents indicating that solvents polarity significantly affects the antioxidant capacity [34].

3.3. Characterization of Lipophilic Antioxidant Compounds by LC-ESI-MS/MS

The most active extract recovered from Mix 4 solvent system was used for the identification of lipophilic antioxidant compounds from all the seaweed studied. The selected extracts were characterized by liquid chromatography coupled with mass spectrometry using positive electrospray ionization mode (LC-ESI-MS). The identification of bioactive compounds in the extracts was carried out by comparing retention time, characteristic UV/visible (UV/vis) spectra and ESI-MS fragmentation data of each separated peak with that of the authentic standard. The UV/vis spectra provide characteristic chromophore information in pigments which cannot be obtained from MS data [39]. Therefore, chlorophyll and carotenoid pigments which could not be differentiated by only MS, were characterized by a combination of UV/vis spectral data with ESI-MS.

The selected extracts exhibited good separation by reverse phase (RP) HPLC and showed 12 distinct peaks in *H. elongata*, 13 peaks in *L. saccharina* and 12 peaks in *L. digitata*. The UV-vis absorption maxima (λ_{max}) recorded by online HPLC-PDA analyses of each peak are shown in Table 2. The absorption maxima (λ_{max}) of peaks recorded at 280 and 532 nm corresponds to anthocyanin pigments (flavonoid derivatives) in all the extracts [40]. Compounds with typical absorptions between 400 and 500 nm with λ_{max} at around 425 nm corresponding to carotenoids. Absorption bands between 400–500 nm and 500–600 nm with λ_{max} at 430 nm and 660 nm (chlorophyll *a* derivatives) and at 450 nm and 640 nm (chlorophyll *b* derivatives) representing chlorophylls [39,41]. The characteristic UV spectra revealed the presence of 8 carotenoid derivatives, 2 chlorophyll derivatives and 1 anthocyanin pigment while 1 peak was unidentified in *H. elongata*. Similarly, *L. saccharina* extract showed the presence of 9 carotenoid derivatives, 2 chlorophyll derivatives while 2 peaks were unidentified. UV spectral data from *L. digitata* extract exhibited the occurrence of 7 carotenoid derivatives, 2 chlorophyll derivatives and 1 anthocyanin pigment while 2 peaks were unidentified. The pattern of the absorption spectrum, as well as corresponding λ_{max}, was similar for numerous compounds extracted among 3 seaweed species studied which indicates that the tested seaweed may have a few similar compound compositions. Due to the presence of the long chromophore of conjugated double bonds, carotenoid pigments can absorb UV and visible light and provide precious information about their structure [42]. Hence, characteristic UV-visible maxima (λ_{max}) of each individual peak of HPLC-PDA profile of selected extracts were recorded. On the basis of UV-visible spectra, these pigments can be summarized under three categories i.e., tetrapyrroles (chlorophyll derivatives), carotenoids (carotene and xanthophyll derivatives) and flavonoids (anthocyanin derivatives). Generally, both chlorophylls and carotenoids show absorption maxima within the region of 400–500 nm but only chlorophyll derivatives show an additional band within the region of 550–700 nm, which differentiate them from carotenoid derivatives [43].

Table 2. UV/visible (λ_{max}) and characteristic mass spectra (MS/MS) of the compounds isolated from lipophilic extracts of brown seaweeds *H. elongata*, *L. saccharina* and *L. digitata*.

Peak No	t_R [min]	λ_{max} [nm]	Molecular Ion Species M⁺ [m/z]	Fragment Ions (MS–MS) [m/z]	Identification
			H. elongata		
1	2.1	269,424	–	–	Unidentified
2	2.5	282,532	449 [M + H]⁺	287 [M + H − 162]⁺	Cyanidin-3-*O*-glucoside
3	3.2	326,425	–	–	Carotenoid
4	3.8	453,480	536.9 [M + H]⁺	444.2 [M + H − 92]⁺ 430.3 [M + H − 106]⁺	β-carotene
5	5.3	272,408,505	601.5 [M + H]⁺	583.5 [M + H − 18]⁺ 565.5 [M + H − 18 − 18]⁺	Violaxanthin
6	6.2	278,430,620,662	893.5 [M + H]⁺	615.2 [M + H − 278]⁺	Chlorophyll *a* derivative
7	8.5	276,420,446	–	–	Carotenoid
8	9.8	275,430,592,664	–	–	Chlorophyll
9	11.5	273,423,513	–	–	Carotenoid
10	13.5	327,420,472,505	–	–	Carotenoid
11	15.4	266,332,448	659.6 [M + H]⁺	641.6 [M + H − 18]⁺ 581.5 [M + H − 78]⁺	Fucoxanthin
12	24.1	278,422,508	–	–	Carotenoid
			L. saccharina		
1	1.9	278,424	–	–	Unidentified
2	2.5	326,425	–	–	Carotenoid
3	3.0	269,425	–	–	Unidentified
4	3.4	424,572	–	–	Carotenoid
5	3.8	430,620,662	893.5 [M + H]⁺	615.2 [M + H − 278]⁺	Chlorophyll *a* derivative
6	4.2	272,425,532	–	–	Carotenoid
7	5.0	276,413,504	601 [M + H]⁺	583 [M + H − 18]⁺ 565 [M + H − 18 − 18]⁺	Violaxanthin
8	5.9	422,532	–	–	Carotenoid
9	8.3	276,424,504	–	–	Carotenoid
10	8.9	431,483,665	–	–	Chlorophyll
11	10.9	421,572	–	–	Carotenoid
12	12.6	266,332,448	659.2 [M + H]⁺	641.2 [M + H − 18]⁺ 581.5 [M + H − 78]⁺	Fucoxanthin
13	19.7	276,429,527	–	–	Carotenoid
			L. digitata		
1	1.8	282,532	449 [M + H]⁺	287 [M + H − 162]⁺	Cyanidin-3-*O*-glucoside
2	4.4	425,572	–	–	Carotenoid
3	5.6	273,410,505	601.5 [M + H]⁺	583.5 [M + H − 18]⁺ 565.5 [M + H − 18 − 18]⁺	Violaxanthin
4	7.4	320,531	–	–	Unidentified
5	8.1	425,483,529	–	–	Carotenoid
6	9.4	451,484,507,641	906.2 [M + H]⁺	628.2 [M + H − 278]⁺	Chlorophyll *b* derivative
7	10.4	275,430,620,662	893.5 [M + H]⁺	615.2 [M + H − 278]⁺	Chlorophyll *a* derivative
8	11.1	328,536	–	–	Unidentified
9	13.0	277,359,420	–	–	Carotenoid
10	13.7	425,572	–	–	Carotenoid
11	15.9	274,376,427,527	–	–	Carotenoid
12	18.8	274,399,429,528	–	–	Carotenoid

Isolated lipophilic compounds from each extract were submitted for LC-ESI-MS/MS analysis. HPLC coupled to mass spectrometry with ESI proved extremely useful for peak assignment and gives a great deal of structural information and characterization of individual substances. Table 2 shows the typical ions resulting from mass spectra of lipophilic compounds obtained by LC-ESI-MS and MS/MS fragmentation. The ESI-MS spectra produced 5 protonated ([M + H]⁺) molecules at *m/z* 449 (peak 2), 536.9 (peak 4), 891.2 (peak 6), 601.5 (peak 7) and 659.6 (peak 11) in *H. elongata*; 3 protonated molecules at *m/z* 891.2 (peak 5), 601.5 (peak 7) and 659.6 (peak 12) in *L. saccharina* and 4 protonated molecules at *m/z* 449 (peak 1), 601.5 (peak 3), 891.2 (peak 6) and 905.5 (peak 7) in *L. digitata* (Table 2). However, MS spectra did not show any other protonated molecules from the remaining peaks of tested seaweed extracts.

Furthermore, all protonated ions were submitted for MS/MS fragmentation and their major fragmented ions are presented in Table 2. Results indicated that MS-MS fragmentation of peak 2 (t_R 2.5 min) in *H. elongata* and peak 1 (t_R 1.8 min) in *L. digitata* produced a major fragmented ion at

m/z 287 [M + H − 162]$^+$ due to loss of a glucose molecule from the base peak ion m/z 449 (Table 2), suggesting the presence of cyanidin-3-O-glucoside, which corresponds to aglycone cyaniding [44]. Anthocyanin derivatives exhibit the characteristic UV-visible maxima at a range of 515–550 nm (band I) and 275–285 nm (band II) whereas, these compounds do not show any absorption at around 400 nm [23]. Characteristic UV spectra recorded for peak 2 (*H. elongata*) and peak 1 (*L. digitata*) which showed a λ_{max} at 282 nm and 532 nm are in agreement with reported literature [23].

β-carotene, a carotenoid pigment, was identified only in *H. elongata* extract. A characteristic UV spectrum of peak 4 (t_R 3.8 min) showed a λ_{max} at 453 nm and 480 nm while MS data exhibited a molecular ion m/z 536.9 and upon MS/MS fragmentation, the major fragments were produced at m/z 444.2 and 430.3 corresponding to the elimination of toluene (92 u, atomic mass unit) and xylene (106 u), part of the central acyclic chain of the β-carotene skeleton, respectively (Table 2). This fragmentation pattern indicates the presence of extensive conjugation within the molecule or the cyclization of fragments of the polyene chain of the β-carotene skeleton [45]. The β-carotene is identified in accordance with the published results [41,46,47].

Peak 5 (t_R 5.3 min) in *H. elongata*, Peak 7 (t_R 5.0 min) in *L. saccharina* and Peak 3 (t_R 5.6 min) in *L. digitata* extracts were identified as violaxanthin according to the λ_{max} and its molecular ions. From MS analysis of these peaks, protonated molecular ion [M + H]$^+$ was detected at m/z 601.5 and fragment ions at m/z 583.5 and 565.5 corresponding to the loss of one (18 u) and two water molecules (36 u) from the protonated ion respectively (Table 2). These assignments are consistent with the ESI-MS/MS fragmentation pattern of violaxanthin standard and are also in agreement with the mass fragmentation data described by Rivera et al. [45] wherein similar MS/MS fragmented ions (m/z 583 and 565) were recorded for violaxanthin pigment.

Peaks 11 in *H. elongata* and Peak 12 in *L. saccharina* extracts showed the same absorption spectra with the λ_{max} at 266 nm, 332 nm and 448 nm, but have the different retention times (t_R 15.4 and 12.6 min respectively). The MS data showed a molecular ion m/z 659.6, suggesting the presence of fucoxanthin pigment, which was confirmed by the fragment ions at m/z 641.6 and 581.5 due to the loss of water (18 u) and acetic acid along with water (78 u) from the base precursor ion respectively (Table 2). A similar ESI-MS/MS fragmentation pattern was recorded with fucoxanthin standard which confirmed the presence of fucoxanthin pigment in both seaweed extracts [14].

Identification of chlorophyll in all 3 tested extracts was confirmed by characteristic λ_{max}, MS and MS/MS fragmentation data. Peak 6 (t_R 6.2 min) in *H. elongata*, peak 5 (t_R 3.8 min) in *L. saccharina* and peak 7 (t_R 9.4 min) in *L. digitata* extracts exhibited the same absorption spectra with the λ_{max} at 430 nm, 620 nm and 662 nm which corresponds to chlorophyll *a* derivatives. Different retention time of chlorophyll *a* derivative in different tested seaweeds are probably due to the presence of different epimers of chlorophyll *a* molecule. Chlorophyll epimers exhibit identical absorption spectra to the chlorophyll molecule but show different chromatographic abilities [48]. For instance, chlorophyll *a'*, an epimer of chlorophyll *a*, is less polar and appears on the longer retention time than chlorophyll *a*, because the –CHOOCH$_3$ group at the C-13^2 position in the chlorophyll a molecule is on a different plane of the C-17^3 phytyl chain and is therefore less hindered, thus more polar than chlorophyll *a'* [49]. Epimers of chlorophyll and its derivatives are mostly naturally present but sometimes chlorophylls can be converted into its epimers during the extraction process. Therefore, it is anticipated that different seaweed extracts had different epimers of chlorophyll *a* derivative thus eluted at different time intervals. The most abundant product ions in ESI positive ion mass spectra of chlorophyll and its derivatives, usually relate to the dissociation of a quite weak esterifying phytyl linkage at the C-17 position of chlorophyll skeleton resulting in a fragmentation with the loss of the phytyl chain (as the phytadiene, C$_{20}$H$_{38}$) which appeared in the mass spectrum at the m/z value corresponding to [M + H − 278]$^+$ [48,50]. The MS spectra showed the precursor ion [M + H]$^+$ at m/z 893.5 and the fragment ions detected at m/z 615.2 correlating to the loss of the phytyl chain [M − 278]+ (Table 2). On the contrary, chlorophyll *b* derivative was detected only in *L. digitata* extract which was identified by absorption spectra of peak 6 (t_R 10.4 min) with the λ_{max} at 411 nm, 484 nm and 507 nm, and protonated molecular ion [M + H]$^+$ at *m/z* 905.5. The presence of chlorophyll *b* derivative was confirmed by the fragment ions *m/z* 629.2 correlating to the removal of the phytyl chain from the chlorophyll skeleton (Table 2). Chlorophyll *b* has 14 u higher molecular weight than chlorophyll *a* because of the presence of formyl group (–CHO) instead of a methyl (–CH$_3$) group at the C-7 position in chlorophyll skeleton. The presence of aldehyde group increases the polarity of chlorophyll *b* thus elutes prior to chlorophyll *a* on a non-polar C-18 column [49]. The identification of chlorophyll compounds was carried out as reported by Zvezdanović et al. [50] who described a similar fragmentation pattern of chlorophyll derivatives using ESI-MS/MS.

Brown seaweeds are a valuable source of lipophilic antioxidants and these compounds have a tendency to dissolve in low polarity solvents and are considered to be lipophilic in nature [43]. Our results revealed that the extraction yield in the extracts from *n*-hexane (least polar) was significantly higher in all the seaweed, however, the same extracts exhibited the lowest antioxidant capacity and phytochemical constituents. Furthermore, extracts from Mix 4 showed lower extraction yield but displayed the highest antioxidant capacity and phytochemical constituents. This indicated that polarity of an extraction solvent has no direct relation with the extraction yield and antioxidant activity, and a selective solvent system (with optimum polarity) is required to extract lipophilic antioxidant compounds from seaweed. On a contrary, Matanjun [26] reported that more polar compounds were found in seaweed extracts and increasing solvent polarity increased the extraction yield.

It was observed that *H. elongata* was better seaweed than *L. saccharina* and *L. digitata* as a source of antioxidants. Results interpret that all extracts from *H. elongata* exhibited highest antioxidant capacity (DPPH and FRAP), total phenol and flavonoid content compared to *L. saccharina* and *L. digitata*. Previous studies also reported that *Fucoid* species (*H. elongata*) contained higher phytochemical constituents and antioxidant activity than kelps (*L. saccharina* and *L. digitata*) which is in agreement with the present results [22,37,46]. The high antioxidant activities of HE may be due to the high phenolic, flavonoid and carotenoid content. The results also indicated a strong correlation between the antioxidant activity (DPPH, FRAP) and total phenolic content, which agree with study of Duan et al. [36]. On a contrary, the metal-ion chelating ability was detected higher in *L. saccharina* and *L. digitata* as compared to *H. elongata* which are in agreement with our previous findings wherein methanolic extracts from *Laminaria* species exhibited higher chelating ability than *H. elongata* [22]. Metal chelating ability in terms of ferrous ion chelating capacity is claimed as one of the important mechanisms of antioxidant activity. The ferrous ions are the most powerful pro-oxidants among various species of transition metals present in food systems [51]. Antioxidants from seaweed could either act as free radical scavengers and mitigate the ROS/free radicals [52] or could prevent the formation of hydroxyl radicals by either deactivating free metal ions through chelation or converting H_2O_2 to other harmless compounds (such as water and oxygen) [11].

Previous studies have reported many compounds in seaweed, for example zeaxanthin, fucoxanthin, violaxanthin, β-carotene, phlorotannins, anthocyanin, gallic acid, kaempferol, gallic acid 4-*O*-glucoside, cirsimaritin, carnosic acid, epigallocatechin gallate, epicatechin and fatty acids, which are strong antioxidant components [11,14,39–41,45,53–55]. In this study, the antioxidant capacity in lipophilic extract were the result of pigments and phenolic compounds. Compounds such as cyanidin-3-*O*-glucoside, β-carotene, violaxanthin and fucoxanthin were identified in the Mix 4 extract of *H. elongata* which could be the reason that the selected seaweed exhibited the highest antioxidant capacity. Carotenoids compounds such as violaxanthin and fucoxanthin were identified in the *L. saccharina* extract while violaxanthin and cyanidin-3-*O*-glucoside were identified in the *L. digitata* extract. The extract from *H. elongata* exhibited more antioxidant compounds than *L. saccharina* and *L. digitata*, and the antioxidant capacity in 3 species follow the following order: *H. elongata* > *L. saccharina* > *L. digitata*. It is also anticipated that chlorophyll compounds were least responsible for the antioxidant capacity as Mix 4 extracts from tested species showed moderate total chlorophyll content but exhibited the highest antioxidant capacity. Lanfer-Marquez et al. [56] reported that chlorophyll derivatives shows antioxidant capacity at very high concentration by behaving as pro-oxidants. However, they do not seem to donate hydrogen when exhibiting antioxidant capacity but may be involved in protection of linoleic acid against oxidation or by preventing breakdown of hydroperoxides. The study screened a selective solvent system for extracting lipophilic antioxidants and identified a range of antioxidant compounds. The identification of these lipophilic antioxidant compounds in selected brown seaweeds, can constitute a new move in the understanding of the health benefits of Irish brown seaweed as functional ingredients in food, cosmetics and medicinal preparation.

4. Conclusions

In conclusion, lipophilic extracts from Irish brown seaweed *H. elongata*, *L. saccharina* and *L. digitata* exhibit strong antioxidant property and metal-ion chelating ability. The phytochemical content and antioxidant capacity were majorly affected by the polarity or dielectric constant of extraction solvents. The highest phytochemical content and antioxidant capacity were achieved by an equal volume mixture of *n*-hexane, diethyl ether and chloroform (Mix 4) in all the seaweed studied. Among all the tested species, *H. elongata* was the most potent species which contained the highest antioxidant capacity followed by *L. saccharina* and *L. digitata*. The antioxidant capacity of *H. elongata* was comparable with that of reference ascorbic acid. A total of 10–11 lipophilic compounds with potential antioxidant capacity across the tested seaweed were identified by comparing retention times and UV spectral data. LC-ESI-MS/MS based characterization of lipophilic extracts confirmed the presence of fucoxanthin, violaxanthin, β-carotene, cyanidin-3-*O*-glucoside and other carotenoid and chlorophyll derivatives in the extracts. This suggests that algal derived lipophilic antioxidants may be the principal constituents responsible for the antioxidant properties from these species. These findings indicate that there may be a potential to further characterize these compounds in such extracts which can be used in pharmaceuticals, foods and cosmetics to act as antioxidants thus enhancing the quality and nutritive value of such products. Although seaweed has a great potential to be used as a source of natural antioxidant in food and cosmetics, their application as a dietary supplement or as a food ingredient should not be based only on in-vitro analysis which is just a preliminary screening tool. More research focusing on mechanisms of antioxidant action and activity against various free radicals will be advantageous in leading to the development of food and medicinal products to protect against certain age-related diseases. The identified lipophilic compounds/extracts should also be screened for their toxicity as well as for bioavailability and bioaccessibility in an in-vivo system prior to their application in commercial products.

Author Contributions: G.R. designed the work, performed the experiments, the statistical treatment of the data and wrote the manuscript.

Funding: This work was partly supported by Science Foundation Ireland (SFI) [grant number: 14/IA/2548].

Acknowledgments: The author would like to thank Prof. John O'Doherty for providing consumables for this work.

Conflicts of Interest: The author declares no conflict of interest.

References

1. Shahidi, F.; Naczk, M. *Phenolics in Food and Nutraceuticals*; CRC Press: Boca Raton, FL, USA, 2004.
2. Prior, R.; Wu, X.; Schaich, K. Standardized methods for the determination of antioxidant capacity and phenolics in foods and dietary supplements. *J. Agric. Food Chem.* **2005**, *53*, 4290–4302. [CrossRef]
3. Lee, H.-H.; Lin, C.-T.; Yang, L.-L. Neuroprotection and free radical scavenging effects of Osmanthus fragrans. *J. Biomed. Sci.* **2007**, *14*, 819–827. [CrossRef]
4. Augustyniak, A.; Bartosz, G.; Čipak, A.; Duburs, G.; Horáková, L.U.; Łuczaj, W.; Majekova, M.; Odysseos, A.D.; Rackova, L.; Skrzydlewska, E. Natural and synthetic antioxidants: An updated overview. *Free Radic. Res.* **2010**, *44*, 1216–1262. [CrossRef]
5. Shahidi, F. Nutraceuticals and functional foods: Whole versus processed foods. *Trends Food Sci. Technol.* **2009**, *20*, 376–387. [CrossRef]

6. Rice-Evans, C.A.; Miller, N.J.; Paganga, G. Structure-antioxidant activity relationships of flavonoids and phenolic acids. *Free Radic. Biol. Med.* **1996**, *20*, 933–956. [CrossRef]
7. Lesser, M.P. Oxidative stress in marine environments: Biochemistry and physiological ecology. *Annu. Rev. Physiol.* **2006**, *68*, 253–278. [CrossRef]
8. Plaza, M.; Santoyo, S.; Jaime, L.; Garcia-Blairsy Reina, G.; Herrero, M.; Senorans, F.J.; Ibanez, E. Screening for bioactive compounds from algae. *J. Pharm. Biomed. Anal.* **2010**, *51*, 450–455. [CrossRef]
9. Ganesan, P.; Kumar, C.S.; Bhaskar, N. Antioxidant properties of methanol extract and its solvent fractions obtained from selected Indian red seaweeds. *Bioresour. Technol.* **2008**, *99*, 2717–2723. [CrossRef]
10. Herrero, M.; Jaime, L.; Martín-Álvarez, P.J.; Cifuentes, A.; Ibáñez, E. Optimization of the Extraction of Antioxidants from Dunaliella salina Microalga by Pressurized Liquids. *J. Agric. Food Chem.* **2006**, *54*, 5597–5603. [CrossRef]
11. Huang, H.-L.; Wang, B.-G. Antioxidant Capacity and Lipophilic Content of Seaweeds Collected from the Qingdao Coastline. *J. Agric. Food Chem.* **2004**, *52*, 4993–4997. [CrossRef]
12. Maeda, H.; Tsukui, T.; Sashima, T.; Hosokawa, M.; Miyashita, K. Seaweed carotenoid, fucoxanthin, as a multi-functional nutrient. *Asia Pac. J. Clin. Nutr.* **2008**, *17*, 196–199.
13. Balboa, E.M.; Conde, E.; Moure, A.; Falqué, E.; Domínguez, H. In vitro antioxidant properties of crude extracts and compounds from brown algae. *Food Chem.* **2013**, *138*, 1764–1785. [CrossRef]
14. Rajauria, G.; Foley, B.; Abu-Ghannam, N. Characterization of dietary fucoxanthin from Himanthalia elongata brown seaweed. *Food Res. Int.* **2017**, *99*, 995–1001. [CrossRef]
15. Focsan, A.L.; Polyakov, N.E.; Kispert, L.D. Photo protection of Haematococcus pluvialis algae by astaxanthin: Unique properties of astaxanthin deduced by EPR, optical and electrochemical studies. *Antioxidants* **2017**, *6*, 80. [CrossRef]
16. Zaragozá, M.C.; López, D.; Sáiz, M.P.; Poquet, M.; Pérez, J.; Puig-Parellada, P.; Marmol, F.; Simonetti, P.; Gardana, C.; Lerat, Y.; et al. Toxicity and antioxidant activity in vitro and in vivo of two Fucus vesiculosus extracts. *J. Agric. Food Chem.* **2008**, *56*, 7773–7780. [CrossRef]
17. Naczk, M.; Shahidi, F. Extraction and analysis of phenolics in food. *J. Chromatogr. A* **2004**, *1054*, 95–111. [CrossRef]
18. Çelik, S.E.; Özyürek, M.; Güçlü, K.; Apak, R. Solvent effects on the antioxidant capacity of lipophilic and hydrophilic antioxidants measured by CUPRAC, ABTS/persulphate and FRAP methods. *Talanta* **2010**, *81*, 1300–1309. [CrossRef]
19. Rajauria, G.; Jaiswal, A.K.; Abu-Ghannam, N.; Gupta, S. Antimicrobial, antioxidant and free radical-scavenging capacity of brown seaweed Himanthalia elongata from western coast of Ireland. *J. Food Biochem.* **2013**, *37*, 322–335. [CrossRef]
20. Rajauria, G.; Abu-Ghannam, N. Isolation and partial characterization of bioactive fucoxanthin from Himanthalia elongata brown seaweed: A TLC-based approach. *Int. J. Anal. Chem.* **2013**, *2013*, 802573. [CrossRef]
21. Liu, S.; Lin, J.; Wang, C.; Chen, H.; Yang, D. Antioxidant properties of various solvent extracts from lychee (Litchi chinenesis Sonn.) flowers. *Food Chem.* **2009**, *114*, 577–581. [CrossRef]
22. Rajauria, G.; Jaiswal, A.K.; Abu-Ghannam, N.; Gupta, S. Effect of hydrothermal processing on colour, antioxidant and free radical scavenging capacities of edible Irish brown seaweeds. *Int. J. Food Sci. Technol.* **2010**, *45*, 2485–2493. [CrossRef]
23. Jaiswal, A.K.; Rajauria, G.; Abu-Ghannam, N.; Gupta, S. Effect of Different Solvents on Polyphenolic Content, Antioxidant Capacity and Antibacterial Activity of Irish York Cabbage. *J. Food Biochem.* **2012**, *36*, 344–358. [CrossRef]
24. Decker, E.A.; Welch, B. Role of ferritin as a lipid oxidation catalyst in muscle food. *J. Agric. Food Chem.* **1990**, *38*, 674–677. [CrossRef]
25. Sugawara, T.; Baskaran, V.; Tsuzuki, W.; Nagao, A. Brown algae fucoxanthin is hydrolyzed to fucoxanthinol during absorption by Caco-2 human intestinal cells and mice. *J. Nutr.* **2002**, *132*, 946–951. [CrossRef] [PubMed]
26. Matanjun, P.; Mohamed, S.; Mustapha, N.M.; Muhammad, K.; Ming, C.H. Antioxidant activities and phenolics content of eight species of seaweeds from north Borneo. *J. Appl. Phycol.* **2008**, *20*, 367–373. [CrossRef]

27. Pangestuti, R.; Kim, S.-K. Biological activities and health benefit effects of natural pigments derived from marine algae. *J. Funct. Foods* **2011**, *3*, 255–266. [CrossRef]
28. Peng, J.; Yuan, J.-P.; Wu, C.-F.; Wang, J.-H. Fucoxanthin, a marine carotenoid present in brown seaweeds and diatoms: Metabolism and bioactivities relevant to human health. *Mar. Drugs* **2011**, *9*, 1806–1828. [CrossRef]
29. Chandini, S.K.; Ganesan, P.; Bhaskar, N. In vitro antioxidant activities of three selected brown seaweeds of India. *Food Chem.* **2008**, *107*, 707–713. [CrossRef]
30. Hosokawa, M.; Okada, T.; Mikami, N.; Konishi, I.; Miyashita, K. Bio-functions of marine carotenoids. *Food Sci. Biotechnol.* **2009**, *18*, 1–11.
31. Mhadhebi, L.; Mhadhebi, A.; Robert, J.; Bouraoui, A. Antioxidant, anti-inflammatory and antiproliferative effects of aqueous extracts of three mediterranean brown seaweeds of the genus cystoseira. *Iran. J. Pharm. Res. IJPR* **2014**, *13*, 207–220.
32. Gammone, M.A.; D'Orazio, N. Anti-obesity activity of the marine carotenoid fucoxanthin. *Mar. Drugs* **2015**, *13*, 2196–2214. [CrossRef] [PubMed]
33. Abdul, F.; Singh, I.M.P. Effect of ternary solvent system on the permeability of lisinopril across rat skin in vitro. *Int. J. Drug Dev. Res.* **2009**, *1*, 67–74.
34. Sahreen, S.; Khan, M.R.; Khan, R.A. Evaluation of antioxidant activities of various solvent extracts of Carissa opaca fruits. *Food Chem.* **2010**, *122*, 1205–1211. [CrossRef]
35. Sun, T.; Ho, C.T. Antioxidant activities of buckwheat extracts. *Food Chem.* **2005**, *90*, 743–749. [CrossRef]
36. Duan, X.-J.; Zhang, W.-W.; Li, X.-M.; Wang, B.-G. Evaluation of antioxidant property of extract and fractions obtained from a red alga, Polysiphonia urceolata. *Food Chem.* **2006**, *95*, 37–43. [CrossRef]
37. Jiménez-Escrig, A.; Jiménez-Jiménez, I.; Pulido, R.; Saura-Calixto, F. Antioxidant activity of fresh and processed edible seaweeds. *J. Sci. Food Agric.* **2001**, *81*, 530–534. [CrossRef]
38. Gordon, M.H.; Kourimská, L. Effect of antioxidants on losses of tocopherols during deep-fat frying. *Food Chem.* **1995**, *52*, 175–177. [CrossRef]
39. Maoka, T.; Fujiwara, Y.; Hashimoto, K.; Akimoto, N. Rapid Identification of Carotenoids in a Combination of Liquid Chromatography/UV-Visible Absorption Spectrometry by Photodiode-Array Detector and Atmospheric Pressure Chemical Ionization Mass Spectrometry (LC/PAD/APCI-MS). *J. Oleo Sci.* **2002**, *51*, 1–9. [CrossRef]
40. Schütz, K.; Persike, M.; Carle, R.; Schieber, A. Characterization and quantification of anthocyanins in selected artichoke (Cynara scolymus L.) cultivars by HPLC–DAD–ESI–MS n. *Anal. Bioanal. Chem.* **2006**, *384*, 1511–1517. [CrossRef]
41. Heriyanto, J.A.; Shioi, Y.; Limantara, L.; Brotosudarmo, T. Analysis of pigment composition of brown seaweeds collected from Panjang Island, Central Java, Indonesia. *Philipp. J. Sci.* **2017**, *146*, 323–330.
42. Meléndez-Martínez, A.J.; Britton, G.; Vicario, I.M.; Heredia, F.J. Relationship between the colour and the chemical structure of carotenoid pigments. *Food Chem.* **2007**, *101*, 1145–1150. [CrossRef]
43. Schoefs, B. Chlorophyll and carotenoid analysis in food products. Properties of the pigments and methods of analysis. *Trends Food Sci. Technol.* **2002**, *13*, 361–371. [CrossRef]
44. Gouvêa, A.C.; Araujo, M.C.; Schulz, D.F.; Pacheco, S.; Godoy, R.L.; Cabral, L.M. Anthocyanins standards (cyanidin-3-O-glucoside and cyanidin-3-O-rutinoside) isolation from freeze-dried açaí (*Euterpe oleraceae* Mart.) by HPLC. *Food Sci. Technol.* **2012**, *32*, 43–46. [CrossRef]
45. Rivera, S.M.; Christou, P.; Canela-Garayoa, R. Identification of carotenoids using mass spectrometry. *Mass Spectrom. Rev.* **2014**, *33*, 353–372. [CrossRef]
46. De Quiros, A.R.-B.; Frecha-Ferreiro, S.; Vidal-Pérez, A.M.; López-Hernández, J. Antioxidant compounds in edible brown seaweeds. *Eur. Food Res. Technol.* **2010**, *231*, 495–498. [CrossRef]
47. Enzell, C.; Francis, G.; Liaaen-Jensen, S. Mass spectrometric studies of carotenoids. I. Occurrence and intensity ratios of M–92 and M–106 peaks. *Acta Chem. Scand.* **1968**, *22*, 1054–1055. [CrossRef]
48. Milenković, S.M.; Zvezdanović, J.B.; Anđelković, T.D.; Marković, D.Z. The identification of chlorophyll and its derivatives in the pigment mixtures: HPLC-chromatography, visible and mass spectroscopy studies. *Adv. Technol.* **2012**, *1*, 16–24.
49. Lim, C.K. *High-Performance Liquid Chromatography and Mass Spectrometry of Porphyrins, Chlorophylls and Bilins*; World Scientific Publishing Co.: Singapore, 2009; Volume 2, p. 177.

50. Zvezdanović, J.B.; Petrović, S.M.; Marković, D.Z.; Andjelković, T.D.; Andjelković, D.H. Electrospray ionization mass spectrometry combined with ultra high performance liquid chromatography in the analysis of in vitro formation of chlorophyll complexes with copper and zinc. *J. Serb. Chem. Soc.* **2014**, *79*, 689–706. [CrossRef]
51. Hultin, H. Oxidation of lipids in seafoods. In *Seafoods: Chemistry, Processing Technology and Quality*; Springer: Dordrecht, The Netherlands, 1994; pp. 49–74.
52. Molyneux, P. The use of the stable free radical diphenylpicrylhydrazyl (DPPH) for estimating antioxidant activity. *Songklanakarin J. Sci. Technol.* **2004**, *26*, 211–219.
53. Santoso, J.; Yoshie, Y.; Suzuki, T. Polyphenolic compounds from seaweeds: Distribution and their antioxidative effect. *Dev. Food Sci.* **2004**, *42*, 169–177.
54. Takeshi, S.; Yumiko, Y.-S.; Joko, S. Mineral components and anti-oxidant activities of tropical seaweeds. *J. Ocean Univ. China* **2005**, *4*, 205–208. [CrossRef]
55. Rajauria, G.; Foley, B.; Abu-Ghannam, N. Identification and characterization of phenolic antioxidant compounds from brown Irish seaweed Himanthalia elongata using LC-DAD–ESI-MS/MS. *Innov. Food Sci. Emerg. Technol.* **2016**, *37*, 261–268. [CrossRef]
56. Lanfer-Marquez, U.M.; Barros, R.M.; Sinnecker, P. Antioxidant activity of chlorophylls and their derivatives. *Food Res. Int.* **2005**, *38*, 885–891. [CrossRef]

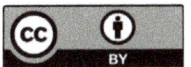

© 2019 by the author. Licensee MDPI, Basel, Switzerland. This article is an open access article distributed under the terms and conditions of the Creative Commons Attribution (CC BY) license (http://creativecommons.org/licenses/by/4.0/).

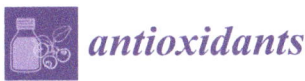

Article

Genome–Scale Metabolic Networks Shed Light on the Carotenoid Biosynthesis Pathway in the Brown Algae *Saccharina japonica* and *Cladosiphon okamuranus*

Delphine Nègre [1,2,3], Méziane Aite [4], Arnaud Belcour [4], Clémence Frioux [4,5], Loraine Brillet-Guéguen [1,2], Xi Liu [2], Philippe Bordron [2], Olivier Godfroy [1], Agnieszka P. Lipinska [1], Catherine Leblanc [1], Anne Siegel [4], Simon M. Dittami [1], Erwan Corre [2] and Gabriel V. Markov [1,*]

[1] Sorbonne Université, CNRS, Integrative Biology of Marine Models (LBI2M), Station Biologique de Roscoff (SBR), 29680 Roscoff, France; delphine.negre@sb-roscoff.fr (D.N.); loraine.gueguen@sb-roscoff.fr (L.B.-G.); olivier.godfroy@sb-roscoff.fr (O.G.); alipinska@sb-roscoff.fr (A.P.L.); catherine.leblanc@sb-roscoff.fr (C.L.); simon.dittami@sb-roscoff.fr (S.M.D.)
[2] Sorbonne Université, CNRS, Plateforme ABiMS (FR2424), Station Biologique de Roscoff, 29680 Roscoff, France; xi.liu@sb-roscoff.fr (X.L.); philippe.bordron@univ-nantes.fr (P.B.); erwan.corre@sb-roscoff.fr (E.C.)
[3] Groupe Mer, Molécules, Santé-EA 2160, UFR des Sciences Pharmaceutiques et Biologiques, Université de Nantes, 9, Rue Bias, 44035 Nantes, France
[4] Université de Rennes 1, Institute for Research in IT and Random Systems (IRISA), Equipe Dyliss, 35052 Rennes, France; meziane.aite@inria.fr (M.A.); arnaud.belcour@irisa.fr (A.B.); clemence.frioux@quadram.ac.uk (C.F.); anne.siegel@irisa.fr (A.S.)
[5] Quadram Institute, Colney Lane, Norwich NR4 7UQ, UK
* Correspondence: gabriel.markov@sb-roscoff.fr

Received: 14 October 2019; Accepted: 15 November 2019; Published: 16 November 2019

Abstract: Understanding growth mechanisms in brown algae is a current scientific and economic challenge that can benefit from the modeling of their metabolic networks. The sequencing of the genomes of *Saccharina japonica* and *Cladosiphon okamuranus* has provided the necessary data for the reconstruction of Genome–Scale Metabolic Networks (GSMNs). The same in silico method deployed for the GSMN reconstruction of *Ectocarpus siliculosus* to investigate the metabolic capabilities of these two algae, was used. Integrating metabolic profiling data from the literature, we provided functional GSMNs composed of an average of 2230 metabolites and 3370 reactions. Based on these GSMNs and previously published work, we propose a model for the biosynthetic pathways of the main carotenoids in these two algae. We highlight, on the one hand, the reactions and enzymes that have been preserved through evolution and, on the other hand, the specificities related to brown algae. Our data further indicate that, if abscisic acid is produced by *Saccharina japonica*, its biosynthesis pathway seems to be different in its final steps from that described in land plants. Thus, our work illustrates the potential of GSMNs reconstructions for formalizing hypotheses that can be further tested using targeted biochemical approaches.

Keywords: genome–scale metabolic networks (GSMNs); data integration; brown algae; oxygenated carotenoid biosynthesis; fucoxanthin; abscisic acid; *Saccharina japonica*; *Cladosiphon okamuranus*

1. Introduction

Saccharina japonica and *Cladosiphon okamuranus* are two brown algal species widely used in Asian aquaculture, known, respectively, as kombu and mozuku. *S. japonica* is the most important edible alga from an economic viewpoint. Its production was multiplied by 8 over the last 40 years: 0.8 million tons harvested in 1976 against 4.5 million tons in 2004 [1]. The annual production of *C. okamuranus* is estimated to be 20,000 tons [2,3]. Thus, studying the mechanisms of biomass production of those organisms through their Genome–Scale Metabolic Networks (GSMNs) may have a direct interest for algoculture [4]. Indeed, to produce molecules with high added value through biotechnological engineering, one first needs to understand their biosynthetic pathways. Brown algae produce specific carotenoids, some of them having potentially positive effects on human health, in particular, due to their antioxidant properties [5–10]. Some cleaved carotenoid derivatives are also signaling molecules and important phytohormones in land plants, like strigolactones or abscisic acid (ABA) [11–13].

Carotenoids are a ubiquitous class of molecules found in many organisms, such as plants, fungi, algae, and even metazoans. They are membrane–stabilizing hydrophobic molecules that also play a crucial role as photoprotective pigments in photosynthetic organisms [11,12,14,15]. Some carotenoids have been preserved through evolution, such as violaxanthin, which is detected in plants, green algae, and brown algae, among other organisms. This molecule is, on the one hand, the entry point for the biosynthesis of xanthophylls specific to brown algae, like fucoxanthin, which is the main marine carotenoid of this lineage [16–18] and, on the other hand, one of the precursors in the biosynthesis of ABA. Except for Laminariales [19], nothing is known about ABA in brown algae, including Ectocarpales like the model species *Ectocarpus siliculosus* or *C. okamuranus*. Given the potential importance of this signaling molecule in the biology of brown algae, one of our objectives when reconstructing the GSMNs of *S. japonica* and *C. okamuranus* was to clarify the possible contribution of land plant-like biosynthetic enzymes to the production of ABA in brown algae.

There have been extensive efforts to improve GSMN reconstructions from a computational perspective [20,21]. One current challenge is to integrate the knowledge of genome-based evidence and the knowledge coming from metabolome-based evidence, which is usually much more heterogeneous [22]. Following the protocol recommended in Palsson and Thiele [23] and in line with previous work on the model algae *E. siliculosus* [24], *Tisochrysis luteae* [21] and *Chondrus crispus* [25], the automated reconstruction methods and labor-intensive manual curation were combined to build a genome–scale metabolic model in the brown algae *S. japonica* and *C. okamuranus*, with a specific focus on the carotenoid biosynthesis pathway.

2. Materials and Methods

2.1. Data Sources and Cleaning

Genome and protein sequences of *S. japonica* and *C. okamuranus* are freely available, respectively, in references [26] and [3]. These algae are usually grown in non-axenic media, and the presence of contaminating sequences was demonstrated in the published genome of *S. japonica* [27]. Therefore, Taxoblast analysis (version 1.21beta) was carried out to discriminate prokaryote and eukaryote in order to filter out all prokaryotic sequences from the genome of *S. japonica*. Blast analyses were performed using diamond blastx (version 0.9.18) [28] against the nr database (downloaded on 13 August 2016) and the nodes.dmp (downloaded on 23 March 2018) from https://ftp.ncbi.nlm.nih.gov/pub/taxonomy/. The cleaned version of the *S. japonica* genome is available under the following link: http://abims.sb-roscoff.fr/resources/genomic_resources.

2.2. Reconstruction of Genome–Scale Metabolic Networks

AuReMe (AUtomatic REconstruction of MEtabolic models—version 1.2.4) dedicated to "à la carte" reconstruction of GSMNs [21] was used to reconstruct the GSMNs of *S. japonica* and *C. okamuranus*. This workflow was installed locally from a docker image. As suggested for state-of-the-art GSMN reconstruction methods [23], this workflow allowed, through the encapsulation of several tools and the local installation of specialized tools in the docker container, to create a high-quality GSMNs based on genomic and metabolic profiling data. It combined 2 complementary approaches to extract information from the genome sequences. One results from the functional annotation of the genome (see Table S1 and Figure S1 of Supplementary Materials), and the other is derived from the comparison with

GSMNs and protein sequences of organisms selected as templates. These intermediate networks were then merged, analyzed both qualitatively (topological analysis) and quantitatively (constraint-based analysis), refined by manual curation and enriched with metabolic profiling data extracted from the literature (see Table S2 and Table S3 of Supplementary Materials).

To reconstruct the intermediate annotation-based network, predicted coding regions in transcripts were functionally annotated using the Trinotate pipeline (version 3.0.1) [29]. An internal Trinotate script extracted the Gene Ontology Terms (GOT) [30,31]. The Kyoto Encyclopedia of Genes and Genomes identifiers (KEGG) [32] from the annotation file were used to retrieve the EC numbers associated with the genes. This step was performed via the KEGG–APi REST (REpresentational State Transfer) application programming interface (http://www.kegg.jp/kegg/rest/keggapi.html). The annotation concerning *S. japonica* was enriched by further analyses carried out with Kobas [33] and Blast2GO [34] with an e-value cutoff of 1e−05. A file created in the GenBank format, containing all the available data, was then generated using the following script: https://github.com/ArnaudBelcour/gbk_from_gff. This GenBank file was used as an input to the PathoLogic software from the Pathway Tools suite (version 20.5, default settings) [35]. The database containing the information from the annotation was then exported in attribute-value flat files, which were necessary for further analysis in the AuReMe workspace.

To reconstruct the intermediate orthology–supported network, templates from 3 model organisms were used: *Arabidopsis thaliana* [36], *E. siliculosus* [24], and *Nannochloropsis salina* [37]. Those templates were chosen according to the quality of their GSMNs or their phylogenetic proximity to the 2 studied algae. Orthology searches between the 2 studied algae, and these 3 templates were carried out using the OrthoMCL (version 1.4) [38] and Inparanoid (version 4.0) [39]. The results of the latter were combined using the pantograph (version 0.2) [37]. Since the *S. japonica* GSMN was the first to be generated, it was added to the 3 previous templates during the reconstruction of the *C. okamuranus* GSMN. As the *A. thaliana* and *N. salina* data refer to the KEGG [32] and BIGG [40] databases, respectively, a mapping operation, intrinsic to AuReMe, against the MetaCyc database (version 20.5) [41–43] was performed to standardize the identifiers with the MetaNetX dictionary [44].

Once the networks resulting from the annotation-based and orthology-based approaches were merged, an automatic gap-filling step was conducted using Meneco (version 1.5.0) [45]. This tool first tests the ability of the topological GSMNs to produce a set of metabolite targets defined by metabolite occurrences from the literature (Tables S2 and S3 of the Supplementary Materials) according to a Boolean abstraction of the metabolic network expansion [46]. We tested here whether or not metabolic paths existed between specific compounds known to be present in the studied algae. When one or more target(s) was (were) not reachable in the GSMNs, Meneco proposed a list of missing reactions to complete the GSMNs. For this qualitative analysis, it was necessary to provide 2 lists, one containing the target metabolites and the other containing a description of the culture medium, including the cofactors (seeds) essential for biochemical reactions (Table S4 of the Supplementary Materials).

One established criterion to consider the GSMN functional was the production of biomass with balanced growth. Flux Balance Analysis (FBA) is a widely used method to quantitatively model the behavior of the system under given conditions. This optimization problem was based on the principle of mass conservation and considered the steady state assumption (intracellular metabolites at equilibrium). Mathematically, this reaction was modeled by a linear function to be optimized. This point was tested using the quantitative FBA python scripts from the Padmet toolbox, based on the CobraPy package [47] and provided in AuReMe. To do this, the same production reactions, transport, and exchange of biomass used in the reconstruction of *E. siliculosus* GSMN [24] were added to our GSMNs (Table S5 of the Supplementary Materials). Biologically, the biomass reaction modeled the synthesis of essential amino acids, membrane lipids, and sugars by the organism. When the flux associated with a metabolite was nil, this implied the incompleteness of the GSMNs resulting either from missing reactions in the biosynthesis pathway or from an accumulation of one or more reaction products due to the absence of a degradation reaction for those metabolites. To overcome this issue, manual analysis was then carried out, either by adding outward transport reactions or by determining the reactions missing through the analysis of GSMNs of similar organisms. This manual analysis was guided by the predictions performed by the Fluto gap-filling tool [48].

The Venn diagrams presented in the results section illustrating the comparison between *S. japonica*, *C. okamuranus*, and *E. siliculosus* GSMNs were obtained using http://bioinformatics.psb.ugent.be/webtools/Venn/. The final versions of those GSMNs are available through their respective Wiki–websites: https://gem-aureme.genouest.org/sjapgem and https://gem-aureme.genouest.org/cokagem. They are designed to allow the visualization and specific search of the different components of a GSMN (pathways, metabolites, reactions, genes) [21]. The traceability of the reconstruction procedure was ensured by the display of the source(s) of each reaction: Annotations, orthology, and manual curation or gap-filling. These user-friendly wiki websites allow semantic searches according to the W3C standards, and they are designed to enable updates according to the expertise of the scientific community.

2.3. Exploration and Assessment of Carotenoid Biosynthesis Pathways in Brown Algae

The manual exploration of the carotenoid biosynthesis pathway (CAROTENOID–PWY) and the first cycle of xanthophylls (PWY–5945) was conducted starting from the pathways encoded in the MetaCyc database (version 22.6) [43] and completed by further literature searches. These 2 pathways encoded the activity of 10 enzymes whose protein sequences were selected, when identified, in *E. siliculosus* or, if not available, in *A. thaliana* (sometimes supplemented with other terrestrial plants). These protein sequences are accessible either via the Uniprot database (https://www.uniprot.org) or via the Online Resource for Community Annotation of Eukaryotes (ORCAE) website for *E. siliculosus* (https://bioinformatics.psb.ugent.be/orcae/overview/EctsiV2) [49]. Sequences homologous to these enzymes were then searched for in the proteomes of 3 green algae *Chlamydomonas reinhardtii*, *Volvox carteri*, *Ulva mutabilis*, 3 red algae *Chondrus crispus*, *Porphyra umbilicalis*, *Galdieria sulphuraria* and 6 stramenopiles *Nannochloropsis gaditana*, *N. salina*, *Phaeodactylum tricornutum*, *C. okamuranus*, *S. japonica*. With the exception of *Ulva mutabilis* and *E. siliculosus*, for which homology searches were carried out through the ORCAE portal [49], all proteomes are accessible in the Genome database (https://www.ncbi.nlm.nih.gov/genome) of the NCBI. All accession numbers used are available as Table S6 in Supplementary Materials. Proteome indexing was performed using formatdb (version 2.2.16), then homology searches were done with blastp (version 2.7.1+). Hits with an e-value of less than 1e–5 were selected for alignment after checking the organization of their protein domains (HmmerWeb [50] version 2.30.0—https://www.ebi.ac.uk/Tools/hmmer/search/phmmer). The sequence files previously obtained were aligned using the Muscle algorithm implemented in the Seaview software (version 4.4.2) [51]. The associated phylogenetic trees were generated in Seaview using maximum likelihood (PhyML) with the LG (Le et Gascuel) model, the BIONJ algorithm (BIO Neighbor–joining) for the starting tree, and 100 bootstrap replicates. The 5 trees presented in the supplementary data have been edited with Figtree (version 1.4.4). The modifications made to the GSMNs are detailed in Appendix A. Some of them are related to the second cycle of xanthophylls (PWY–7949), and fucoxanthin biosynthesis pathway (PWY–7950) encoded in MetaCyc.

3. Results

3.1. Genome–Scale Metabolic Network Reconstructions

Presented here are the functional GSMNs for *S. japonica* and *C. okamuranus*, both of which are of similar size. The *S. japonica* GSMN is composed of 3345 reactions and 2211 metabolites, and the *C. okamuranus* GSMN comprises of 3390 reactions, 2255 metabolites. Both GSMNs were expected to sustain biomass production since Flux Balance Analysis (FBA) analyses evidenced that their maximal growth rates were 3.67 mmol·gDW^{-1}·h^{-1} and 3.56 mmol·gDW^{-1}·h^{-1} (millimole per gram dry weight per hour), respectively. They constituted valuable tools for assessing and visualizing the currently available knowledge on the metabolism of these organisms.

Both GSMNs were compared with the one from *E. siliculosus* [24], which was a brown algal model more closely related to *C. okamuranus* than to *S. japonica*. This was intended to test, at the global scale, if the differences between closely related species can be attributed to biological factors, or if they were merely due to technical differences in the reconstruction procedure. The results are shown in Figure 1.

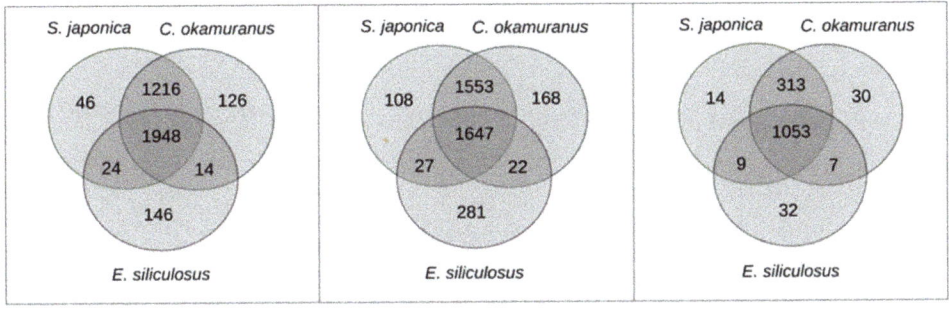

Figure 1. Comparison of the content of genome–scale metabolic networks of the three brown algae *S. japonica*, *C. okamuranus*, and *E. siliculosus*.

Strikingly, there were more reactions, metabolites, and pathways shared exclusively between *S. japonica* and *C. okamuranus* (1553 reactions) than exclusively between *E. siliculosus* and *C. okamuranus* (22 reactions), although the latter were phylogenetically closer. This was explained by examining the sources of reactions in the GSMNs (Figure 2). Of the reactions resulting from the annotations, 52% (*S. japonica*) and 44% (*C. okamuranus*) were not supported by the orthology with *E. siliculosus*. These differences were partly due to recent improvements in databases and annotation methods. The functional annotation of *E. siliculosus* that we used was done manually 10 years ago by an expert consortium [52], whereas we used Trinotate for *S. japonica* and *C. okamuranus* GSMNs. Therefore, the strong differences between *E. siliculosus* and the two other algae did not reflect biological differences, but different ways of annotation. One crucial point for the quality check was to build strong pathway-by-pathway expertise by scrutinizing them. AuReMe enabled the curation work to be stored and to reiterated on later versions of the GSMNs. To illustrate these points, intense manual curation centralized on the carotenoid biosynthesis pathway was performed.

3.2. Focused Exploration of GSMNs Regarding the Carotenoid Biosynthesis Pathway, Generalities, and Specificities

In order to facilitate the reading and understanding of the following sections, all the details related to the manual curation of GSMNs (names of enzymes or reactions, modifications of gene-reaction associations, adding or removing reactions, etc.) are available in Appendix A. Based on known pathways in terrestrial plants [53] and MetaCyc pathways (CAROTENOID-PWY), we conducted our exploration of the carotenoid pathway by starting with the transformation of geranylgeranyl diphosphate.

It should be noted, however, that this essential metabolic component was derived from isopentyl diphosphate (IPP). This fundamental and ubiquitous building block of the metabolism was itself obtained by the biosynthetic pathways methylerythritol phosphate pathway (MEP) and/or the mevalonate pathway (MVA) [54] (Figures S2 and S3 and Tables S7 and S8 of the Supplementary Materials). These pathways belonged to a set of reactions preserved through evolution that we will call core reactions. These reactions were easily and quickly identifiable within the GSMNs since they corresponded to those that have been inferred from the orthological search with a phylogenetically distant organism (here *A. thaliana*). In other words, these reactions were supported by all the components (orthology and annotations—square in Figure 2) that were used to build the GSMNs.

Reactions associated with the enzyme, common to terrestrial plants and various algal phyla, which catalyzed the transformation of lycopene into β–carotene, also belonged to this set of core reactions.

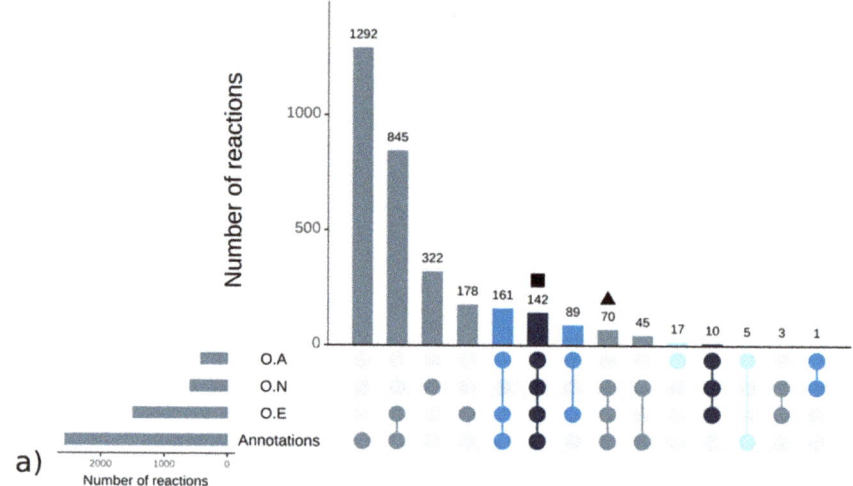

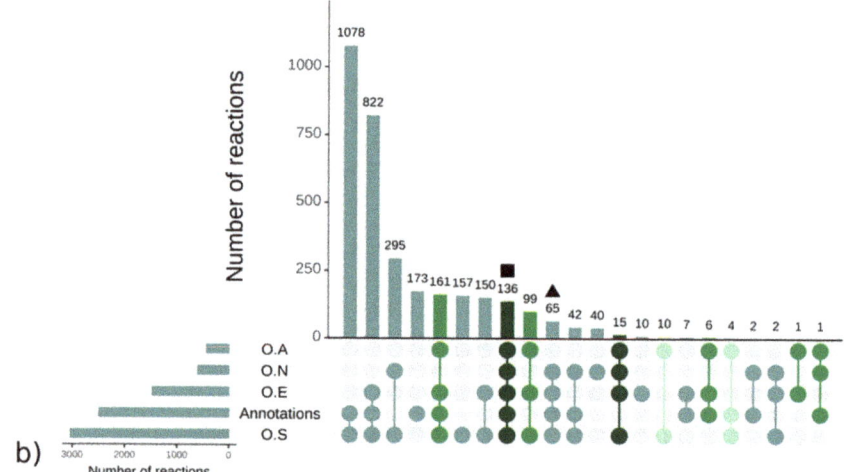

Figure 2. Sources of reactions in the *S. japonica* (**a**) and *C. okamuranus* (**b**) genome—scale metabolic networks. Reactions supported by orthology with *A. thaliana* (O.A), *E. siliculosus* (O.E), *N. salina* (O.N), and *S. japonica* (O.S). The different colors refer to the core reactions (blue and green gradient, from darkest to lightest). The square and triangle shapes are the examples corresponding to the mevalonate pathway (MVA), methylerythritol phosphate pathway (MEP), and the geranylgeranyl diphosphate pathways presented in the main text.

From geranylgeranyl diphosphate, five conserved enzymes were involved in producing lycopene (Figure 3). The genes of these enzymes have been characterized in green, red, and brown algae [55]. Homology searches based on *E. siliculosus* proteins coupled with network annotations confirmed the accuracy of the enzymes associated with those reactions (triangle in Figure 2) in *S. japonica* and *C. okamuranus*.

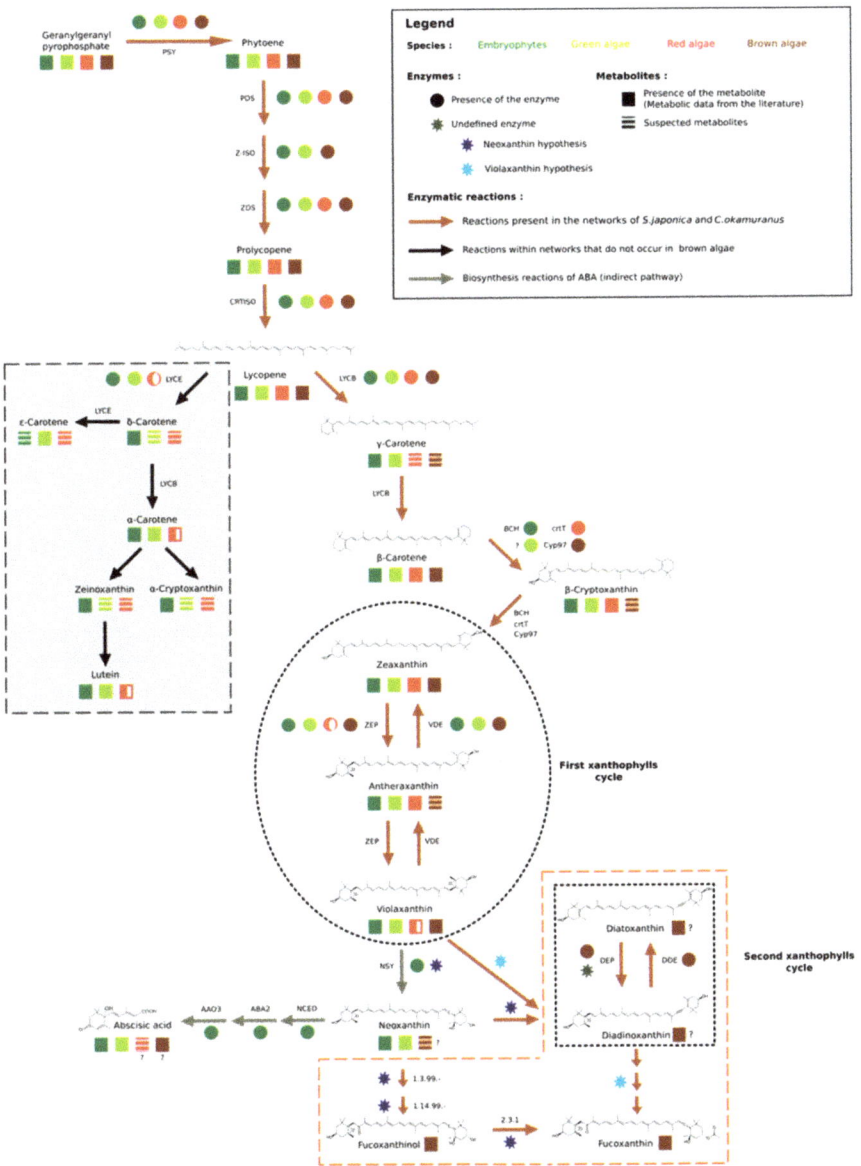

Figure 3. Carotenoid biosynthesis. The mechanisms of carotenoid synthesis seem to be common to all algae and terrestrial plants. The first connection point is made from lycopene. The synthesis of δ-carotene and its derivatives is absent in red microalgae and brown algae (grey insert), while the synthesis of β-carotene is also common to all organisms. The second point of divergence appears during the first xanthophyll cycle (black circle) partially found in red algae. In terrestrial plants, violaxanthin is transformed into neoxanthin, the starting point for the synthesis of abscisic acid (ABA), among other metabolites. Nevertheless, if this step exists in various algal groups, it seems to be carried out by different enzymes. Finally, stramenopiles have a second xanthophyll cycle (black square), for which one of the supposed precursors is also neoxanthin and whose enzymes remain to be determined (brown insert). Since pathways have been hypothesized for diatoms, we extended this hypothesis to brown algae. The figure is based on our results and the following references [5,53,55–62].

Among the terrestrial plants, red, green, and brown algae, lycopene was the first point of connection in the synthesis of carotenoids, since it offered two possible routes: The one of α–carotene and the one of β–carotene. These pathways started respectively, with the action of lycopene ε–cyclase (LYCE) for α–carotene and lycopene β–cyclase (LYCB) for β–carotene [63]. β–carotene is a carotene present in the majority of photosynthetic organisms, while α–carotene seems to be absent in stramenopiles and red microalgae [56]. These results were confirmed manually by our homology search. This search also allowed us to identify a single sequence containing one lycopene cyclase domain (PF05834) within the proteomes of brown algae: The lycopene β–cyclase [55,56,64] (Figure S4 of the Supplementary Materials). Nevertheless, within the GSMNs of the two brown algae, all the reactions leading to the synthesis of α–carotene and its derivatives (the grey part of Figure 3) were wrongly predicted and supported by this lycopene β–cyclase. Manual curation, therefore, led us to correct and suppress the reactions associated with α–carotene synthesis within the GSMNs.

The topology of the GSMNs, and in particular the presence of gaps, also revealed the specificities of the lineages. For instance, within the initially reconstructed GSMNs, no reaction allowing β–carotene transformation into zeaxanthin was automatically inferred. However, we know that this transformation involved different enzymes in different lineages, and in stramenopile species. Recent studies have suggested that this modification was catalyzed by an enzyme belonging to the P450 monooxygenase family [58,64]. During a homology search within the proteomes of *S. japonica* and *C. okamuranus*, we found two CYP97 contiguous paralogs sequences that we associated with this transformation (Figure 3).

3.3. No Plant-Like Abscisic Acid Synthesis Pathway in Brown Algae

Because ABA has been reported in various kelp species [19] and associated with biological effects on kelp growth and maturation [65,66], we thought it would be important to clarify if both *S. japonica* and *C. okamuranus* can produce it. The enzymes responsible for the synthesis of ABA from violaxanthin have been identified and characterized in embryophytes [67]. According to the MetaCyc pathway PWY–695, five enzymes are essential for the biosynthesis of ABA [67–70] (Figure 4a). We searched for orthologs of these five proteins in the brown algal genomes, but only paralogs were found (Figure 4b). All of them are members of large multigenic families whose conserved domains are general and, therefore, prevent the inference of their precise catalytic activities (Figure 4b and Figures S4–S7, and Table S9 of the Supplementary Materials).

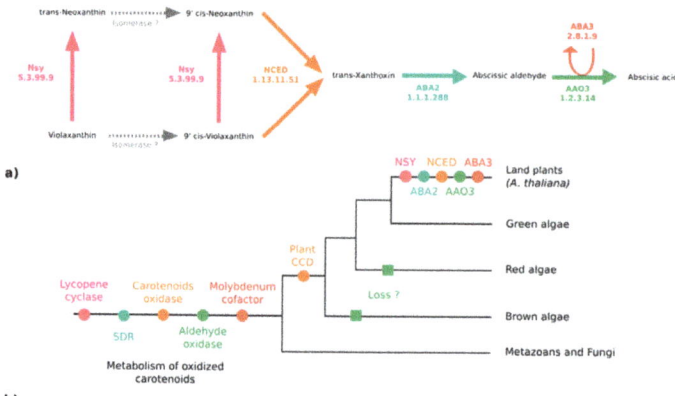

Figure 4. Enzymes of the abscisic acid biosynthesis pathway. (**a**) The ABA biosynthesis pathway in embryophytes (*A. thaliana*) [67]. (**b**) Phylogenetic tree representing the putative apparition and loss of the biosynthetic enzymes. NSY: Neoxanthin synthase; NCED: Abscisic–aldehyde oxidase; ABA2: Xanthoxin dehydrogenase; ABA3: Molybdenum cofactor sulfurase; AAO3: Abscisic–aldehyde oxidase; SDR: Short-chain alcohol dehydrogenase/reductase; CCD: Carotenoid cleavage dioxygenase.

We also examined two reactions involved in the regulation of ABA availability through its conjugation with glucose by an ABA glucosyltransferase (AOG — RXN-8155). Glycosylated ABA is inactive and can be stored for regulatory purposes. The activation of glycosylated ABA pools was performed by glucosidase (BG1 or BG2 — RXN-11469) [71,72]. However, a homology search carried out on these enzymes in predicted brown algal proteomes did not reveal any homologous sequences either.

3.4. Extending the Fucoxanthin Biosynthesis Models from Diatoms to Brown Algae

With the exception of the interconversion of zeaxanthin, antheraxanthin, and violaxanthin, violaxanthin was not consumed and corresponds at the GSMN level, to a dead end [73]. This, in silico dead end does not represent a biological reality since we know that this molecule is the entry point for the biosynthesis of fucoxanthin, but also of diatoxanthin and diadinoxanthin, two xanthophylls strongly suspected of being present in brown algae [56,59]. The reconstruction of the GSMNs was based, among other things, on the functional annotation of their genome, but on average, 35% of the predicted coding sequences in the two algae were devoid of annotations (See Figure S1 of Supplementary Materials). Among the sequences without any type of annotation, 28% (1984 *S. japonica* sequences) and 22% (1015 *C. okamuranus* sequences) can be considered as taxonomically restricted or orphan genes (sequences from one species not homologous to the other species). They represent on average, 11% and 7% of all predicted coding sequences. The other sequences without annotation 5088 and 3640 sequences in *S. japonica* and *C. okamuranus*, respectively, represent conserved proteins of unknown function. These unannotated sequences constitute a protein reservoir with unknown biochemical functions, probably including these sought enzymes.

The number and nature of cycling xanthophylls, metabolites involved in photoprotection and which depend on light conditions, differ among the algal lineages (black insert Figure 3) [59,60,74,75]. Based on previous studies, two distinct cycles have been described in stramenopiles: The zeaxanthin to violaxanthin interconversion cycle [74,75] and the diatoxanthin to diadinoxanthin interconversion cycle [59]. The enzymes involved in the first cycle are zeaxanthin epoxidase (ZEP) and violaxanthin de-epoxidase (VDE). The sequences corresponding to those involved in the second cycle, diadinoxanthin de-epoxidase (DDE) and diatoxanthin–epoxidase (DEP), have not yet been identified. However, it would appear that these enzymes are very close to ZEP and VDE since they catalyze the same type of reaction (opening or epoxide formation on the cyclic ends of molecules) [5,18,60]. Indeed, it has previously been suggested that one copy of the VDE gene, identified as VDL, could correspond to the DDE enzyme [5,60]. Within the various algal proteomes queried, we found only one sequence associated with the ZEP and, as expected, three known out–paralogues of VDE: VDE, VDR-related, and VDL-like (Figure S8 of the Supplementary Materials). Consistent with the absence of a xanthophyll cycle, no copy of the VDE gene was found in red algal proteomes, and the presence of a VDL appeared to be a specificity of stramenopiles [5,61]. We decided to associate this sequence with the reaction catalyzed by the DDE within our reconstructions

Finally, a hypothetical pathway leading to the production of fucoxanthin has been proposed in *P. tricornutum* (diatoms), but the enzymes are not yet known biochemically [60]. Nevertheless, two production hypotheses exist: Either through neoxanthin, whose presence is discussed in the literature [5,56,60,76] or directly through violaxanthin [18,60,61]. However, the investigation of the proteomes of the two brown algae has shown that the conversion of violaxanthin to neoxanthin, if it takes place, cannot be performed by neoxanthin synthase (NSY), as in terrestrial plants [53,77]. Whatever the hypothesis considered, in view of molecular structures, these biosynthetic steps require the intervention of at least three enzymes. It is likely that the latter, if they exist, are in the set of non-annotated sequences. Awaiting biological confirmation, we propose these two pathways in our reconstructions (brown insert in Figure 3).

4. Discussion

The use of automatic or semi-automatic, GSMN reconstruction workflows allows efficient and rapid modeling of GSMNs, even for emerging model organisms, as is the case for *S. japonica* and *C. okamuranus*. The theoretical biomass reaction we have tested here is mainly composed of the list of amino acids and some essential sugars. All these compounds were predicted to be producible, and our GSMNs are considered functional. In fine, for instance, adding compounds such as fucoxanthin, a molecule with pharmaceutical interest [17], could make it possible to understand and improve their production in the coming years

The reconstruction of the GSMNs is partially based on the assumption that two orthologous sequences, resulting from a speciation event, share the same function. Such reactions, called core reactions, reflect an ancient evolutionary origin and indicate which metabolites are preserved through the various kingdoms of life. For the most part, they correspond to metabolites historically qualified as primary (amino acids, essential sugars, ATP, ADP) but also ubiquitous secondary metabolites such as lycopene. The preliminary steps to the IPP synthesis are highlighted by the orthology component of the reconstruction, suggesting and confirming their ancestral origin. In general, all the reactions present within the GSMNs that are supported by orthology with *A. thaliana* illustrate this phenomenon. However, the list proposed based on this criterion is not exhaustive since, on the one hand, the *A. thaliana* GSMN preferentially targets "primary metabolites" and, on the other hand, some reactions may have been lost during the mapping steps between the various databases. This point is illustrated by the reactions allowing the synthesis of lycopene from geranylgeranyl diphosphate (triangle in Figure 2). They belong to the core reaction set (similar enzymes in plants and various algal lineages) but are not supported by the *A. thaliana* component. In contrast, reactions supported only by annotation may indicate a specificity of the species or lineage.

A contrario, the presence of gaps, and *a fortiori* dead ends within GSMNs has a high predictive power by informing either on the computational limit and/or biological specificity related to one species. From a purely bioinformatic point of view, the presence of gaps is directly related to the quality and quantity of data present in the databases. Apart from encoding issues of some metabolites, there is currently little *Phaeophyceae* referenced data. As such, a gap in the GSMNs may be a direct reflection of the biological specificities of the studied lineages and open up to new questions and biological investigations (i.e., identification of fucoxanthin biosynthesis enzymes). The first source of answers is probably to be found in the set of unannotated sequences, which are not taken into account in the reconstruction of the GSMNs. Indeed, the reconstruction is based on the functional annotation of coding sequences. Among all sequences, about 35% of them do not have any annotation and are of sufficient size to encode functional enzymes (average of 525 amino acids — see Figure S9 of the Supplementary Materials). There is no doubt that these sequences constitute a reservoir/pool of candidates for the shadows that persist within the current knowledge of brown algae. Moreover, diversifying the tools used during the annotation step could be considered in order to compensate slightly for computational artifacts listed above. Indeed, using Kobas and Blast2GO on *S. japonica* data allow finding 3.2% additional GO terms and 6.0% Kegg identifiers, which are necessary to track EC numbers (Figure S10 of the Supplementary Materials) Among the unannotated sequences, some may be candidates to be assigned to a reaction inferred by gap-filling without any known associated enzymes. Correlating gene expression data, targeted chemical profiling can help to narrow down candidates for full biochemical characterization, as already done in some model bacteria [78].

The GSMNs have been tested and enriched with targeted metabolic profiling data from the literature. Few or none of these targets were reachable before the gap-filling stage. The effectiveness of this step, more than two-thirds of the targets are now achievable, allowing us to propose a better topology of the GSMNs that can mimic the biological behavior of the brown algae (see Appendix A). Nevertheless, despite the presence of a positive flux under constraint-based modeling, some of the target metabolites are topologically not structurally producible in the GSMNs. These problems of unproducible compounds within bacterial and eukaryotic GSMNs are known [22,25]. The first intuitive constatation is that if the targets are not found during the topological analysis, this implies that at least some genomic data (e.g., an enzyme) is missing and that there is a need for further development of functional approaches. However, among the 12 and 7 unreachable targets—in *S. japonica* and *C. okamuranus* GSMNs, respectively—we found mainly fatty acids, which are rarely found in their free forms. By focusing on conjugated forms, particularly with acetyl–CoA, we realize that some of these compounds are present in the GSMNs thanks to the addition of gap-filling reactions. To summarize, the non-producibility of these targets can also come from the encoding choice of the referenced metabolites, and in this case, the GSMNs already reflect the biochemical reality of fatty acid metabolism. An additional category of metabolites is those that could even not be incorporated as targets for gap filling because they are not yet connected to biochemical reaction models and thus not incorporated in the Metacyc database. For such molecules, specific tools have been developed to infer new reaction models using detailed comparisons of already known reactions and molecules substructures or to infer the precise structures of the unknown intermediates leading to known metabolites [25].

The curation of the carotenoid pathway has pointed out one of the limits of automatic GSMN reconstructions with the proposal of genes and reactions leading to the synthesis of α–carotene and its derivatives. This point highlights the need for manual curation steps since, in this specific case, only the user's expertise could make it possible not to infer these reactions. Indeed, the in silico proposal of these pathways is not aberrant since the enzyme that catalyzes the transformation of lycopene into α–carotene, LYCE, is very similar to LYCB, which transforms the same substrate into β–carotene [57,77,79]. The approaches used here are based on the EC numbers of enzymes, and in this case, the proximity of their EC numbers (EC 5.5.1.18 and EC 5.5.1.19 respectively) explains why these undesired reactions were added and associated with the LYCB sequence.

In any case, as we have seen, these two in silico reconstructions of GSMNs provide a satisfactory model of the carotenoid biosynthesis pathway. We highlighted, on the one hand, the common skeleton (reactions and enzymes) that have been preserved through evolution and, on the other hand, the specificities related to brown algae. One of them corresponds to the presence of a second cycle of xanthophylls, and even if we are not able to propose a synthesis pathway with certainty, we propose a candidate for one of the two enzymes involved in the interconversion of diatoxanthin and diadinoxanthin. Another major point is the production of fucoxanthin. Here, we extend the biosynthetic hypotheses that were previously formulated in diatoms to brown algae.

On the contrary, there is not enough knowledge yet to identify the ABA synthesis pathway in filamentous brown algae from the kelp data for a number of reasons. In the European kelp species *Laminaria hyperborea*, *Laminaria digitate*, and *Saccharina latissima*, the presence of ABA in sporophytic tissues were reported about 20 years ago [19]. The characterization of this phytohormone has been performed by GC–MS (gas chromatography coupled with mass spectrometry). It has been reported that ABA concentration varies according to the seasons, with a maximum peak around November, and that a negative correlation exists between the increase in ABA concentration and vegetative growth of sporophytes [19]. Later, the presence of ABA was also detected in *S. japonica* by LC–MS/MS analysis (liquid chromatography coupled with two tandem mass spectrometers) [80]. In addition, it has been shown that the application of exogenous ABA may inhibit sporophyte growth and induce the accelerated formation of reproductive tissues called *sori* [65]. ABA has also been proposed to play a role in the control of elicitor-induced oxidative bursts [66].

Two pathways for the biosynthesis of ABA are known in the literature: The direct pathway and the indirect pathway. Chemically, two other pathways related to the regulation of ABA production have been proposed, but they are not supported by characterized enzymes thus far. ABA could be obtained by transformation of acid xanthoxin resulting from the oxidation of xanthoxin or by abscisic alcohol resulting from the oxidation of abscisic aldehyde [69]. In fungi, ABA is produced by the direct pathway within the cytoplasm from farnesyl diphosphate with ionylidene derivatives. In terrestrial plants, the existence of a pathway derived from farnesyl diphosphate is assumed but has not yet been identified [67]. The indirect pathway, the one explored here (see Figure 4a), is carried out in the plastids of the photosynthetic organisms following carotenoid cleavage [72,77,81]. Violaxanthin is transformed into neoxanthin by an intramolecular oxidoreductase, neoxanthin synthase (NSY). A series of structural modifications likely carried out by isomerases produces the 9-cis forms of the epoxycarotenoids (C40) violaxanthin or neoxanthin (main epoxycarotenoid) [67]. These two molecules undergo oxidative cleavage by a 9-cis-epoxycarotenoid dioxygenase belonging to the NCED family to form xanthoxin (C15). After the export of xanthoxin to the cytosol, an enzyme (ABA2) of the SDR family (short-chain alcohol dehydrogenase/reductase) oxidises this molecule. The opening of the epoxy forms the abscisic aldehyde. Finally, an abscisic aldehyde oxidase acid (AAO3) oxidises the abscisic aldehyde to ABA. This transformation is only achievable in the presence of a molybdenum cofactor sulfurase (MoCo - ABA3) that catalyzes the sulfarylation of a dioxo form of MoCo into a mono-oxo sulfide form necessary for the activation of abscisic aldehyde oxidase acid [82,83]. Homology searches did not allow us to find any orthologs of the corresponding genes in brown algae (see Figure 4b, Figures S4–S7, and Table S9 of Supplementary Materials). Thus, the paralogue sequences identified during the homology searches may be involved in the metabolism of carotenoids, but not specifically in the metabolism of plant-like intermediates in the ABA synthesis pathway from violaxanthin and this pathway, therefore, probably emerged in terrestrial plants.

To conclude, if brown algae are able to synthesize ABA, the corresponding pathway is either unknown at the moment or it could be close to that of fungi. Collecting metabolic data about biosynthetic intermediates would be key to discriminate between both hypotheses. Another possibility is that the metabolite reported as ABA is another structurally close oxidized carotenoid, like β–ionone, which could have an equivalent role [84]. Aside from ABA, there is a huge diversity of oxidized carotenoids involved in signaling processes [85], which gives ample room for possible structural variation in signaling molecules across lineages. Facing such diversity, integrative approaches through genome–scale metabolic models should be helpful tools to prioritize further experimental efforts, in a context where the discovery of drugs coming from natural products is experiencing a revival, fuelled by an increasing integration with genomics data [86].

Supplementary Materials: The following are available online at http://www.mdpi.com/2076-3921/8/11/564/s1. **Table S1:** Data from the annotation of algal protein–coding genes, **Figure S1:** Source of the *S. japonica* (**a**) and *C. okamuranus* (**b**) annotations, **Table S2:** Targets for *S. japonica* from metabolic data in the literature [19,87–95], **Table S3:** Targets for *C. okamuranus* from metabolic data in the literature [2,96–99], **Table S4:** List of cofactors (seeds) added to the *S. japonica* and *C. okamuranus* GSMNs, **Table S5:** List of biomass reactions added to the *S. japonica* and *C. okamuranus* GSMNs [24], **Table S6:** Accession numbers of enzymes and protein sequences used, **Figure S2:** Pathways of methylerythritol phosphate (MEP) within the *S. japonica* and *C. okamuranus* GSMNs [43,54], **Table S7:** List of reactions and genes associated with the MEP pathways [43,54], **Figure S3:** Pathways of mevalonate (MVA) within the *S. japonica* and *C. okamuranus* GSMNs [43,54], **Table S8:** List of reactions and genes associated with the MVA pathways [43,54], **Figure S4:** Maximum likelihood tree of the lycopene cyclase family [57,77,100], **Figure S5:** Maximum likelihood tree of the NCED family [12,14,101–105], **Figure S6:** Maximum likelihood tree of the xanthine oxidase family [106,107], **Table S9:** Type of SDR found in the genomes of *S. japonica* and *C. okamuranus* [108], **Figure S7:** Maximum likelihood tree of the Mocos family [109–113], **Figure S8:** Maximum likelihood tree of the VDE [5,18,60,61], **Figure S9:** Amino acid length of unannotated *S. japonica* and *C. okamuranus* coding sequences, **Figure S10:** Enrichment of the annotation in GO terms and KEGG identifiers: data fusion. The wiki–website is available under the following links: https://gem-aureme.genouest.org/sjapgem/index.php/Main_Page and https://gem-aureme.genouest.org/cokagem/index.php/Main_Page.

Author Contributions: Conceptualization, S.M.D., E.C. and G.V.M.; data curation, D.N., A.P.L., C.L., S.M.D., E.C., and G.V.M.; formal analysis, D.N., C.F., X.L., and A.P.L.; funding acquisition, C.L., A.S., S.M.D., and E.C.; investigation, D.N.; methodology, A.S.; resources, L.B.-G., P.B., O.G.; software, M.A., A.B., C.F., and A.S.; supervision, E.C. and G.V.M.; writing—original draft, D.N., E.C., and G.V.M.; Writing—review and editing, D.N., C.F., A.P.L., C.L., A.S., S.M.D., E.C., and G.V.M. All authors approved the submitted version and agreed to be personally accountable for the authors' own contributions.

Funding: This research received funding from the French Government via the National Research Agency investment expenditure program IDEALG (ANR–10–BTBR–04) and from Région Bretagne via the grant « SAD 2016 – METALG (9673) ».

Acknowledgments: The authors thank Catherine Boyen, Jonas Collén, and Philippe Potin for their comments and suggestions. We acknowledge the GenOuest bioinformatics core facility (https://www.genouest.org) for providing the computing infrastructure.

Conflicts of Interest: The authors declare no conflict of interest

Appendix A

A.1. Qualitative Analysis of Genome–Scale Metabolic Networks and Gap-Filling

Lists of 61 and 29 metabolites were compiled for *S. japonica* and *C. okamuranus* (Tables S1 and S2 of Supplementary Materials) and used to test the topology of the GSMNs. According to topological criteria modeling the Boolean behavior of the system dynamics and before the gap-filling step conducted by Meneco, five targets (L–α–alanine, mannose–1–phosphate, GDP–mannose, D–mannitol 1–phosphate, GDP–mannuronate) were reachable in the *S. japonica* GSMN. The topological gap-filling allowed reaching 45 and 22 additional metabolites by adding 90 and 67 gap-filling reactions, respectively, in *S. japonica* and *C. okamuranus* GSMNs, including 46 common reactions to both algae. The targets that could not be reached were mainly fatty acids. From a dynamic point of view, the presence of a target was then verified and supported by the possibility of producing a flux. This means that all import, export, and production reactions of these compounds were present in the GSMNs. In our analyses, all targets had a positive flux.

A.2. Manual Curation Made to the S. japonica and C. okamuranus Genome–Scale Metabolic Networks

All modifications are reported in Table A1 and Figure A1.

Carotenoids (xanthophylls and carotenes) are synthesized from geranylgeranyl diphosphate, which was transformed into phytoene and then into lycopene under the action of five enzymes, three of them being common to all photosynthetic organisms: Phytoene synthase (PSY — EC 2.5.1.32), phytoene desaturase (PDS — EC 1.3.5.5) and ζ–carotene desaturase (ZDS — EC 1.3.5.6). As the genes of these enzymes are known in algae [55], a homology search based on *E. siliculosus* proteins coupled with annotations from the GSMNs have made it possible to identify one candidate for PSY (SJ02885 and g11610), one candidate for PDS (SJ08891 and g10852), and one to two candidates for ZDS (SJ05680, SJ05681 and g16199) in *S. japonica* and *C. okamuranus*, respectively.

The two other steps in the synthesis of all-trans lycopene were either catalyzed by ζ–carotene isomerase (Z–iso — EC 5.2.1.12) and prolycopene isomerase (crtISO — EC 5.2.1.13) or compensated by photoisomerization [53,62,102]. Based on the results published in reference [55], annotations, and homology searches, it appeared that one copy of the Z–iso gene (SJ04715 and g9721) was found in the brown algae. However, two and three copies of crtISO were found in *S. japonica* and *C. okamuranus*, respectively. According to the evolutionary history of these sequences, the most likely hypothesis would be the loss of the copy annotated as amine oxidase in *S. japonica* after a successive triple duplication [55]. Therefore, we propose two potential candidates for this gene for each of the algae, one of which is annotated with the expected EC number (SJ05083 and g8850) and the other without EC annotation (SJ22161 and g4521).

All-trans lycopene is the first carotenoid from which the biosynthesis pathway diverges since it allows forming both β–carotene and α–carotene. The cyclization of lycopene is ensured by a lycopene cyclase, which adds one β–ring (lycopene β–cyclase — EC 5.5.1.19) or one ε–ring (lycopene ε–cyclase — EC 5.5.1.18) at the extremity of the molecule [63]. The α–carotene, composed of a ε–ring and a β–ring is the precursor of lutein while the β–carotene, composed of two β–rings is the entry point for xanthophylls biosynthesis. The search for proteins homologous to lycopene β–cyclase (LYCB) and lycopene ε–cyclase (LYCE) of *A. thaliana* coupled with the check for the presence of the lycopene cyclase protein domain PF05834 made it possible to identify a lycopene cyclase sequence for each of the studied algae (SJ04962 and g10898). The reconstruction of the phylogenetic tree (see Figure S4 of the Supplementary Materials for more details) of the previously selected sequences allows linking these sequences to the lycopene β–cyclase, thus confirming the absence of α–carotene and its derivatives in these two brown algae [55–57]. However, all these reactions were inferred from the GSMNs and were supported, among other things, by the gene identified as LYCB (EC 5.5.1.19).

This point, therefore, led us to remove from the GSMNs reactions associated with the synthesis of δ–carotene (RXN1F–147), α–carotene (RXN1F–148), ε–carotene (RXN–8028), zeinoxanthin (RXN–5961), α–cryptoxanthin (RXN–12226—only for *C. okamuranus* GSMNs) and lutein (RXN–8962).

The addition of a hydroxyl group at each end of the β–carotene forms zeaxanthin. Within the reconstructed *S. japonica* and *C. okamuranus* GSMNs, no reaction allows this modification. However, there are two reactions (RXN–8025 and RXN–8026) within the MetaCyc database that ensure this transformation using an intermediate, β–cryptoxanthin. The enzyme responsible for this transformation in algae is probably a monooxygenase belonging to the P450 family and more particularly of the CYP97B type [58,64]. In each of the genomes, two genes (SJ07227 and SJ07228 for *S. japonica*; g4983 and g4984 for *C. okamuranus*) were identified as such and one of them could ensure the hydroxylation of β–carotene to zeaxanthin [58].

The first cycle of xanthophylls in brown algae involves two enzymes and allows, depending on light conditions, the interconversion of zeaxanthin to violaxanthin through antheraxanthin [59,74]. In poor light conditions, a zeaxanthin epoxidase (ZEP — EC 1.14.15.21) causes the opening of the cycles positioned at the ends of zeaxanthin and then antheraxanthin to form epoxides. Within the algal genomes, there is a copy of this enzyme (SJ19373 and g5910), but only one reaction, that corresponding to the transformation of antheraxanthin into violaxanthin (RXN–7979) appears within the GSMNs. As a result, the reaction allowing the transformation of zeaxanthin into antheraxanthin (RXN–7978) was added manually to the GSMNs. In excess light, violaxanthin de–epoxidase (VDE — EC 1.23.5.1) converts violaxanthin into antheraxanthin (RXN–7984), which is then further modified to create zeaxanthin (RXN–7985). Within the GSMNs obtained, there is also a reversible reaction (RXN–13185) allowing the direct conversion of violaxanthin to zeaxanthin. For each of the algae, three sequences are associated with these reactions and the analysis of their phylogeny makes it possible to identify the three known out–paralogs: VDE (SJ03764 and g11316), VDL (VDE–like SJ20456 and g16187), and VDR (VDE–related, SJ19927 and g4586). The second cycle of xanthophylls, known in diatoms [60,61], and suspected in brown algae [56,59] operates on the same principle as the first cycle. Thus, the reactions linked to the interconversion of diatoxanthin into diadinoxanthin (RXN–19200 and RXN–19202) were added to the GSMNs. VDL (SJ20456 and g16187) has been associated with the reaction that converts diadinoxanthin to diatoxanthin (RXN–19202) [5,61] (see Figure S8 of the Supplementary Materials for more details).

According to the two hypotheses reviewed in reference [18], we have added seven reactions related to the synthesis of fucoxanthin and diadinoxanthin. According to the violaxanthin hypothesis [59], we created two reactions to allow the transformation of violaxanthin into diadinoxanthin (opening of the epoxide and formation of a triple bond—probably related to the action of a single enzyme) and the transformation of diadinoxanthin into fucoxanthin (reactions probably carried out by three independent enzymes). According to the neoxanthin hypothesis, we have added the three reactions presented in reference [60] (RXN–19203, RXN–19197 and RXN–19196) and also chose to add the reaction related to the transformation of violaxanthin into neoxanthin (RXN1F–155), even if there is no NSY in the two brown algae. Finally, a reaction allowing the transformation of neoxanthin into diadinoxanthin having been proposed by reference [60], we also added it to the GSMNs.

Table A1. List of manual modifications made to the GSMNs of *S. japonica* and *C. okamuranus*.

Enzymes	ID Reactions (MetaCyc)	Publication	S. japonica (Associated Genes)	C. okamuranus (Associated Genes)
Carotenoid biosynthesis and first xanthophyll cycle, well-known reactions whose genes are characterized in brown algae				
PSY (phytoene synthase)	RXN-13323	[11,53,55,61,62,104]	SJ02885	g11610
	2.5.1.32-RXN			
	RXNARA-8002			
PDS (phytoene desaturase)	RXN-12243	[11,53,55,61,62,104]	SJ08891	g10852
	RXN-12244			
	RXN-11355			
Z-iso (ζ-carotene isomerase)	RXN-11354	[55,104]	SJ04715	g9721
ZDS (ζ-carotene desaturase)	RXN-12242	[11,53,55,61,62,104]	SJ05680	g16199
	RXN-11356		SJ05681	
	RXN-11357			
crtISO (prolycopene isomerase)	RXN-8042	[55,56,61,62,104]	SJ05083	g8850
LycB (lycopene β-cyclase)	RXN1F-150	[11,53,55–57,61–63,104]	SJ04962	g10898
	RXN1F-151			
Cyp97B	RXN-8025	[12,58,62,64,104]	SJ07227	g4983
	RXN-8026		SJ07228	g4984
	RXN1F-152			
ZEP (zeaxanthin epoxidase)	RXN-7979	[11,18,53,55,56,62,74,104]	SJ19373	g5910
	RXN-7978			
VDE (violaxanthin de-epoxidase)	RXN-7984	[11,18,53,56]	SJ03764	g11316
			SJ20456 VDL (VDE-like ~ DDE)	g16187 VDL (VDE-like ~ DDE)
	RXN-7985		SJ19927 VDR (VDE-related)	g4586 VDR (VDE-related)

Table A1. *Cont.*

Enzymes	ID Reactions (MetaCyc)	Publication	*S. japonica* (Associated Genes)	*C. okamuranus* (Associated Genes)
		Reactions removed		
phytoene desaturase (fungi – al-1 or crtI)	RXN-12413		SJ18358 (ANNOTATION)	g18971.t1 (ORTHOLOGY)
	RXN-11974			
	RXN-8023			
	RXN-8024			
	RXN-8022			
	RXN-12412			
LycE (lycopene ε-cyclase)	RXN-8040			
LycB (lycopene β-cyclase)	RXN-8038			
LycE (lycopene ε-cyclase)	RXN1F-147		7 sequences (ORTHOLOGY x2)	18 sequences (ORTHOLOGY x3)
	RXN-8028			
LycB (lycopene β-cyclase)	RXN1F-148			
	RXN-5961		5 sequences (ORTHOLOGY)	7 sequences (ORTHOLOGY x2)
Carotene epsilon monooxygenase	RXN-5962		6 sequences (ORTHOLOGY)	8 sequences (ORTHOLOGY x2)
	RXN-12226		—	g13263.t1 (ANNOTATION)
		Reactions added manually		
DDE (diadinoxanthin de-epoxidase)	RXN-19200	[12,59,61]	SJ20456 (VDE-like ~ DDE)	g16187 (VDE-like ~ DDE)
DEP (diatoxanthin-epoxidase)	RXN-19202		—	—
1.3.99. –	RXN-19203		—	—
1.14.99.M8	RXN-19197	[5,18,60]	—	—
2.3.1. –	RXN-19196		—	—
—	RXN-19184	[60]	—	—
—	RXN1F-155		—	—
—	ConversionViolaxanthinToDiadinoxanthin	[18]	—	—
—	ConversionDiadinoxanthinToFucoxanthin	[18]	—	—

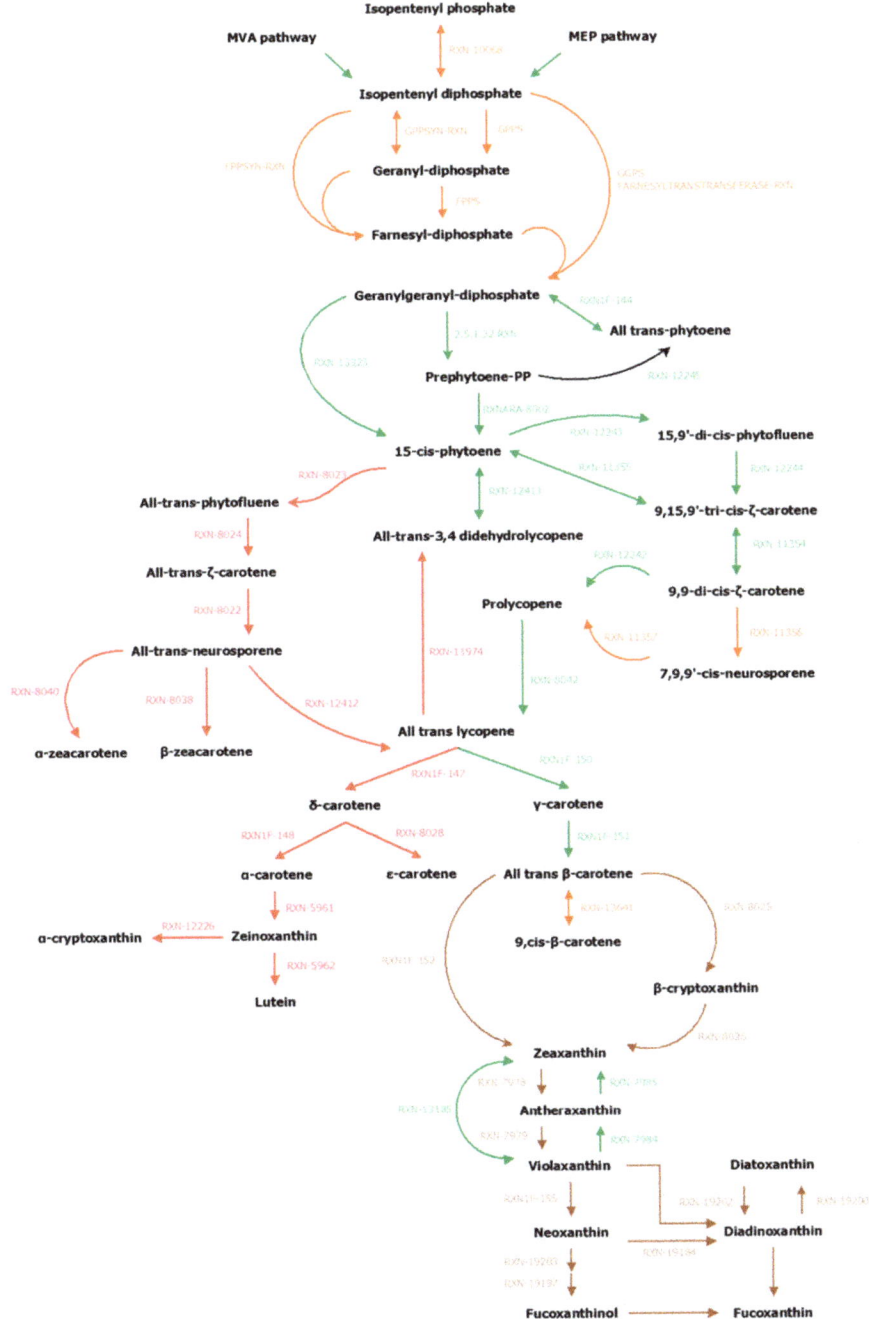

Figure A1. Reconstruction and manual curation of the genome–scale metabolic networks of *S. japonica* and *C. okamuranus*. In green, the reactions present initially in the GSMNs, in red those that were deleted, in brown those added, and in orange those to be checked.

References

1. Bartsch, I.; Wiencke, C.; Bischof, K.; Buchholz, C.M.; Buck, B.H.; Eggert, A.; Feuerpfeil, P.; Hanelt, D.; Jacobsen, S.; Karez, R.; et al. The genus *Laminaria sensu lato*: Recent insights and developments. *Eur. J. Phycol.* **2008**, *43*, 1–86. [CrossRef]
2. Cheng, K.-C.; Kuo, P.-C.; Hung, H.-Y.; Yu, K.-H.; Hwang, T.-L.; Shieh, P.-C.; Chang, J.-S.; Wu, T.-S. Four new compounds from edible algae *Cladosiphon okamuranus* and *Chlorella sorokiniana* and their bioactivities. *Phytochem. Lett.* **2016**, *18*, 113–116. [CrossRef]
3. Nishitsuji, K.; Arimoto, A.; Iwai, K.; Sudo, Y.; Hisata, K.; Fujie, M.; Arakaki, N.; Kushiro, T.; Konishi, T.; Shinzato, C.; et al. A draft genome of the brown alga, *Cladosiphon okamuranus*, S-strain: A platform for future studies of 'mozuku' biology. *DNA Res.* **2016**, *23*, 561–570. [CrossRef]
4. Bleakley, S.; Hayes, M. Algal Proteins: Extraction, Application, and Challenges Concerning Production. *Foods* **2017**, *6*, 33. [CrossRef]
5. Mikami, K.; Hosokawa, M. Biosynthetic Pathway and Health Benefits of Fucoxanthin, an Algae-Specific Xanthophyll in Brown Seaweeds. *Int. J. Mol. Sci.* **2013**, *14*, 13763–13781. [CrossRef]
6. Christaki, E.; Bonos, E.; Giannenas, I.; Florou-Paneri, P. Functional properties of carotenoids originating from algae. *J. Sci. Food Agric.* **2013**, *93*, 5–11. [CrossRef]
7. Álvarez, R.; Vaz, B.; Gronemeyer, H.; de Lera, Á.R. Functions, Therapeutic Applications, and Synthesis of Retinoids and Carotenoids. *Chem. Rev.* **2014**, *114*, 1–125. [CrossRef] [PubMed]
8. Bohn, T. Carotenoids and Markers of Oxidative Stress in Human Observational Studies and Intervention Trials: Implications for Chronic Diseases. *Antioxidants* **2019**, *8*, 179. [CrossRef] [PubMed]
9. Amengual, J. Bioactive Properties of Carotenoids in Human Health. *Nutrients* **2019**, *11*, 2388. [CrossRef] [PubMed]
10. Mounien, L.; Tourniaire, F.; Landrier, J.-F. Anti-Obesity Effect of Carotenoids: Direct Impact on Adipose Tissue and Adipose Tissue-Driven Indirect Effects. *Nutrients* **2019**, *11*, 1562. [CrossRef]
11. Esteban, R.; Moran, J.F.; Becerril, J.M.; García-Plazaola, J.I. Versatility of carotenoids: An integrated view on diversity, evolution, functional roles and environmental interactions. *Environ. Exp. Bot.* **2015**, *119*, 63–75. [CrossRef]
12. Rodriguez-Concepcion, M.; Avalos, J.; Bonet, M.L.; Boronat, A.; Gomez-Gomez, L.; Hornero-Mendez, D.; Limon, M.C.; Meléndez-Martínez, A.J.; Olmedilla-Alonso, B.; Palou, A.; et al. A global perspective on carotenoids: Metabolism, biotechnology, and benefits for nutrition and health. *Prog. Lipid Res.* **2018**, *70*, 62–93. [CrossRef] [PubMed]
13. Sandmann, G. Antioxidant Protection from UV- and Light-Stress Related to Carotenoid Structures. *Antioxidants* **2019**, *8*, 219. [CrossRef] [PubMed]
14. Sui, X.; Kiser, P.D.; von Lintig, J.; Palczewski, K. Structural basis of carotenoid cleavage: From bacteria to mammals. *Arch. Biochem. Biophys.* **2013**, *539*, 203–213. [CrossRef]
15. Firn, R.D.; Jones, C.G. A Darwinian view of metabolism: Molecular properties determine fitness. *J. Exp. Bot.* **2009**, *60*, 719–726. [CrossRef]
16. Mise, T.; Ueda, M.; Yasumoto, T. Production of Fucoxanthin-Rich Powder from *Cladosiphon okamuranus*. *Adv. J. Food Sci. Technol.* **2011**, *3*, 73–76.
17. Kanazawa, K.; Ozaki, Y.; Hashimoto, T.; Das, S.K.; Matsushita, S.; Hirano, M.; Okada, T.; Komoto, A.; Mori, N.; Nakatsuka, M. Commercial-Scale Preparation of Biofunctional Fucoxanthin from Waste Parts of Brown Sea Algae *Laminaria japonica*. *FSTR* **2008**, *14*, 573–582. [CrossRef]
18. Kuczynska, P.; Jemiola-Rzeminska, M.; Strzalka, K. Photosynthetic Pigments in Diatoms. *Mar. Drugs* **2015**, *13*, 5847–5881. [CrossRef]
19. Schaffelke, B. Abscisic Acid in Sporophytes of Three Laminaria Species (Phaeophyta). *J. Plant Physiol.* **1995**, *146*, 453–458. [CrossRef]
20. Ebrahim, A.; Almaas, E.; Bauer, E.; Bordbar, A.; Burgard, A.P.; Chang, R.L.; Dräger, A.; Famili, I.; Feist, A.M.; Fleming, R.M.; et al. Do genome-scale models need exact solvers or clearer standards? *Mol. Syst. Biol.* **2015**, *11*, 831. [CrossRef]
21. Aite, M.; Chevallier, M.; Frioux, C.; Trottier, C.; Got, J.; Cortés, M.P.; Mendoza, S.N.; Carrier, G.; Dameron, O.; Guillaudeux, N.; et al. Traceability, reproducibility and wiki-exploration for "à-la-carte" reconstructions of genome-scale metabolic models. *PLoS Comput. Biol.* **2018**, *14*, e1006146. [CrossRef] [PubMed]

22. Frainay, C.; Schymanski, E.; Neumann, S.; Merlet, B.; Salek, R.; Jourdan, F.; Yanes, O. Mind the Gap: Mapping Mass Spectral Databases in Genome-Scale Metabolic Networks Reveals Poorly Covered Areas. *Metabolites* **2018**, *8*, 51. [CrossRef] [PubMed]
23. Thiele, I.; Palsson, B.Ø. A protocol for generating a high-quality genome-scale metabolic reconstruction. *Nat. Protoc.* **2010**, *5*, 93–121. [CrossRef] [PubMed]
24. Prigent, S.; Collet, G.; Dittami, S.M.; Delage, L.; Ethis de Corny, F.; Dameron, O.; Eveillard, D.; Thiele, S.; Cambefort, J.; Boyen, C.; et al. The genome-scale metabolic network of *Ectocarpus siliculosus* (EctoGEM): A resource to study brown algal physiology and beyond. *Plant J.* **2014**, *80*, 367–381. [CrossRef]
25. Belcour, A.; Girard, J.; Aite, M.; Delage, L.; Trottier, C.; Marteau, C.; Leroux, C.; Dittami, S.M.; Sauleau, P.; Corre, E.; et al. Inferring biochemical reactions and metabolite structures to cope with metabolic pathway drift. *bioRxiv* **2018**, 462556. [CrossRef]
26. Ye, N.; Zhang, X.; Miao, M.; Fan, X.; Zheng, Y.; Xu, D.; Wang, J.; Zhou, L.; Wang, D.; Gao, Y.; et al. Saccharina genomes provide novel insight into kelp biology. *Nat. Commun.* **2015**, *6*, 1–11. [CrossRef]
27. Dittami, S.M.; Corre, E. Detection of bacterial contaminants and hybrid sequences in the genome of the kelp *Saccharina japonica* using Taxoblast. *PeerJ* **2017**, *5*, e4073. [CrossRef]
28. Buchfink, B.; Xie, C.; Huson, D.H. Fast and sensitive protein alignment using DIAMOND. *Nat. Methods* **2015**, *12*, 59–60. [CrossRef]
29. Bryant, D.M.; Johnson, K.; DiTommaso, T.; Tickle, T.; Couger, M.B.; Payzin-Dogru, D.; Lee, T.J.; Leigh, N.D.; Kuo, T.-H.; Davis, F.G.; et al. A Tissue-Mapped Axolotl De Novo Transcriptome Enables Identification of Limb Regeneration Factors. *Cell Rep.* **2017**, *18*, 762–776. [CrossRef]
30. Ashburner, M.; Ball, C.A.; Blake, J.A.; Botstein, D.; Butler, H.; Cherry, J.M.; Davis, A.P.; Dolinski, K.; Dwight, S.S.; Eppig, J.T.; et al. Gene Ontology: Tool for the unification of biology. *Nat. Genet.* **2000**, *25*, 25–29. [CrossRef]
31. The Gene Ontology Consortium. The Gene Ontology Resource: 20 years and still GOing strong. *Nucleic Acids Res.* **2019**, *47*, D330–D338. [CrossRef] [PubMed]
32. Kanehisa, M.; Goto, S. KEGG: Kyoto Encyclopedia of Genes and Genomes. *Nucleic Acids Res.* **2000**, *28*, 27–30. [CrossRef] [PubMed]
33. Xie, C.; Mao, X.; Huang, J.; Ding, Y.; Wu, J.; Dong, S.; Kong, L.; Gao, G.; Li, C.-Y.; Wei, L. KOBAS 2.0: A web server for annotation and identification of enriched pathways and diseases. *Nucleic Acids Res.* **2011**, *39*, W316–W322. [CrossRef] [PubMed]
34. Götz, S.; García-Gómez, J.M.; Terol, J.; Williams, T.D.; Nagaraj, S.H.; Nueda, M.J.; Robles, M.; Talón, M.; Dopazo, J.; Conesa, A. High-throughput functional annotation and data mining with the Blast2GO suite. *Nucleic Acids Res.* **2008**, *36*, 3420–3435. [CrossRef]
35. Karp, P.D.; Paley, S.; Romero, P. The Pathway Tools Software. *Bioinformatics* **2002**, *18*, S225–S232. [CrossRef]
36. De Oliveira Dal'Molin, C.G.; Quek, L.-E.; Palfreyman, R.W.; Brumbley, S.M.; Nielsen, L.K. AraGEM, a Genome-Scale Reconstruction of the Primary Metabolic Network in Arabidopsis. *Plant Physiol.* **2010**, *152*, 579–589. [CrossRef]
37. Loira, N.; Mendoza, S.; Paz Cortés, M.; Rojas, N.; Travisany, D.; Genova, A.D.; Gajardo, N.; Ehrenfeld, N.; Maass, A. Reconstruction of the microalga Nannochloropsis salina genome-scale metabolic model with applications to lipid production. *BMC Syst. Biol.* **2017**, *11*, 66. [CrossRef]
38. Li, L.; Stoeckert, C.J.; Roos, D.S. OrthoMCL: Identification of Ortholog Groups for Eukaryotic Genomes. *Genome Res.* **2003**, *13*, 2178–2189. [CrossRef]
39. O'Brien, K.P.; Remm, M.; Sonnhammer, E.L.L. Inparanoid: A comprehensive database of eukaryotic orthologs. *Nucleic Acids Res.* **2005**, *33*, D476–D480. [CrossRef]
40. King, Z.A.; Lu, J.; Dräger, A.; Miller, P.; Federowicz, S.; Lerman, J.A.; Ebrahim, A.; Palsson, B.O.; Lewis, N.E. BiGG Models: A platform for integrating, standardizing and sharing genome-scale models. *Nucleic Acids Res.* **2016**, *44*, D515–D522. [CrossRef]
41. Caspi, R.; Foerster, H.; Fulcher, C.A.; Kaipa, P.; Krummenacker, M.; Latendresse, M.; Paley, S.; Rhee, S.Y.; Shearer, A.G.; Tissier, C.; et al. The MetaCyc Database of metabolic pathways and enzymes and the BioCyc collection of Pathway/Genome Databases. *Nucleic Acids Res.* **2008**, *36*, D623–D631. [CrossRef] [PubMed]
42. Caspi, R.; Dreher, K.; Karp, P.D. The challenge of constructing, classifying and representing metabolic pathways. *FEMS Microbiol. Lett.* **2013**, *345*, 85–93. [CrossRef] [PubMed]

43. Caspi, R.; Billington, R.; Fulcher, C.A.; Keseler, I.M.; Kothari, A.; Krummenacker, M.; Latendresse, M.; Midford, P.E.; Ong, Q.; Ong, W.K.; et al. The MetaCyc database of metabolic pathways and enzymes. *Nucleic Acids Res.* **2018**, *46*, D633–D639. [CrossRef] [PubMed]
44. Moretti, S.; Martin, O.; Van Du Tran, T.; Bridge, A.; Morgat, A.; Pagni, M. MetaNetX/MNXref—Reconciliation of metabolites and biochemical reactions to bring together genome-scale metabolic networks. *Nucleic Acids Res.* **2016**, *44*, D523–D526. [CrossRef] [PubMed]
45. Prigent, S.; Frioux, C.; Dittami, S.M.; Thiele, S.; Larhlimi, A.; Collet, G.; Gutknecht, F.; Got, J.; Eveillard, D.; Bourdon, J.; et al. Meneco, a Topology-Based Gap-Filling Tool Applicable to Degraded Genome-Wide Metabolic Networks. *PLoS Comput. Biol.* **2017**, *13*, e1005276. [CrossRef]
46. Ebenhöh, O.; Handorf, T.; Heinrich, R. Structural analysis of expanding metabolic networks. *Genome Inform.* **2004**, *15*, 35–45.
47. Ebrahim, A.; Lerman, J.A.; Palsson, B.O.; Hyduke, D.R. COBRApy: COnstraints-Based Reconstruction and Analysis for Python. *BMC Syst. Biol.* **2013**, *7*, 74. [CrossRef]
48. Frioux, C.; Schaub, T.; Schellhorn, S.; Siegel, A.; Wanko, P. Hybrid metabolic network completion. *Theory Pract. Log. Program.* **2019**, *19*, 83–108. [CrossRef]
49. Sterck, L.; Billiau, K.; Abeel, T.; Rouzé, P.; Van de Peer, Y. ORCAE: Online resource for community annotation of eukaryotes. *Nat. Methods* **2012**, *9*, 1041. [CrossRef]
50. Potter, S.C.; Luciani, A.; Eddy, S.R.; Park, Y.; Lopez, R.; Finn, R.D. HMMER web server: 2018 update. *Nucleic Acids Res.* **2018**, *46*, W200–W204. [CrossRef]
51. Gouy, M.; Guindon, S.; Gascuel, O. SeaView version 4: A multiplatform graphical user interface for sequence alignment and phylogenetic tree building. *Mol. Biol. Evol.* **2010**, *27*, 221–224. [CrossRef] [PubMed]
52. Cock, J.M.; Sterck, L.; Rouzé, P.; Scornet, D.; Allen, A.E.; Amoutzias, G.; Anthouard, V.; Artiguenave, F.; Aury, J.-M.; Badger, J.H.; et al. The *Ectocarpus* genome and the independent evolution of multicellularity in brown algae. *Nature* **2010**, *465*, 617–621. [CrossRef] [PubMed]
53. Hirschberg, J. Carotenoid biosynthesis in flowering plants. *Curr. Opin. Plant Biol.* **2001**, *4*, 210–218. [CrossRef]
54. Zhao, L.; Chang, W.; Xiao, Y.; Liu, H.; Liu, P. Methylerythritol Phosphate Pathway of Isoprenoid Biosynthesis. *Annu. Rev. Biochem.* **2013**, *82*, 497–530. [CrossRef] [PubMed]
55. Wang, S.; Zhang, L.; Chi, S.; Wang, G.; Wang, X.; Liu, T.; Tang, X. Phylogenetic analyses of the genes involved in carotenoid biosynthesis in algae. *Acta Oceanol. Sin.* **2018**, *37*, 89–101. [CrossRef]
56. Takaichi, S. Carotenoids in Algae: Distributions, Biosyntheses and Functions. *Mar. Drugs* **2011**, *9*, 1101–1118. [CrossRef]
57. Cui, H.; Wang, Y.; Qin, S. Molecular Evolution of Lycopene Cyclases Involved in the Formation of Carotenoids in Eukaryotic Algae. *Plant Mol. Biol. Rep.* **2011**, *29*, 1013–1020. [CrossRef]
58. Teng, L.; Fan, X.; Nelson, D.R.; Han, W.; Zhang, X.; Xu, D.; Renault, H.; Markov, G.V.; Ye, N. Diversity and evolution of cytochromes P450 in stramenopiles. *Planta* **2019**, *249*, 647–661. [CrossRef]
59. Lohr, M.; Wilhelm, C. Algae displaying the diadinoxanthin cycle also possess the violaxanthin cycle. *Proc. Natl. Acad. Sci. USA* **1999**, *96*, 8784–8789. [CrossRef]
60. Dambek, M.; Eilers, U.; Breitenbach, J.; Steiger, S.; Büchel, C.; Sandmann, G. Biosynthesis of fucoxanthin and diadinoxanthin and function of initial pathway genes in *Phaeodactylum tricornutum*. *J. Exp. Bot.* **2012**, *63*, 5607–5612. [CrossRef]
61. Coesel, S.; Oborník, M.; Varela, J.; Falciatore, A.; Bowler, C. Evolutionary Origins and Functions of the Carotenoid Biosynthetic Pathway in Marine Diatoms. *PLoS ONE* **2008**, *3*, e2896. [CrossRef] [PubMed]
62. Frommolt, R.; Werner, S.; Paulsen, H.; Goss, R.; Wilhelm, C.; Zauner, S.; Maier, U.G.; Grossman, A.R.; Bhattacharya, D.; Lohr, M. Ancient Recruitment by Chromists of Green Algal Genes Encoding Enzymes for Carotenoid Biosynthesis. *Mol. Biol. Evol.* **2008**, *25*, 2653–2667. [CrossRef] [PubMed]
63. Cunningham, F.X.; Pogson, B.; Sun, Z.; McDonald, K.A.; DellaPenna, D.; Gantt, E. Functional analysis of the beta and epsilon lycopene cyclase enzymes of *Arabidopsis* reveals a mechanism for control of cyclic carotenoid formation. *Plant Cell* **1996**, *8*, 1613–1626. [CrossRef] [PubMed]
64. Cui, H.; Yu, X.; Wang, Y.; Cui, Y.; Li, X.; Liu, Z.; Qin, S. Evolutionary origins, molecular cloning and expression of carotenoid hydroxylases in eukaryotic photosynthetic algae. *BMC Genom.* **2013**, *14*, 457. [CrossRef]
65. Nimura, K.; Mizuta, H. Inducible effects of abscisic acid on sporophyte discs from *Laminaria japonica* Areschoug (Laminariales, Phaeophyceae). *J. Appl. Phycol.* **2002**, *14*, 159–163. [CrossRef]

66. Shimizu, K.; Uji, T.; Yasui, H.; Mizuta, H. Control of elicitor-induced oxidative burst by abscisic acid associated with growth of *Saccharina japonica* (Phaeophyta, Laminariales) sporophytes. *J. Appl. Phycol.* **2018**, *30*, 1371–1379. [CrossRef]
67. Nambara, E.; Marion-Poll, A. Abscisic acid biosynthesis and catabolism. *Annu. Rev. Plant Biol.* **2005**, *56*, 165–185. [CrossRef]
68. Xiong, L.; Zhu, J.-K. Regulation of Abscisic Acid Biosynthesis. *Plant Physiol.* **2003**, *133*, 29–36. [CrossRef]
69. Seo, M.; Koshiba, T. Complex regulation of ABA biosynthesis in plants. *Trends Plant Sci.* **2002**, *7*, 41–48. [CrossRef]
70. Finkelstein, R.R.; Rock, C.D. Abscisic Acid Biosynthesis and Response. *Arab. Book* **2002**, *1*, e0058. [CrossRef]
71. Lee, K.H.; Piao, H.L.; Kim, H.-Y.; Choi, S.M.; Jiang, F.; Hartung, W.; Hwang, I.; Kwak, J.M.; Lee, I.-J.; Hwang, I. Activation of Glucosidase via Stress-Induced Polymerization Rapidly Increases Active Pools of Abscisic Acid. *Cell* **2006**, *126*, 1109–1120. [CrossRef] [PubMed]
72. Hauser, F.; Waadt, R.; Schroeder, J.I. Evolution of Abscisic Acid Synthesis and Signaling Mechanisms. *Curr. Biol.* **2011**, *21*, R346–R355. [CrossRef] [PubMed]
73. Mackie, A.; Keseler, I.M.; Nolan, L.; Karp, P.D.; Paulsen, I.T. Dead End Metabolites—Defining the Known Unknowns of the *E. coli* Metabolic Network. *PLoS ONE* **2013**, *8*, e75210. [CrossRef] [PubMed]
74. Sajilata, M.G.; Singhal, R.S.; Kamat, M.Y. The Carotenoid Pigment Zeaxanthin—A Review. *Compr. Rev. Food Sci. Food Saf.* **2008**, *7*, 29–49. [CrossRef]
75. Jahns, P.; Latowski, D.; Strzalka, K. Mechanism and regulation of the violaxanthin cycle: The role of antenna proteins and membrane lipids. *Biochim. Biophys. Acta (BBA)-Bioenerg.* **2009**, *1787*, 3–14. [CrossRef]
76. Haugan, J.A. Algal carotenoids 54. Carotenoids of brown algae (Phaeophyceae). *Biochem. Syst. Ecol.* **1994**, *22*, 31–41. [CrossRef]
77. Bouvier, F.; D'Harlingue, A.; Backhaus, R.A.; Kumagai, M.H.; Camara, B. Identification of neoxanthin synthase as a carotenoid cyclase paralog: Plastid neoxanthin synthase. *Eur. J. Biochem.* **2000**, *267*, 6346–6352. [CrossRef]
78. Pan, S.; Reed, J.L. Advances in gap-filling genome-scale metabolic models and model-driven experiments lead to novel metabolic discoveries. *Curr. Opin. Biotechnol.* **2018**, *51*, 103–108. [CrossRef]
79. Cunningham, F.X.; Gantt, E. One ring or two? Determination of ring number in carotenoids by lycopene epsilon-cyclases. *Proc. Natl. Acad. Sci. USA* **2001**, *98*, 2905–2910. [CrossRef]
80. Wang, X.; Zhao, P.; Liu, X.; Chen, J.; Xu, J.; Chen, H.; Yan, X. Quantitative profiling method for phytohormones and betaines in algae by liquid chromatography electrospray ionization tandem mass spectrometry: Determination of phytohormones and betaines in algae by LC-MS/MS. *Biomed. Chromatogr.* **2014**, *28*, 275–280. [CrossRef]
81. Schwartz, S.H.; Qin, X.; Zeevaart, J.A. Elucidation of the Indirect Pathway of Abscisic Acid Biosynthesis by Mutants, Genes, and Enzymes. *Plant Physiol.* **2003**, *131*, 1591–1601. [CrossRef] [PubMed]
82. Bittner, F.; Oreb, M.; Mendel, R.R. ABA3 Is a Molybdenum Cofactor Sulfurase Required for Activation of Aldehyde Oxidase and Xanthine Dehydrogenase in *Arabidopsis thaliana*. *J. Biol. Chem.* **2001**, *276*, 40381–40384. [CrossRef] [PubMed]
83. Kaufholdt, D.; Baillie, C.-K.; Meinen, R.; Mendel, R.R.; Hänsch, R. The Molybdenum Cofactor Biosynthesis Network: In Vivo Protein-Protein Interactions of an Actin Associated Multi-Protein Complex. *Front. Plant Sci.* **2017**, *8*, 1946. [CrossRef] [PubMed]
84. Salt, S.D.; Tuzun, S.; Kuć, J. Effects of β-ionone and abscisic acid on the growth of tobacco and resistance to blue mold. Mimicry of effects of stem infection by *Peronospora tabacina* Adam. *Physiol. Mol. Plant Pathol.* **1986**, *28*, 287–297. [CrossRef]
85. Havaux, M. Carotenoid oxidation products as stress signals in plants. *Plant J.* **2014**, *79*, 597–606. [CrossRef]
86. Harvey, A.L.; Edrada-Ebel, R.; Quinn, R.J. The re-emergence of natural products for drug discovery in the genomics era. *Nat. Rev. Drug Discov.* **2015**, *14*, 111–129. [CrossRef]
87. Chi, S.; Liu, T.; Wang, X.; Wang, R.; Wang, S.; Wang, G.; Shan, G.; Liu, C. Functional genomics analysis reveals the biosynthesis pathways of important cellular components (alginate and fucoidan) of *Saccharina*. *Curr. Genet.* **2018**, *64*, 259–273. [CrossRef]
88. Park, J.-N.; Ali-Nehari, A.; Woo, H.-C.; Chun, B.-S. Thermal stabilities of polyphenols and fatty acids in *Laminaria japonica* hydrolysates produced using subcritical water. *Korean J. Chem. Eng.* **2012**, *29*, 1604–1609. [CrossRef]

89. Getachew, P.; Kang, J.-Y.; Choi, J.-S.; Hong, Y.-K. Does bryozoan colonization alter the biochemical composition of *Saccharina japonica* affecting food safety and quality? *Bot. Mar.* **2015**, *58*, 267–274. [CrossRef]
90. Patterson, G.W. Sterols of Laminaria. *Comp. Biochem. Physiol.* **1968**, *24*, 501–505. [CrossRef]
91. Zhang, P.; Shao, Z.; Jin, W.; Duan, D. Comparative Characterization of Two GDP-Mannose Dehydrogenase Genes from *Saccharina japonica* (Laminariales, Phaeophyceae). *BMC Plant Biol.* **2016**, *16*, 62. Available online: https://bmcplantbiol.biomedcentral.com/articles/10.1186/s12870-016-0750-3 (accessed on 9 January 2018). [CrossRef] [PubMed]
92. Duan, D.; Liu, X.; Pan, F.; Liu, H.; Chen, N.; Fei, X. Extraction and Identification of Cytokinin from *Laminaria japonica* Aresch. *Bot. Mar.* **1995**, *38*, 409–412. [CrossRef]
93. Honya, M.; Kinoshita, T.; Ishikawa, M.; Mori, H.; Nisizawa, K. Seasonal variation in the lipid content of cultured *Laminaria japonica*: Fatty acids, sterols, β-carotene and tocopherol. *J. Appl. Phycol.* **1994**, *6*, 25–29. [CrossRef]
94. Hwang, J.-H.; Kim, N.-G.; Woo, H.-C.; Rha, S.-J.; Kim, S.-J.; Shin, T.-S. Variation in the chemical composition of *Saccharina japonica* with harvest area and culture period. *J. Aquac. Res. Dev.* **2014**, *5*, 286.
95. Groisillier, A.; Shao, Z.; Michel, G.; Goulitquer, S.; Bonin, P.; Krahulec, S.; Nidetzky, B.; Duan, D.; Boyen, C.; Tonon, T. Mannitol metabolism in brown algae involves a new phosphatase family. *J. Exp. Bot.* **2014**, *65*, 559–570. [CrossRef]
96. Saito, H.; Xue, C.; Yamashiro, R.; Moromizato, S.; Itabashi, Y. High Polyunsaturated Fatty Acid Levels in Two Subtropical Macroalgae, *Cladosiphon Okamuranus* and *Caulerpa Lentillifera*. *J. Phycol.* **2010**, *46*, 665–673. [CrossRef]
97. Tako, M.; Yoza, E.; Tohma, S. Chemical Characterization of Acetyl Fucoidan and Alginate from Commercially Cultured *Cladosiphon okamuranus*. *Bot. Mar.* **2005**, *43*, 393–398. [CrossRef]
98. Lim, S.J.; Wan Aida, W.M.; Schiehser, S.; Rosenau, T.; Böhmdorfer, S. Structural elucidation of fucoidan from *Cladosiphon okamuranus* (Okinawa mozuku). *Food Chem.* **2019**, *272*, 222–226. [CrossRef]
99. Kakisawa, H.; Asari, F.; Kusumi, T.; Toma, T.; Sakurai, T.; Oohusa, T.; Hara, Y.; Chiharai, M. An allelopathic fatty acid from the brown alga *Cladosiphon okamuranus*. *Phytochemistry* **1988**, *27*, 731–735. [CrossRef]
100. Al-Babili, S.; Hugueney, P.; Schledz, M.; Welsch, R.; Frohnmeyer, H.; Laule, O.; Beyer, P. Identification of a novel gene coding for neoxanthin synthase from *Solanum tuberosum*. *FEBS Lett.* **2000**, *485*, 168–172. [CrossRef]
101. Tan, B.-C.; Joseph, L.M.; Deng, W.-T.; Liu, L.; Li, Q.-B.; Cline, K.; McCarty, D.R. Molecular characterization of the Arabidopsis 9-cis epoxycarotenoid dioxygenase gene family. *Plant J.* **2003**, *35*, 44–56. [CrossRef] [PubMed]
102. Walter, M.H.; Strack, D. Carotenoids and their cleavage products: Biosynthesis and functions. *Nat. Prod. Rep.* **2011**, *28*, 663–692. [CrossRef] [PubMed]
103. Priya, R.; Siva, R. Phylogenetic analysis and evolutionary studies of plant carotenoid cleavage dioxygenase gene. *Gene* **2014**, *548*, 223–233. [CrossRef] [PubMed]
104. Ahrazem, O.; Gómez-Gómez, L.; Rodrigo, M.J.; Avalos, J.; Limón, M.C. Carotenoid Cleavage Oxygenases from Microbes and Photosynthetic Organisms: Features and Functions. *Int. J. Mol. Sci.* **2016**, *17*, 1781. [CrossRef]
105. Harrison, P.J.; Bugg, T.D.H. Enzymology of the carotenoid cleavage dioxygenases: Reaction mechanisms, inhibition and biochemical roles. *Arch. Biochem. Biophys.* **2014**, *544*, 105–111. [CrossRef]
106. Seo, M.; Aoki, H.; Koiwai, H.; Kamiya, Y.; Nambara, E.; Koshiba, T. Comparative Studies on the Arabidopsis Aldehyde Oxidase (AAO) Gene Family Revealed a Major Role of AAO3 in ABA Biosynthesis in Seeds. *Plant Cell Physiol.* **2004**, *45*, 1694–1703. [CrossRef]
107. Rodríguez-Trelles, F.; Tarrío, R.; Ayala, F.J. Convergent neofunctionalization by positive Darwinian selection after ancient recurrent duplications of the xanthine dehydrogenase gene. *Proc. Natl. Acad. Sci. USA* **2003**, *100*, 13413–13417. [CrossRef]
108. Moummou, H.; Kallberg, Y.; Tonfack, L.B.; Persson, B.; van der Rest, B. The Plant Short-Chain Dehydrogenase (SDR) superfamily: Genome-wide inventory and diversification patterns. *BMC Plant Biol.* **2012**, *12*, 219. [CrossRef]
109. Peng, T.; Xu, Y.; Zhang, Y. Comparative genomics of molybdenum utilization in prokaryotes and eukaryotes. *BMC Genom.* **2018**, *19*, 691. [CrossRef]

110. Filiz, E.; Distelfeld, A.; Fahima, T.; Metin, Ö.K.; Nevo, E.; Weining, S.; Uncuoğlu, A.A. Barley molybdenum cofactor sulfurase (MCSU): Sequencing, modeling, and its comparison to other higher plants. *Turk. J. Agric. For.* **2015**, *39*, 786–796. [CrossRef]
111. Mendel, R.R. The Molybdenum Cofactor. *J. Biol. Chem.* **2013**, *288*, 13165–13172. [CrossRef] [PubMed]
112. Hille, R.; Nishino, T.; Bittner, F. Molybdenum enzymes in higher organisms. *Coord. Chem. Rev.* **2011**, *255*, 1179–1205. [CrossRef] [PubMed]
113. Mendel, R.R.; Hänsch, R. Molybdoenzymes and molybdenum cofactor in plants. *J. Exp. Bot.* **2002**, *53*, 1689–1698. [CrossRef] [PubMed]

© 2019 by the authors. Licensee MDPI, Basel, Switzerland. This article is an open access article distributed under the terms and conditions of the Creative Commons Attribution (CC BY) license (http://creativecommons.org/licenses/by/4.0/).

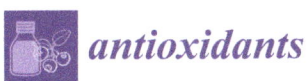

Communication

Promises and Challenges of Microalgal Antioxidant Production

Clementina Sansone * and Christophe Brunet

Stazione Zoologica Anton Dohrn, Istituto Nazionale di Biologia, Ecologia e Biotecnologie marine, Villa Comunale, 80121 Napoli, Italy
* Correspondence: clementina.sansone@szn.it; Tel.: +39-0815833262

Received: 3 June 2019; Accepted: 25 June 2019; Published: 27 June 2019

Abstract: The exploration of natural antioxidants for nutraceuticals and pharmaceuticals industries has recently increased. This communication aims to grasp the relevance of microalgae in the panorama of natural antioxidant molecules supply to industrial applications as alternatives and/or complements to those typically used from higher plants. Microalgal richness in antioxidant compounds and scavenging ability compared to higher plants is discussed in the context of microalgal biodiversity. We mainly focus on families of powerful antioxidant compounds that have been scarcely investigated in microalgae, such as phenolic compounds, sterols, or vitamins, discussing the promise and challenges of microalgae as providers of health benefits, for instance, through their use as functional food ingredients.

Keywords: microalgae; antioxidant; biodiversity

1. Antioxidants and the Ability of Organisms to Finely Balance Oxygen between Cell Life and Death

Oxygen is essential but can be harmful for life on Earth, causing oxidative stress in cells and tissues through the development of ROS (reactive oxygen species) [1]. Lipids, nucleic acids (RNA and DNA), and proteins represent the main targets of ROS, reactive nitrogen species (RNS), and reactive sulfur species (RSS) [2].

Antioxidants, scavengers of ROS, are substances able to protect, scavenge, and repair oxidative damage, thereby protecting target structures or molecules from oxidative injuries [3]. In protecting against ROS, antioxidants help optimize human physiological functions, thus helping to maintain a healthy state and protect against diseases. Numerous compounds, such as some vitamins, carotenoids, and polyphenols (such as flavonoids), play a relevant role in preventing oxidative damages caused by free radicals by scavenging activity, and/or have a key role in the prevention of degenerative neuropathies or diabetes or in preventing cardiovascular diseases or cancers, as well as exerting anti-inflammatory, anti-viral, or anti-ageing activities [4–9].

The antioxidant endogenous machinery in humans, although highly efficient, is not enough by itself to counteract the development or harmful effects of ROS, thus requiring a supplement of exogenous antioxidant molecules. Indeed, recent studies report that human longevity is also related to the ingestion of food with high content of antioxidants, which help in protecting the body against ROS [10]. Exogenous antioxidants are mainly derived from photosynthetic organisms and belong to different families such as polyphenols (phenolic acids, flavonoids, anthocyanins, lignans, and stilbenes), carotenoids (xanthophylls and carotenes), sterols, or vitamins (vitamins B, D, E, and C) [11]. Some of them are only synthesized in vegetables and bio-accumulate in animals [10] and along ecosystem trophic web, such as in marine systems [12]. The sea is a rich source of antioxidants, such as vitamins B_{12}, C, D, E, peptides, amino acids, chitooligosaccharide derivatives, astaxanthin and generally carotenoids, sulphated polysaccharides, sterols, phlorotannins, phenolic compounds, and flavones [13–18].

Investigating new natural antioxidants for nutraceuticals and pharmaceuticals industries is a relevant key-research topic [19]; microalgae are highly promising in this context [11–20].

2. The Small Size of the Bioactive Power: Promises of Microalgae as Antioxidant Providers

Microalgae are characterized by a high biodiversity (Table 1) and richness in terms of adaptive traits allowing them to colonize all kind of aquatic ecosystems.

Table 1. Principal marine microalgal classes (ca. 50,000 known species, estimated to be 200,000–800,000 species [21]; microalgal biomass represents ca. one-quarter of the total vegetation biomass in the world) and their potential in antioxidant biotechnology.

Classes	Species Number Estimation	Distribution	Forms	Known Interests for Bioactive Families	Applications	Expectations
Bacillariophyceae	10,000 [22]	ubiquitous	single, filament colonial	carotenoids	little	polyphenols, vitamins [23]; sterols [16]
Chlorophyceae	8000 [21]	ubiquitous	flagellate single	PUFAs, carotenoids	yes	vitamin B12 [26] vitamin E [27] MAAs [29] DMSP [30] carotenoids sterols [16,31]
Cyanophyceae	2000 [24,25]	oligotrophic, coastal	filament, colonial single	phycobiliproteins proteins carotenoids	yes	
Dinophyceae	1500 [28]	ubiquitous	flagellate	sterols [16]	little	
Prymnesiophyceae Pavlovophyceae	500 [21]	ubiquitous	single, filament flagellate	DMSP	little	
Crysophyceae	400 [21]	mostly ubiquitous	filament, colonial single	-	no	
Cryptophyceae	200 [32]	ubiquitous	Often flagellate	phycobiliproteins	little	
Prasinophyceae	100 [21]	mostly ubiquitous	flagellate	-	no	
Pelagophyceae	10 [21]	oligotrophic, coastal	single	-	no	
Bolidophyceae	15 [21]	oligotrophic	single	-	no	

PUFAs = polyunsaturated fatty acids; MAAs = mycosporine-like amino acids; DMSP = dimethylsulphoniopropionate.

The metabolic diversity of microalgae, stemming from the adaptive flexibility of the microalgal world, makes them promising candidates to be exploited in biotechnological applications [33]. The advantages of microalgae compared to higher plants or fruits—the actual main source of antioxidants for human—derive from the combination of being photosynthetic, mainly unicellular, displaying high growth rate, and occupying reduced space for their large cultivation.

In Table 2, we report data from literature comparing the antioxidant activity of microalgae vs. higher plants or fruits.

Table 2. Antioxidant activity (Trolox equivalents, µmol (g^{-1}DM)) of different higher plants and microalgal classes.

Species	Trolox Equivalents µ mol (g^{-1}DM)	References
Rubus sp.	~224.80	[34]
Rosmarinus sp.	~116.00	[35,36]
Zataria multiflora Boiss	~108.00	[35,37]
Perlagonium graveolens L'Hér.	~36.00	[35,38]
Chamaemelum nobile L.	~7.60	[35,39]
Achillea wilhelmsii C. Koch	~3.00	[35,40]
Carthamus tinctorius L.	~1.80	[35,41]
Eustigmatophyceae	46.16–258.20	[42,43]
Chlorophyceae	5.50–214.34	[42–44]
Xanthophyceae	~122.52	[42,43]
Cryptophyceae	30.44–110.42	[42,43]
Pavlophyceae	24.19–94.19	[43,45]
Euglenoidea	~86.99	[42,43]
Different classes of Rhodophyta	16.61–67.95	[42,43]
Chrysophyceae	~57.35	[42,43]
Bacillariophyceae	4.55–48.90	[42–46]
Cyanophyceae	2.40–38.90	[42–47]
Dinophyceae	2.20–6.30	[42]

The antioxidant power of microalgae is comparable, and even higher than, the antioxidative activity of higher plants or fruits (Table 2). In both cases, the variability is high (ranging from ≈4 to 260 Trolox equivalents µmol g^{-1}DM). Interestingly, the antioxidant potential of some classes of microalgae such as *Chlorophyta* and *Eustigmatophyceae* (Table 2, highest values ranged from 214 to 258 Trolox equivalents µmol g^{-1}DM) is comparable to the antioxidant activity displayed by *Rubus* sp. (raspberry) fruits (224 Trolox equivalents µmol g^{-1}DM [34]). These results point to the reason that there is such great interest in the highly promising microalgae as antioxidant providers for nutraceuticals and human wellness, and invoke the necessity of further exploring this great potential. The relevant antioxidant activity is probably related to the high content and diversity of antioxidant molecules in microalgae, which are a source of a wide range of antioxidant molecules [42–48] (Figure 1), some of which are aquatic-specific, while others are shared with terrestrial plants.

Astaxanthin, an "aquatic" carotenoid, is one of the most known for its health properties [49]. Among carotenoids, many are shared with higher plants [50], while algae (micro- and macro-) contain peculiar ones, such as fucoxanthin, which is well known for its bioactivity [51], and many others, such as diatoxanthin, diadinoxanthin, siphonein, or siphonaxanthin, with potentially interesting bioactivity [21,52]. Also, aquatic protein pigments such as phycobiliproteins are of great interest for their antioxidant and pharmaceutical activity [53]. Aquatic organisms, like microalgae, can also be providers of other sources of antioxidant molecules, such as the mycosporine-like amino acids (MAAs, [29]), which act as sunscreens against UVs and also possess antioxidant and osmoprotectant activities [54]. Moreover, the osmolyte dimethylsulphoniopropionate (DMSP) and its enzymatic cleavage product dimethylsulphide (DMS), produced in some microalgae have also been shown to display antioxidant activity [30].

Other families with powerful antioxidant activity that are well known in higher plants are also present in microalgae, although they tend to be far less studied in microalgae than in terrestrial plants (e.g., phenolic compounds, sterols and vitamins). Phenolic compounds, including several classes of flavonoids, such as isoflavones, flavanones, flavonols, and dihydrochalcones, have a protective effect on the liver, which is one of the principal targets of ROS-related diseases [55]. *Spirulina* sp., aquatic cyanobacteria, are a rich source of phenolic compounds including gallates, chlorogenates, cinnamates, pinostrobates, and p-hydroxybenzoates [56] as well as salicylic, trans-cinnamic, synapic, chlorogenic, and caffeic acids [57]. Previous studies have looked at the content and diversity of sterols in microalgae (see [16] and references therein) and have reported that microalgae can be relevant producers of sterols. Microalgal sterols have beneficial health effects in diseases such as hypocholesterolemia and neurological diseases like Parkinson illness, and also possess anticancer and anti-inflammatory activities [17].

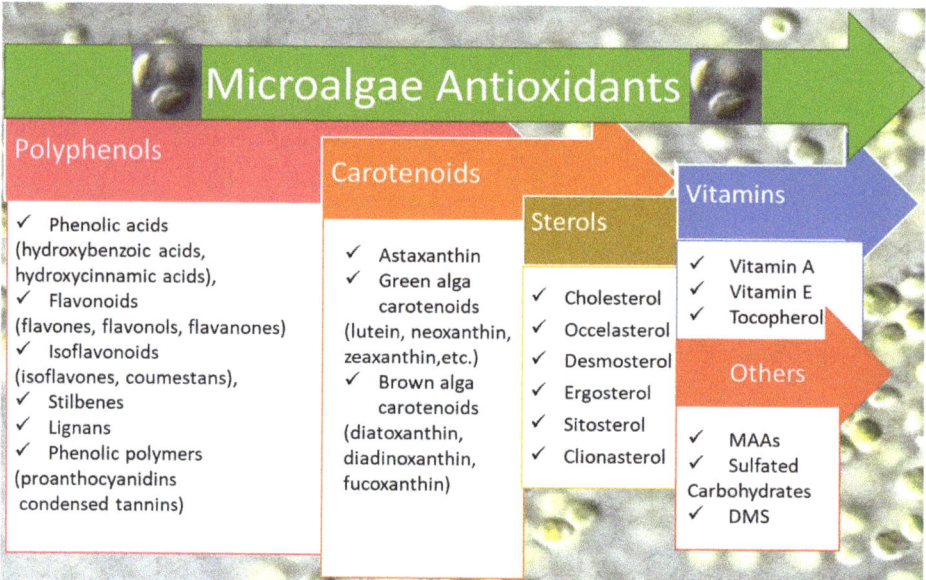

Figure 1. Challenging microalgal antioxidants of interest for biotechnological issues. DMS: dimethylsulphide.

Together with phenols and sterols, microalgae are also a rich source of vitamins, such as vitamin E (tocopherols), D, and C, as well as β-carotene (pro-vitamin A), pyridoxine, nicotinamide (vitamin B_3), thiamine (vitamin B_1), riboflavin, and biotin [58]. Sulfated polysaccharides isolated from microalgae also display relevant antioxidant properties with effective scavenging abilities on superoxide radicals, hydroxyl radicals, and hydroxyl peroxide [59]. Furthermore, microalgae are also a rich source of protein enzymes, peptides, and amino acids [60], which are necessary for the normal physiological activities of cells and tissues and have strong health-protecting effects [60].

3. BioDivAct (Biodiversity and Bioactivity): A Microalgal Antioxidant Challenging Project

Activation of physiological regulation pathways induced by environmental stress generates the synthesis of molecules that are able to react against ROS. These bioactive molecules are of strong interest for biotechnological applications, especially for nutraceuticals and cosmetics. Investigating natural sources of bioactive molecules and enhancing their synthetic yield are biotechnological requirements for further addressing societal needs in terms of human wellness. Marine microalgae, which represent a reservoir of known and unknown biodiversity, can majorly contribute to this goal [61]. Indeed, microalgal diversity (Table 1) offers a broad range of adaptive biological features (which may be fruitful for biotechnological applications [48]) related to their growth in the most varied marine systems, from intertidal sediments, polar or ultra-oligotrophic systems, to coastal ecosystems. Yet, a lack of information on regulative processes and their variability among biodiversity is notable, except on what is regarding the photoprotective responses such as the xanthophyll cycle and NPQ activation [62].

The challenge is to investigate the diversity of bioactive molecules and its modulation along the microalgal biodiversity scale.

The steps to reach the "microalgal antioxidant illuminated life" are defined below:

1) Deeply investigate the content and diversity of the least known families of microalgal bioactive molecules. Phenolics, flavonoids, and vitamins (A, B, C, D, and E) have been scarcely documented in microalgae [16–20,23,63–77]. Compared to these families, microalgal sterols have been more documented thanks to the pioneering works of Volkman [16,63]. These groups of biotechnologically appealing bioactive molecules require deep investigations in microalgae. Also, other promising bioactive molecules such as the mycosporine-like amino acids [29,78] have to be further investigated.

2) Deploy a large screening of the little-known antioxidant molecules/families among the microalgal biodiversity, as recently conducted by Volkman on microalgal sterols [16]. One of the aims of this action is to generate a crossed biodiversity (*BioDivAct*) matrix providing information on the relationship between taxa/groups and the concentrations and relative contributions of the diverse families. From this, the "key molecule concept" can be proposed for the different microalgal groups (i.e., with "key" defined as molecules present in high quantity in cells, or by their high and/or peculiar bioactivity interest.).

3) Understand the role of these key molecules and their place in cells (e.g., chloroplasts, mitochondria, etc.).

4) Decipher the main biosynthetic pathways of these molecules.

5) Assess and compare the antioxidant activities of single molecules or families harvested from the microalgal diversity. These data must thus be included in the *BioDivAct* matrix. It is expected that some single molecules or subfamilies of molecules display greater activity of scavenging and/or repairing than others, as it is generally found in higher plants/fruits.

6) Investigate the regulative properties driving the synthesis of bioactive molecules in the different microalgal groups in relation to the functional groups they belong. This approach was already carried out by Dimier et al. [79] on the xanthophyll cycling pigments modulation with respect to the ecosystem properties where the microalgae come from. This can be done on cells grown under different environmental conditions, mainly by manipulating light (intensity, daily light dose, spectral composition [16,23,78]), or through others forms of manipulations [16], such as temperature, salinity, nutrient concentrations, and water movement during cultivation. Spectral light modulation, mainly varying the red:blue ratio, is of great interest for manipulating microalgal physiology and regulative properties [23].

7) Assess the antioxidative power of mixes of molecules/families harvested from mono-microalgal cultures. This feature is relevant since one way to enhance bioactivity concerns the synergism between different molecules/groups extracted together [80].

8) Optimize protocols to maximize the harvested yield of the targeted compounds and investigate procedures to maximize the extraction efficiency of bioactive mixtures from microalgae.

9) Investigate the biological and environmental conditions for developing the co-cultivation of different microalgal groups in order to provide an efficient complementary of the bioactive molecules.

The microalgal antioxidant challenge, with the specific aims described previously, will enhance the added value of microalgal harvested biomass in terms of bioactivity and thus its role in nutraceutics and/or cosmetics. Indeed, this will help to lower the cost of the production rate for obtaining a high-quality biomass. The costs of microalgal growth for cosmetics or nutraceutical applications (i.e. using them for bioactive compounds) have not yet been estimated. Attempts on comparing the costs of microalgal production vs. terrestrial plants production have been carried out [81], especially for energetics application, such as lipid production. The results of the previous study suggested that the production of algal biomass can be profitable, compared to higher plants, but requires a maximization of yields, and an optimization of harvesting and processing strategies for microalgal cultivation and for the enhancement of biomass quality (e.g., antioxidant richness for cosmetics or nutraceutical applications).

Author Contributions: C.S. and C.B. equally contributed to this study, and both authors were responsible for preparing, writing, and reviewing the manuscript.

Funding: This research received no external funding.

Acknowledgments: The authors acknowledge the three reviewers for their comments and criticisms on a previous version of the manuscript.

Conflicts of Interest: The authors declare no conflict of interest.

References

1. Lane, N. Elixir of Life and Death. In *Oxygen: The Molecule That Made the World*, 2nd ed.; Oxford Landmark Science: New York, NY, USA, 2002; p. 384.
2. Hultqvust, M.; Olsson, L.A.; Gelderman, K.A.; Holmdah, R. The protective role of ROS in autoimmune disease. *Trends Immunol.* **2009**, *30*, 201–208. [CrossRef] [PubMed]
3. Halliwell, B. Biochemistry of oxidative stress. *Biochem. Soc. Trans.* **2007**, *35*, 1147–1150. [CrossRef] [PubMed]
4. Scalbert, A.; Manach, C.; Morden, C.; Remesy, C.; Jimenez, L. Dietary polyphenols and prevention of diseases. *Crit. Rev. Food Sci. Nutri.* **2005**, *45*, 287–306. [CrossRef] [PubMed]
5. Galasso, C.; Corinaldesi, C.; Sansone, C. Carotenoids from marine organisms: Biological functions and industrial applications. *Antioxidants* **2017**, *6*, 96. [CrossRef] [PubMed]
6. Holick, C.N.; Michaud, D.S.; Stolzenberg Solomon, R.; Mayne, S.T.; Pietinen, P.; Taylor, P.R.; Albanes, D. Dietary carotenoids, serum beta-carotene, and retinol and risk of lung cancer in the alpha-tocopherol, beta-carotene cohort study. *Am. J. Epidemiol.* **2002**, *156*, 536–547. [CrossRef]
7. Gomes, F.S.; Costa, P.A.; Campos, M.B.D.; Tonon, R.V.; Couri, S.; Cabral, L.M.C. Watermelon juice pre-treatment with microfiltration process for obtaining lycopene. *Int. J. Food Sci. Technol.* **2013**, *48*, 601–608. [CrossRef]
8. Gupta, V.K.M.; Shrivastava, R.K.; Singh, N. Status of exogenous antioxidant, total antioxidant capacity and oxidative stress in SCA patients. *Indian J. Appl. Res.* **2018**, *8*, 112–118.
9. Wang, T.Y.; Li, Q.; Bi, K.S. Bioactive flavonoids in medicinal plants: Structure, activity and biological fate. *Asian J. Pharma Sci.* **2018**, *13*, 12–23. [CrossRef]
10. Wilson, D.; Nash, P.; Buttar, H.; Griffiths, K.; Singh, R.; De Meester, F.; Takahashi, T. The role of food antioxidants, benefits of functional foods, and influence of feeding habits on the health of the older person: An overview. *Antioxidants* **2017**, *6*, 81. [CrossRef]
11. Xu, D.P.; Li, Y.; Meng, X.; Zhou, T.; Zhou, Y.; Zheng, J.; Li, H.B. Natural Antioxidants in Foods and Medicinal Plants: Extraction, Assessment and Resources. *Int. J. Mol. Sci.* **2017**, *18*, 96. [CrossRef]
12. Snoeijs, P.; Sylvander, P.; Häubner, N. Aquatic Primary producers as a Driving Force for Ecosystem Responses to Large-Scale Environmental Changes. In *Oxidative Stress in Aquatic Ecosystems*; Abele, D., Vázquez-Medina, J.P., Zenteno-Savín, T., Eds.; Wiley-Blackwell: Oxford, UK, 2011; pp. 72–88.
13. Newman, D.J.; Cragg, G.M. Marine natural products and related compounds in clinical and advanced preclinical trials. *J. Nat. Prod.* **2004**, *67*, 1216–1238. [CrossRef] [PubMed]
14. Aklakur, M. Natural antioxidants from sea: A potential industrial perspective in aquafeed formulation. *Rev. Aquacult.* **2018**, *10*, 385–399. [CrossRef]
15. Al-Saif, S.S.; Abdel-Raouf, N.; El-Wazanani, H.A.; Aref, I.A. Antibacterial substances from marine algae isolated from Jeddah coast of Red sea, Saudi Arabia. *Saudi J. Biol. Sci.* **2014**, *21*, 57–64. [CrossRef] [PubMed]
16. Volkman, J.K. Sterols in microalgae. In *The Physiology of Microalgae*; Borowitzka, M.A., Beardall, J., Raven, J.A., Eds.; Developments in Applied, Phycology; Springer International Publishing: Dordrecht, the Netherlands, 2016; pp. 485–505.
17. Galasso, C.; Gentile, A.; Orefice, I.; Ianora, A.; Bruno, A.; Noonan, D.M.; Sansone, C.; Albini, A.; Brunet, C. Microalgal derivatives as potential nutraceutical and food supplements for human health: A focus on cancer prevention and interception. *Nutrients* **2019**, *11*, 1226. [CrossRef] [PubMed]

18. Ali, H.E.A.; Shanab, S.M.M.; Shalaby, E.A.A.; Eldmerdash, U.; Abdullah, M.A. Screening of microalgae for antioxidant activities, carotenoids and phenolic contents. In *Applied Mechanics and Materials*; Trans Tech Publications: Stafa-Zurich, Switzerland, 2014; Volume 625, pp. 156–159.
19. Asif, M. Chemistry and antioxidant activity of plants containing some phenolic compounds. *Chem. Int.* **2015**, *1*, 35–52.
20. Natrah FM, I.; Yusoff, F.M.; Shariff, M.; Abas, F.; Mariana, N. Screening of Malaysian indigenous microalgae for antioxidant properties and nutritional value. *J. Appl. Phycol.* **2007**, *19*, 711. [CrossRef]
21. Guiry, M.D. How many species of algae are there? *J. Phycol.* **2005**, *48*, 1057–1063. [CrossRef] [PubMed]
22. Norton, T.A.; Melkonian, M.; Andersen, R.A. Algal biodiversity. *Phycologia* **1996**, *35*, 308–326. [CrossRef]
23. Smerilli, A.; Orefice, I.; Corato, F.; Ruban, A.; Brunet, C. Photoprotective and antioxidant responses to light spectrum and intensity variations on a coastal diatom. *Environ. Microbiol.* **2017**, *19*, 611–627. [CrossRef]
24. Mur, L.R.; Skulberg, O.M.; Utkilen, H. Cyanobacteria in the environment. In *Toxic Cyanobacteria in Water: A GUIDE to their Public Health Consequences, Monitoring and Management*; Ingrid Chorus and Jamie Bartram: London, UK, 1999; pp. 25–54.
25. Walter, J.M.; Coutinho, F.H.; Dutilh, B.E.; Swings, J.; Thompson, F.L.; Thompson, C.C. Ecogenomics and Taxonomy of Cyanobacteria Phylum. *Front. Microbiol.* **2017**, *8*, 2132. [CrossRef]
26. Abed, R.M.M.; Dobretsov, S.; Sudesh, K. Applications of cyanobacteria in biotechnology. *J. Appl. Microbiol.* **2009**, *106*, 1–12. [CrossRef] [PubMed]
27. de Morais, M.G.; da Silva, V.B.; de Morais, E.G.; Vieira Costa, J.A. Biologically active metabolites synthesized by microalgae. *BioMed Res. Int.* **2015**, *2015*, 835761. [CrossRef]
28. Gómez, F. A list of free-living dinoflagellate species in the world's oceans. *Acta Bot. Croat.* **2005**, *64*, 129–212.
29. Llewellyn, C.A.; Airs, R.L. Distribution and abundance of MAAs in 33 species of microalgae across 13 classes. *Mar. Drugs* **2010**, *8*, 1273–1291. [CrossRef] [PubMed]
30. Sunda, W.; Kieber, D.J.; Kiene, R.P.; Huntsman, S. An antioxidant function for DMSP and DMS in marine algae. *Nature* **2002**, *418*, 317–320. [CrossRef]
31. Santhosh, S.; Dhandapani, R.; Hemalatha, N. Bioactive compounds from Microalgae and its different applications—A review. *Adv. Appl. Sci. Res.* **2016**, *7*, 153–158.
32. Metfies, K.; Gescher, C.; Frickenhaus, S.; Wichels, R.N.A.; Gerdts, G.; Knefelkamp, B.; Wiltshire, K.; Medlin, L. Contribution of the class cryptophyceae to phytoplankton structure in the German bight. *J. Phycol.* **2010**, *46*, 1152–1160. [CrossRef]
33. Yusoff, F.M.; Nagao, N.; Imaizumi, Y.; Toda, T. Bioreactor for Microalgal Cultivation Systems: Strategy and Development. In *Prospects of Renewable Bioprocessing in Future Energy Systems. Biofuel and Biorefinery Technologies*; Rastegari, A., Yadav, A., Gupta, A., Eds.; Springer: Cham, Switzerland, 2019; p. 10.
34. Chen, L.; Xin, X.L.; Zhang, H.C.; Yuan, Q.P. Phytochemical properties and antioxidant capacities of commercial raspberry varieties. *J. Funct. Foods.* **2013**, *5*, 508–515. [CrossRef]
35. Goodarzi, V.; Zamani, H.; Bajuli, L.; Moradshahi, A. Evaluation of antioxidant potential and reduction capacity of some plant extracts in silver nanoparticles' synthesis. *Mol. Biol. Res. Commun.* **2014**, *3*, 165–174.
36. Zappalà, A.; Vicario, N.; Calabrese, G.; Turnaturi, R.; Pasquinucci, L.; Montenegro, L.; Spadaro, A.; Parenti, R.; Parenti, C. Neuroprotective effects of *Rosmarinus officinalis* L. extract in oxygen glucose deprivation (OGD)-Injured human neural-like cells. *Nat. Prod. Res* **2019**, 1–7. [CrossRef]
37. Mojaddar Langroodi, A.; Tajik, H.; Mehdizadeh, T. Antibacterial and antioxidant characteristics of *Zataria multiflora* Boiss essential oil and hydroalcoholic extract of *Rhus coriaria* L. *J. Food Qual. Hazards Control* **2019**, *6*, 16–24.
38. Lohani, A.; Mishra, A.K.; Verma, A. Cosmeceutical potential of geranium and calendula essential oil: Determination of antioxidant activity and in vitro sun protection factor. *J. Cosmet Dermatol.* **2019**, *18*, 550–557. [CrossRef] [PubMed]
39. Heghes, S.C.; Vostinaru, O.; Rus, L.M.; Mogosan, C.; Iuga, C.A.; Filip, L. Antispasmodic effect of essential oils and their constituents: A review. *Molecules* **2019**, *24*, 1675. [CrossRef] [PubMed]
40. Amiri, M.; Navabi, J.; Shokoohinia, Y.; Heydarpour, F.; Bahrami, G.; Behbood, L.; Derakhshandeh, P.; Momtaz, S.; Farzaei, M.H. Efficacy and safety of a standardized extract from *Achillea wilhelmsii* C. Koch in patients with ulcerative colitis: A randomized double blind placebo-controlled clinical trial. *Complement. Ther. Med* **2019**, in press. [CrossRef]

41. Sharifi, P.; Shorafa, M.; Mohammadi, M.H. Comparison of the effect of Cow manure, Vermicompost, and Azolla on safflower growth in a saline-sodic soil. *Commun. Soil Sci. Plant Anal.* **2019**. [CrossRef]
42. Assunção, M.F.G.; Amaral, R.; Martins, C.B.; Ferreira, J.D.; Ressurreição, S.; Santos, S.D.; Varejão, J.M.T.B.; Santos, L.M.A. Screening microalgae as potential sources of antioxidants. *J. Appl. Phycol.* **2017**, *29*, 865–877. [CrossRef]
43. Banskota, A.H.; Sperker, S.; Stefanova, R.; McGinn, P.J.; O'Leary, S.J.B. Antioxidant properties and lipid composition of selected microalgae. *J. Appl. Phycol.* **2019**, *31*, 309–318. [CrossRef]
44. Li, H.; Cheng, K.; Wong, C.; Fan, K.; Chen, F.; Jiang, Y. Evaluation of antioxidant capacity and total phenolic content of different fractions of selected microalgae. *Food Chem.* **2007**, *102*, 771–776. [CrossRef]
45. Schieler, B.M.; Soni, M.V.; Brown, C.M.; Coolen, M.J.L.; Fredricks, H.; Van Mooy, B.A.S.; Hirsh, D.J.; Bidle, K.D. Nitric oxide production and antioxidant function during viral infection of the coccolithophore *Emiliania huxleyi*. *ISME J.* **2019**, *13*, 1019–1031. [CrossRef]
46. Fimbres-Olivarria, D.; Carvajal-Millan, E.; Lopez-Elias, J.A.; Martinez-Robinson, K.G.; Miranda-Baeza, A.; Martinez-Cordova, L.R.; Valdez-Holguin, J.E. Chemical characterization and antioxidant activity of sulfated polysaccharides from *Navicula* sp. *Food Hydrocoll.* **2018**, *75*, 229–236. [CrossRef]
47. Delfan, P.; Mortazavi, A.; Rad, A.H.E.; Zenoozian, M.S. Measurement of phenolic content and antioxidant capacity of Pennyroyal (*Mentha pulegium* L.) and microalgae *Spirulina platensis* extracted by steeping, ultrasonic and microwave methods. *J. Food Process. Technol* **2019**, *9*, 712.
48. Khan, M.I.; Shin, J.H.; Kim, J.D. The promising future of microalgae: Current status, challenges, and optimization of a sustainable and renewable industry for biofuels, feed, and other products. *Microb. Cell Fact.* **2018**, *17*, 36. [CrossRef] [PubMed]
49. Zhang, D.; Wan, M.; del Rio-Chanona, E.A.; Huang, J.; Wang, W.; Li, Y.; Vassiliadis, V.S. Dynamic modelling of *Haematococcus pluvialis* photoinduction for astaxanthin production in both attached and suspended photobioreactors. *Algal Res.* **2016**, *13*, 69–78. [CrossRef]
50. Barredo, J.L. Microbial Carotenoids from Bacteria and Microalgae. In *Methods and Protocols*; Humana Press: New York, NY, USA, 2012.
51. Xia, S.; Wang, K.; Wan, L.; Li, A.; Hu, Q.; Zhang, C. Production, Characterization, and Antioxidant Activity of Fucoxanthin from the Marine Diatom *Odontella aurita*. *Mar. Drugs* **2013**, *11*, 2667–2681. [CrossRef] [PubMed]
52. Takaichi, S. Carotenoids in algae: Distributions, biosynthesis and functions. *Mar. Drugs* **2011**, *9*, 1101–1118. [CrossRef] [PubMed]
53. Manirafasha, E.; Ndikubwimana, T.; Zeng, X.; Lu, Y.; Jing, K. Phycobiliprotein: Potential microalgae derived pharmaceutical and biological reagent. *Biochem. Eng. J.* **2016**, *109*, 282–296. [CrossRef]
54. Künzel, A. Aharon Oren: Halophilic microorganisms and their environments. *Int. Microbiol.* **2003**, *6*, 151–152. [CrossRef]
55. Sánchez-Salgado, J.C.; Estrada-Soto, S.; García-Jiménez, S.; Montes, S.; Gómez-Zamudio, J.; Villalobos-Molina, R. Analysis of flavonoids bioactivity for cholestatic liver disease: Systematic literature search and experimental approaches. *Biomolecules* **2019**, *9*, 102.
56. Klejdus, B.; Kopeckýb, J.; Benešová, L.; Vaceka, J. Solid-phase/supercritical-fluid extraction for liquid chromatography of phenolic compounds in freshwater microalgae and selected cyanobacterial species. *J. Chromatogr.* **2009**, *1216*, 763–771. [CrossRef]
57. Miranda, M.S.; Cintra, R.G.; Barros, S.B.M.; Mancini-Filho, J. Antioxidant activity of the microalga *Spirulina maxima*. *Braz. J. Med. Biol. Res.* **1998**, *31*, 1075–1079. [CrossRef]
58. Hosseini Tafreshi, A.; Shariati, M. *Dunaliella* biotechnology: Methods and applications. *J. Appl. Microbiol.* **2009**, *107*, 14–35. [CrossRef]
59. Xu, S.Y.; Huang, X.; Cheong, K.L. Recent advances in marine algae polysaccharides: Isolation, structure, and activities. *Mar. Drugs* **2017**, *15*, 388. [CrossRef]
60. Chakrabarti, S.; Guha, S.; Majumder, K. Food-derived bioactive peptides in human health: Challenges and opportunities. *Nutrients* **2018**, *10*, 1738. [CrossRef]
61. Barra, L.; Chandrasekaran, R.; Corato, F.; Brunet, C. The challenge of ecophysiological biodiversity for biotechnological applications of Marine Microalgae. *Mar. Drugs* **2014**, *12*, 1641–1675. [CrossRef]
62. Brunet, C.; Johnsen, G.; Lavaud, J.; Roy, S. Pigments and photoacclimation processes. In *Phytoplankton Pigments, Characterization, Chemotaxonomy and Applications in Oceanography*; Cambridge University Press: Cambridge, UK, 2011; p. 880.

63. Volkman, J.K. Sterols in microorganisms. *Appl. Microbiol. Biotechnol.* **2003**, *60*, 495–506. [CrossRef]
64. Durmaz, Y. Vitamin E (α-tocopherol) production by the marine microalga *Nannochloropsis oculata* (Eustigmatophyceae) in nitrogen limitation. *Aquaculture* **2007**, *272*, 717–722. [CrossRef]
65. Gastineau, R.; Turcotte, F.; Pouvreau, J.-B.; Morançais, M.; Fleurence, J.; Windarto, E.; Prasetiya, F.; Arsad, S.; Jaouen, P.; Babin, M.; et al. Marennine, promising blue pigments from a widespread *Haslea* diatom species complex. *Mar. Drugs* **2014**, *12*, 3161–3189. [CrossRef]
66. Francavilla, M.; Trotta, P.; Luque, R. Phytosterols from *Dunaliella tertiolecta* and *Dunaliella salina*: A potentially novel industrial application. *Bioresour. Technol.* **2010**, *101*, 4144–4150. [CrossRef]
67. Copia, J.; Gaete, H.; Zúñiga, G.; Hidalgo, M.; Cabrera, E. Effect of ultraviolet B radiation on the production of polyphenols in the marine microalga *Chlorella* sp. *Lat. Am. J. Aquat. Res.* **2012**, *40*, 113–123. [CrossRef]
68. Goiris, K.; Van Colen, W.; Wilches, I.; León-Tamariz, W.; De Cooman, L.; Muylaert, K. Impact of nutrient stress on antioxidant production in three species of microalgae. *Algal Res.* **2015**, *7*, 51–57. [CrossRef]
69. Farahin, A.W.; Yusoff, F.M.; Nagao, N.; Basri, M.; Shariff, M. Phenolic content and antioxidant activity of *Tetraselmis tetrathele* (West) Butcher 1959 cultured in annular photobioreactor. *J. Environ. Biol.* **2016**, *37*, 631–639.
70. Morowvat, M.H.; Ghasemi, Y. Evaluation of antioxidant properties of some naturally isolated microalgae: Identification and characterization of the most efficient strain. *Biocatal. Agric. Biotechnol.* **2016**, *8*, 263–269. [CrossRef]
71. Pouvreau, J.B.; Morancais, M.; Taran, F.; Rosa, P.; Dufossé, L.; Guérard, F.; Pin, S.; Fleurence, J.; Pondaven, P. Antioxidant and free radical scavenging properties of marennine, a blue-green polyphenolic pigment from the diatom *Haslea ostrearia* (Gaillon/Bory) Simonsen responsible for the natural greening of cultured oysters. *J. Agric. Food Chem* **2008**, *56*, 6278–6286. [CrossRef]
72. Jerez-Martel, I.; García-Poza, S.; Rodríguez-Martel, G.; Rico, M.; Afonso-Olivares, C.; Gómez-Pinchetti, J.L. Phenolic profile and antioxidant activity of crude extracts from microalgae and cyanobacteria strains. *J. Food Qual.* **2017**, *2017*, 2924508. [CrossRef]
73. Borowitzka, M.A. Commercial-scale production of microalgae for bioproducts. In *Blue Biotechnology: Production and Use of Marine Molecules*; La Barre, S., Bates, S.S., Eds.; Wiley-VCH: Weinheim, Germany, 2018; Volume 1, pp. 33–65.
74. Cirulis, J.T.; Scott, J.A.; Ross, G.M. Management of oxidative stress by microalgae. *Can. J. Physiol. Pharmacol.* **2013**, *9*, 15–21. [CrossRef]
75. Haubrich, B.A. Microbial sterolomics as a chemical biology tool. *Molecules* **2018**, *23*, 2768. [CrossRef]
76. Stonik, V.A.; Stonik, I.A. Sterol and sphingoid glycoconjugates from microalgae. *Mar. Drugs* **2018**, *16*, 514. [CrossRef]
77. Smerilli, A.; Balzano, S.; Maselli, M.; Blasio, M.; Galasso, C.; Sansone, C.; Brunet, C. Antioxidant and photoprotection networking in the coastal diatom *Skeletonema marinoi*. *Antioxidants* **2019**, 8. [CrossRef]
78. de la Coba, F.; Aguilera, J.; Figueroa, F.L.; De Gálvez, M.V.; Herrera, E. Antioxidant activity of mycosporine-like amino acids isolated from three red macroalgae and one marine lichen. *J. Appl. Phycol.* **2009**, *21*, 161–169. [CrossRef]
79. Dimier, C.; Saviello, G.; Tramontano, F.; Brunet, C. Comparative ecophysiology of the xanthophyll cycle in six marine phytoplanktonic species. *Protist* **2009**, *160*, 397–411. [CrossRef]
80. Sansone, C.; Galasso, C.; Orefice, I.; Nuzzo, G.; Luongo, E.; Cutignano, A.; Romano, G.; Brunet, C.; Fontana, A.; Esposito, F.; et al. The green microalga *Tetraselmis suecica* reduces oxidative stress and induces repairing mechanisms in human cells. *Sci. Rep.* **2017**, *7*, 41215. [CrossRef] [PubMed]
81. Williams, P.J.l.B.; Laurens, L.M.L. Microalgae as biodiesel & biomass feedstocks: Review & analysis of the biochemistry, energetics & economics. *Energy Environ. Sci.* **2010**, *3*, 554.

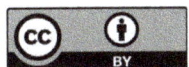

© 2019 by the authors. Licensee MDPI, Basel, Switzerland. This article is an open access article distributed under the terms and conditions of the Creative Commons Attribution (CC BY) license (http://creativecommons.org/licenses/by/4.0/).

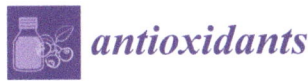

Article

Fucoxanthin, A Carotenoid Derived from *Phaeodactylum tricornutum* Exerts Antiproliferative and Antioxidant Activities In Vitro

Ulrike Neumann [1,†], Felix Derwenskus [2,3,†], Verena Flaiz Flister [1], Ulrike Schmid-Staiger [2], Thomas Hirth [4] and Stephan C. Bischoff [1,*]

1. Institute of Clinical Nutrition, University of Hohenheim, Fruwirthstr. 12, 70593 Stuttgart, Germany; ulrike.neumann@uni-hohenheim.de (U.N.); verena.flister@gmail.com (V.F.F.)
2. Fraunhofer Institute for Interfacial Engineering and Biotechnology IGB, Nobelstr. 12, 70569 Stuttgart, Germany; felix.derwenskus@igb.fraunhofer.de (F.D.); ulrike.schmid-staiger@igb.fraunhofer.de (U.S.-S.)
3. Institute of Interfacial Process Engineering and Plasma Technology IGVP, University of Stuttgart, Nobelstr. 12, 70569 Stuttgart, Germany
4. Karlsruhe Institute for Technology, Kaiserstr. 12, 76131 Karlsruhe, Germany; thomas.hirth@kit.edu
* Correspondence: bischoff.stephan@uni-hohenheim.de; Tel.: +49-711-459-24101
† Contributed equally.

Received: 20 May 2019; Accepted: 17 June 2019; Published: 19 June 2019

Abstract: Microalgae contain a multitude of nutrients and can be grown sustainably. Fucoxanthin, a carotenoid from *Phaeodactylum tricornutum*, could have beneficial health effects. Therefore, we investigated the anti-inflammatory, antioxidative and antiproliferative effects of fucoxanthin derived from this diatom in vitro. The effects of purified fucoxanthin on metabolic activity were assessed in blood mononuclear cells and different cell lines. In cell lines, caspase 3/7 activity was also analyzed. Nitrogen monoxide release and mRNA-expression of proinflammatory cytokines were measured. For antioxidant assays, cell free assays were conducted. Additionally, the antioxidant effect in neutrophils was quantified and glutathione was determined in HeLa cells. The results show that neither did fucoxanthin have anti-inflammatory properties nor did it exert cytotoxic effects on mononuclear cells. However, the metabolic activity of cell lines was decreased up to 58% and fucoxanthin increased the caspase 3/7 activity up to 4.6-fold. Additionally, dose-dependent antioxidant effects were detected, resulting in a 63% decrease in chemiluminescence in blood neutrophils and a 3.3-fold increase in the ratio of reduced to oxidized glutathione. Our studies show that fucoxanthin possesses antiproliferative and antioxidant activities in vitro. Hence, this carotenoid or the whole microalgae *P. tricornutum* could be considered as a food or nutraceutical in human nutrition, showcasing beneficial health effects.

Keywords: microalgae; *Phaeodactylum tricornutum*; fucoxanthin; antioxidative; antiproliferative

1. Introduction

Microalgae are microscopic small unicellular organisms that are abundant in various habitats around the globe. They can be cultured in open ponds or photobioreactors without the use of arable land and thus represent a promising sustainable alternative to plant-based proteins. They do not only produce high amounts of proteins but are also a good source for fatty acids, and vitamins, which can provide health promoting effects in a human diet. Hence, they can serve as novel functional foods or be incorporated into existing food products [1,2].

The unicellular pennate diatom *Phaeodactylum tricornutum* exists in three different morphotypes and its genome has been already fully sequenced [3]. The diatom contains a multitude of different components that could provide health beneficial effects. These include the omega-3 fatty acid eicosapentaenoic acid (EPA), polyphenols like (epi-) catechin and oxygenated carotenoids like fucoxanthin [4–8]. Fucoxanthin, a major marine carotenoid, is located in the thylakoids of chloroplasts and forms a light harvesting complex (LHC) with chlorophyll a/c [9,10]. It was shown in several studies, that fucoxanthin from macroalgae possesses health-conducive effects, including anti-inflammatory, antioxidant, antiobesity and anticancer activities [11–15]. Since most of these studies used fucoxanthin derived from macroalgae, only little is known about the health-beneficial effects of fucoxanthin derived from *P. tricornutum*, although this microalga was shown to have a high content of fucoxanthin between 16.5 to 26.1 mg per gram dry matter (dm) [16,17]. Thus, diatom biomass can contain up to ten times more fucoxanthin than macroalgae. Additionally, diatoms, different from macroalgae, can be cultivated indoors and outdoors not only during specific seasons but all around the year with a high biomass productivity [18]. It is already demonstrated that they can be produced in various types of different closed photobioreactors, like bubble columns and flat panel airlift bioreactors [19–21]. Hence, *P. tricornutum* might be a suitable source for the commercial production of fucoxanthin.

The prevalence of diseases linked to oxidative stress and inflammation is constantly increasing in developed countries [22–24]. The occurrence of those diseases can also be linked to the emergence of cancer [25,26]. Therefore, research is trying to identify new compounds that could be used to reduce inflammation, oxidative stress, and the viability of cancer cells. Fucoxanthin derived from *P. tricornutum* might be used as a new nutraceutical, if it also exhibits the health beneficial effects that were already shown for the carotenoid derived from macroalgae.

2. Materials and Methods

2.1. Cultivation of Microalgae and Fucoxanthin Extraction

P. tricornutum UTEX 640 was cultivated in 180 L Flat-Panel-Airlift photobioreactors in an outdoor pilot scale plant located at the Fraunhofer Center for Chemical-Biotechnological Processes CBP in Leuna, Germany. Modified Mann and Myers medium was used as culture medium as described in Meiser et al. [19,27]. The biomass was disrupted using stirred ball milling (PML-2, Bühler) and freeze-drying prior to fucoxanthin extraction. The cell disruption and extraction method were previously described in detail in Derwenskus et al. [17]. Briefly, Fucoxanthin was extracted from the disrupted biomass by pressurized liquid extraction (ASE 350, Thermo-Fisher) for a static extraction time of 20 min at 100 °C and 100 bar using adequate subcritical organic solvents (described in [28]). Subsequently, the fucoxanthin was purified by multiple separation steps using filters (0.25 µm) consisting of polytetrafluoroethylene to a final purity of 99.2% (w/w) (HPLC). It was compared to a commercial fucoxanthin standard (16337, Sigma-Aldrich) using UHPLC-MS.

It was compared to a commercial fucoxanthin standard (16337, Sigma-Aldrich) using UHPLC-MS.

2.2. Determination of Fucoxanthin by HPLC and UHPLC-MS

Fucoxanthin was quantified using the HPLC method described by Gille et al. [28] with slight modifications. Briefly, the purified fucoxanthin was resolved in pure ethanol with BHT (250 mg/L) and compared to a commercial analytical standard (16337, Sigma-Aldrich, St. Louis, MO, USA) using reverse-phase HPLC with a Suplex pKb 100 column (5 µm, 250 × 4.6mm, Supelco, Bellefonte, PA, USA). Samples (injection volume 5 µL) were analyzed using a HPLC (1200 Infinity, Agilent, Santa Clara, CA, USA) equipped with a multi-wavelength UV detector at 450 nm and a flow rate of 1 mL/min. The gradient used for the method is described in detail elsewhere [29].

Additionally, fucoxanthin from *P. tricornutum* was analyzed and compared to the commercial standard by UHPLC-DAD (1290 Infinity, Agilent Technologies) using a Zorbax Eclipse Plus C18 (2.1 × 50 mm) column with a particle size of 1.8 µm. Mobile phase A contained water with 0.1% formic acid and mobile phase B consisted of methanol with 0.1% formic acid. The gradient used is shown in Table 1. The fucoxanthin was detected at 450 nm and analyzed in a mass spectrometer (LTQ XL, Thermo Scientific) using ESI in full scan mode from 200 to 1000 m/z at a temperature of 275 °C and

−9.0 V. The *m/z* values (see supplementary material, S1) were compared to the analytical standard and to literature [30].

Table 1. Solvent gradient for the UHPLC-MS-Method used in this study. Mobile phase A consisted of water with 0.1% formic acid and mobile phase B was methanol with 0.1% formic acid.

Time [min]	Mobile Phase A [%]	Mobile Phase B [%]
0	70	30
8	3	97
11	3	97
11.1	70	30
14	70	30

2.3. Isolation of Human Primary Blood Cells Band Cell Cultures

Anticoagulated blood was collected from healthy volunteers, approved by the local ethics committee (F-2015-064, Landesärztekammer Baden-Württemberg). Isolation of polymorphonuclear leukocytes (PML) and peripheral blood mononuclear cells (PBMCs) via dextran sedimentation and density gradient centrifugation was conducted as previously described by El Benna & Dang (2007) [30] and Neumann et al. (2018) [31]. PMLs were resuspended in DPBS, PBMCs in RPMI medium with 10% fetal calf serum and 1% penicillin / streptomycin. HepG2 cells were provided by the Max Rubner-Institute (Karlsruhe, Germany). RAW 264.7, HepG2, Caco-2 and HeLa cells were cultured in DMEM with 10% fetal calf serum and 1% penicillin / streptomycin.

2.4. Metabolic Activity

Metabolic activity was assessed using the tetrazolium dye 3-(4,5-dimethylthiazol-2-yl)-2, 5-diphenyltetrazolium bromide (MTT). PBMCs (3×10^5 cells per well) and RAW 264.7 cells (1×10^4 cells per well) were incubated with fucoxanthin (0.1, 1, 10 and 50 µg/mL), β-carotene (1 µg/mL), dimethyl sulfoxide (DMSO, 0.1%) as solvent control or DMSO (5%) as positive control for 24 h. Subsequent, MTT assay was conducted as previously described [31].

2.5. Antiinflammatory Assays

Nitric oxide (NO) production in RAW 264.7 cells was measured using the Griess assay. Therefore, 5×10^5 cells were treated with fucoxanthin (0.1 and 1 µg/mL) or β-carotene (1 µg/mL) and stimulated with lipopolysaccharide (LPS, 1 µg/mL) for 24 h. The level of NO was measured using the Griess reaction, as previously described [32].

The effects of fucoxanthin on the LPS-induced mRNA expression of the cytokines interleukin-(IL-)1β, IL-6, tumor necrosis factor α (TNF-α) and the enzyme cyclooxygenase-2 (COX-2) in PBMCs was measured by quantitative real-time polymerase chain reaction (qRT-PCR). Cells were incubated with fucoxanthin (0.1, 1 or 10 µg/mL), β-carotene (1 µg/mL) or DMSO (0.1%) as solvent control for 24 h. Cells were stimulated with LPS (1 µg/mL) for 6 h. The mRNA expression was measured as formerly described [31].

2.6. Antioxidant Assays

Total phenolics content (TPC) was determined using the Folin-Ciocalteu method [33] with minor modifications. In a 96-well microplate, 30 µL of fucoxanthin (0.1, 1 or 10 µg/mL) were mixed with 150 µL Folin-Ciocalteu reagent (diluted 1/10 in water) and 120 µL sodium carbonate solution (75 g/L). To obtain an individual blank, samples were mixed with 120 µL sodium carbonate solution and 150 µL water. After 2 h in the dark at room temperature, the absorbance was measured at 765 nm with a BioTek Synergy HT plate reader (BioTek Instruments, Winooski, VT, USA). Gallic acid was used to establish a calibration curve (30–580 µM) and results are expressed as gallic acid equivalents (GAE) per gram dry matter (dm).

The ferric reducing antioxidant power (FRAP) assay was performed in accordance to the method of Benzie and Strain [34]. An individual blank was measured for each sample. Ferrous sulphate solutions were used for calibration (50–1000 µM) and the results are expressed as mmol Fe^{2+} per gram dm.

For the 2,2-diphenyl-1-picrylhydrazyl (DPPH) assay a calibration curve was obtained by using DPPH concentrations in the range of 0-100 µM. A DPPH solution was freshly prepared in methanol. 150 µL DPPH (0.1 MM) were mixed with 50 µL fucoxanthin (0.1, 1, 10 or 50 µg/mL), 150 µL methanol instead of DPPH were used for blank measurement. The percentage inhibition was calculated using the following formula:

$$\%\text{Inhibition} = (OD_{DPPH} - OD_{Sample})/OD_{DPPH} \times 100$$

The half maximal inhibitory concentration (IC50) was calculated by linear regression, plotting the percentage inhibition against the different extract concentrations.

The glutathione (GSH) to glutathione disulfide (GSSG) ratio as a marker for oxidative stress was determined using the GSH/GSSG-Glo™ Assay (Promega, Mannheim, Germany). 2×10^4 HeLa cells were incubated with fucoxanthin (0.1, 1, 10 and 50 µg/mL), β-carotene (1 µg/mL), DMSO (0.1%) as solvent control or menadione (40 µM) as control for 24 h.

2′,7′-dichlorofluorescin (DCF) fluorescence and ROS production using luminol chemiluminescence were measured in human PMLs. For DCF fluorescence 100 µL of freshly drawn blood were incubated with 2′,7′-dichlorofluorescin diacetate (20 µM) at 37 °C for 15 min. Lipopolysaccharide (10 ng/mL) and fucoxanthin (0.1, 1, 10 or 50 µg/mL) or β-carotene (1 µg/mL) were added for 1 h at 37 °C. Cells were then stimulated with N-formylmethionyl-leucyl-phenylalanine (fMLP, 500nM). The reaction was stopped after 5 min by placing the samples on ice. After red blood cell lysis using the BD FACS lysing solution according to the manufacturer's instructions, DCF fluorescence was measured with a BD FACS Canto II (BD Biosciences, Becton, Dickinson and Company, San Jose, CA, USA). The percentage of fluorescent PMLs was calculated using the BD FACS Diva Software.

In luminol assays, PMLs were incubated with fucoxanthin (0.1, 1, 10 and 50 µg/mL), β-carotene (1 µg/mL), DMSO (0.1%) as solvent control or menadione (40 µM) as control. The assay was conducted as previously described [35] and cells were stimulated with phorbol 12-myristate 13-acetate (PMA, 100 ng/mL). Chemiluminescence was measured in a Berthold-Biolumat LB937 (Berthold Technologies Co., Bad Wildbad, Germany) at 37 °C for 15 min. Percentage inhibition of luminescence was calculated using the area under the curve (AUC) values.

2.7. Cytotoxic and Apoptotic Assays

MTT assays were conducted with Caco-2, HeLa and Hep G2 cells to assess cytotoxic activity of fucoxanthin on cancer cells. Cells were incubated with fucoxanthin (0.1, 1, 10 and 50 µg/mL), β-carotene (1 µg/mL), DMSO (0.1%) or staurosporine (1 µM) for 48 h, as described elsewhere [32]. For apoptotic properties, the caspase-glo®3/7 assay (Promega, Mannheim, Germany) was conducted according to the manufacturer's instructions.

2.8. Statistics

Data are expressed as mean ± standard error of the mean (SEM) in graphs or ± standard deviation (SD) in tables. Graphs were generated using GraphPad Prism 5 (La Jolla, CA, USA), statistics were done using IBM SPSS Statistics 25 (IBM Corp., Armonk, NY, USA), graphs. Normal distribution was tested using the Shapiro–Wilk test. One-way analysis of variance (ANOVA) was used to evaluate statistic significant differences ($p < 0.05$) between groups. The equality of variances was tested utilizing Levene's test. For equal variances, Tukey's HSD post hoc test was used; for unequal variances, Dunnett's T3 post hoc test3.

3. Results

3.1. Metabolic Activity

For PBMCs, only the positive control with a final concentration of 5% DMSO led to a significant decrease in metabolic activity analyzed using the MTT assay. Fucoxanthin up to a concentration of 50 µg/ml did not influence the metabolic activity (Table 2). For RAW 264.7, however, a decrease in metabolic activity was shown for the positive control and the highest fucoxanthin concentration tested (50 µg/mL, Table 2). Hence, the following anti-inflammatory assays were only conducted with non-cytotoxic concentrations.

Table 2. Effects of fucoxanthin from P. tricornutum, vehicle control (DMSO, 0.1%), positive control (DMSO, 5%) and β-carotene on metabolic activity of PBMCs and RAW 264.7 cells. Data are presented as mean ± SD ($n = 4$–6).

	[µg/mL]	Metabolic Activity [%]	
		PBMCs	RAW 264.7
Vehicle control		100	100
Positive control		54.27 ± 4.23 **	3.39 ± 3.02 ***
Fucoxanthin	50	104.7 ± 14.16	20.88 ± 6.33 **
	10	98.76 ± 5.38	73.28 ± 9.60
	1	95.25 ± 3.84	89.64 ± 13.76
	0.1	88.35 ± 14.13	93.12 ± 5.09
β-carotene	1	87.65 ± 13.47	80.30 ± 13.09

Asterisks mark significant differences to vehicle control as analyzed by ANOVA with Dunnett's T3 post hoc test (*<0.05, ** <0.01, *** <0.001).

3.2. Antiinflammatory Effects

To analyze the anti-inflammatory effects of fucoxanthin, the NO production of RAW 264.7 cells was measured, and mRNA-expressions of inflammatory cytokines were determined in PBMCs (Table 3). Neither fucoxanthin nor β-carotene showed anti-inflammatory effects in the tested concentrations (Table 3). Additionally, no pro-inflammatory effect was seen in unstimulated cells (Table 3).

Table 3. Effects of fucoxanthin from P. tricornutum, vehicle control (DMSO, 0.1%) and β-carotene on relative mRNA expression of pro-inflammatory cytokines in PBMCs and on NO production in RAW 264.7 cells. Data are presented as mean ± SD ($n = 5$–7).

	[µg/mL]	IL-1β [%]	IL-6 [%]	TNFα [%]	NO [µM]
		PBMCs	PBMCs	PBMCs	RAW 264.7
Vehicle control		100	100	100	59.66 ± 7.59
Fucoxanthin	10	110.1 ± 26.55	99.15 ± 26.14	160.4 ± 68.13	56.53 ± 6.58
	1	97.65 ± 18.09	92.10 ± 22.18	133.3 ± 60.35	60.84 ± 7.65
	0.1	101.3 ± 18.29	122.5 ± 32.23	133.9 ± 55.50	59.21 ± 7.69
β-carotene	1	75.07 ± 44.36.	104.2 ± 57.37	158.7 ± 80.90	59.84 ± 7.10
Vehicle control, unstimulated		0.2 ± 0.1	0.1 ± 0.1	5.6 ± 5.7	0.0 ± 0.0
Fucoxanthin, unstimulated	10	0.3 ± 0.5	0.1 ± 0.04	5.1 ± 6.2	0.03 ± 0.1
β-carotene, unstimulated	1	0.2 ± 0.2	0.1 ± 0.2	3.8 ± 2.2	0.0 ± 0.0

No differences between stimulated groups and no differences between unstimulated groups were found by ANOVA ($p < 0.05$). Abbreviations: IL interleukin; TNF tumor necrosis factor, NO nitrogen monoxide.

3.3. Antioxidant Effects

Various assays were conducted to analyze the antioxidant properties of fucoxanthin. In the DPPH assay, fucoxanthin had an IC50 value of 201.2 ± 21.4 µg/mL, while the value for ascorbic acid was 70.3 ± 18.7 µg/mL and for astaxanthin 79.32 ± 18.10 µg/mL. Due to low antioxidant effects, an IC50 for β-carotene could not be calculated. Results of the FRAP assay show that fucoxanthin is equivalent to 64.74 ± 3.93 mmol Fe^{2+} per gram dm, β-carotene to 6.55 ± 0.33 and astaxanthin to 63.97 ± 6.79 mmol Fe^{2+} per gram.

Neither fucoxanthin nor β-carotene showed effects on the DCF fluorescence of PMLs (data not shown). Menadione decreased the GSH/GSSG ratio. However, according to statistical analysis this change was not significant ($p = 0.09$). Fucoxanthin in the highest concentration (50 µg/mL) increased the ratio significantly (Figure 1A). Lower concentrations, however, showed no effects. Luminol chemiluminescence was measured to evaluate the antioxidant properties of fucoxanthin in PMLs. The results are depicted in Figure 1B and show that menadione decreased the luminescence by 96%, fucoxanthin by 63% at 50 µg/mL. The antioxidant effect is dose-response dependent.

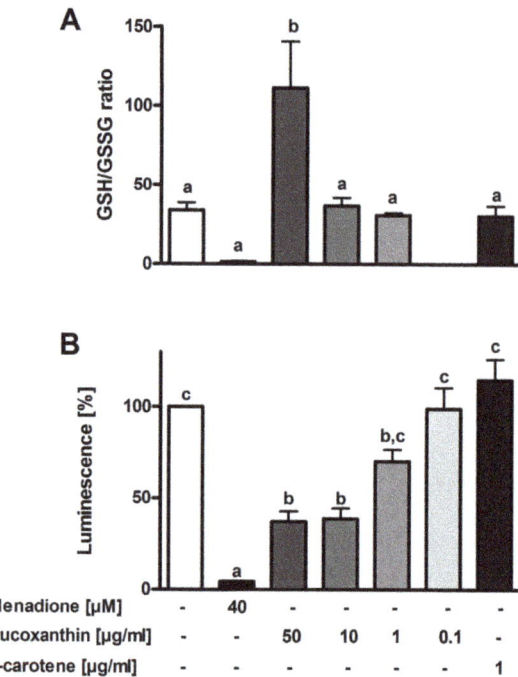

Figure 1. Effects of fucoxanthin from *P. tricornutum* on GSH to GSSG ratio in HeLa cells (**A**) and on luminol chemiluminescence in freshly isolated PMLs (**B**) ($n = 3$–5). Different letters represent significantly different groups (ANOVA followed by Tukey post hoc test for GSH/GSSG assay or with Dunnett's T3 post hoc test for luminol chemiluminescence, $p < 0.05$). Abbreviations: GSH glutathione, GSSG glutathione disulfide.

3.4. Cytotoxic and Apoptotic Effects

Fucoxanthin was able to reduce the metabolic activity of Hep G2, HeLa and Caco-2 cells in a dose-dependent manner (Figure 2A–C). An inhibitory effect of up to 58% was measured in Hep G2 cells. In HeLa and Caco-2 cells, the effect was stronger than that of the positive control with a final concentration of 5% DMSO. In order to evaluate if the decrease in metabolic activity is linked to apoptosis, the caspase 3/7 activity was determined. The results show that fucoxanthin led to a dose-dependent increase in caspase 3/7 activity (Figure 2D–F). A 4.6-fold increase in caspase activity was measured in HeLa cells for the highest fucoxanthin concentration. 50 µg/mL of the carotenoid led to a higher caspase 3/7 activity than 1µM staurosporine in all tested cell cultures.

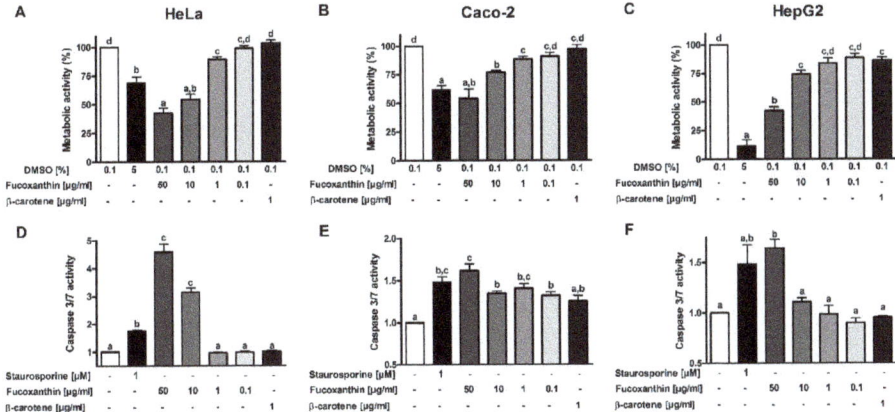

Figure 2. Effects of fucoxanthin from *P. tricornutum* on metabolic activity of HeLa (**A**), Caco-2 (**B**) and HepG2 (**C**) cells (n = 4–6). Cells were incubated for 48 hours, DMSO (5%) was used as a positive control. Caspase 3/7 activity as a marker for apoptosis was assessed in HeLa (**D**), Caco-2 (**E**) and HepG2 (**F**) cells (n = 4). Here, staurosporine (1 μM) was used as a positive control. Different letters mark significant differences (ANOVA followed by Tukey post hoc test for D or with Dunnett's T3 post hoc test, $p < 0.05$).

4. Discussion

Fucoxanthin, a major marine carotenoid that is up to now obtained from macroalgae, was successfully extracted from the microalgae *P. tricornutum*. In this study, we found that fucoxanthin had no influence on the metabolic activity of PBMCs, which was also reported by Ishikawa et al. [36]. This leads to the assumption that fucoxanthin, up to concentrations of 50 μg/mL, has no cytotoxic effects on these cells. However, the carotenoid had a cytotoxic effect on the mouse macrophage cell line RAW 264.7 at 50 μg/mL. This is not concordant to a study by Islam et al. (2013), who only reported a reduced cell viability at much higher doses of fucoxanthin [37].

This study found no effects of fucoxanthin on the NO production of LPS-stimulated RAW 264.7 cells. A study by Islam et al. (2013) supports these findings [37]. Authors showed anti-inflammatory effects only at higher concentrations [37]. However, other studies were able to show a dose-dependent inhibition of NO production by fucoxanthin at lower concentrations [12,38,39]. Here, we also reported that the carotenoid had no effect on the mRNA-expression of pro-inflammatory cytokines in human PBMCs. This is also not concordant to the study by Heo et al. (2010), who showed an inhibitory effect on the mRNA expression in RAW 264.7 cells [12]. Yet, to date, no studies on the anti-inflammatory effects of fucoxanthin on human primary blood cells have been published. It is noteworthy that all mentioned studies utilized fucoxanthin extracted from seaweeds. Therefore, it can be assumed that the carotenoid from *P. tricornutum* might have different effects or that the measured effects in other studies are based on impurities resulting from extraction.

Fucoxanthin showed strong antioxidant effects in cell-free and cell-based assays. The IC50 concentration of fucoxanthin with 201 μg/mL in the DPPH assay was higher than that reported by Sachindra et al. (2007) [40]. The higher values might be caused by differences in extraction or on the origin of the carotenoid. As previously described, β-carotene showed no DPPH radical scavenging activity [41]. Antioxidant effects of ascorbic acid, however, were stronger in FRAP and DPPH assays. The FRAP assay revealed that the antioxidant effects of fucoxanthin extracted from *P. tricornutum* does not significantly differ from that of astaxanthin, a carotenoid with strong antioxidant effects derived from the red algae *Haematococcus pluvialis* which is already successfully commercialized [42,43]. Both, fucoxanthin as well as astaxanthin showed a strong antioxidant effect in the FRAP assay compared to β-carotene.

In the DCF fluorescence assay, neither fucoxanthin nor β-carotene showed antioxidant effects while the luminol assay revealed dose-dependent antioxidant properties of fucoxanthin. The DCF assay is used for the intracellular detection of ROS, especially H2O2 [44]. Luminol, on the other hand, can detect the sum of extra- and intracellular ROS, especially those generated by the myeloperoxidase [45]. Hence, it can be assumed that fucoxanthin is either inhibiting the myeloperoxidase activation or quenching the bactericidal hypochlorite produced by this enzyme. Fucoxanthin was also able to increase the GSH level in HeLa cells, which was already shown by a study in human keratinocytes [46]. GSH as an antioxidant is able to scavenge ROS; the ratio of GSH to GSSG is often used as a marker for oxidative stress. A multitude of diseases is linked to a decreased GSH to GSSG ratio, including Alzheimer's and Parkinson's disease [47–49]. Fucoxanthin could help to increase reduced GSH and hence ameliorate the negative effects of oxidative stress.

Although fucoxanthin had no effect on the metabolic activity of human blood cells, a dose-dependent influence on different carcinoma cell lines was shown. For Caco-2 cells and different cell lines, this was already shown previously [50–52]. To analyze if the reduced metabolic activity is linked to an increased apoptosis of cells, we also measured the caspase 3/7 activity. An increase in activity was shown for all cells, leading to the conclusion that fucoxanthin from P. tricornutum is able to induce apoptosis in different cancer cells. Kim et al. (2010) were able to show, that the induced apoptosis is caused by the formation of ROS by fucoxanthin [51]. The authors state that the production of intracellular H_2O_2 and superoxide in the carcinoma cells triggers the apoptosis. This is, however, inconsistent with the antioxidant effects of the carotenoid that was shown in this study. On the other hand, Kotake-Nara et al. (2005) reported that the induced apoptosis is not accompanied by the production of ROS and caused by the loss of mitochondrial membrane potential [53]. It is assumed that oxidative stress is linked to the initiation and promotion of cancer [25]. ROS might lead to DNA damages and hence lead to uncontrolled cell proliferation and decreased apoptosis in cancer cells. On the other hand, antitumor drugs often function by producing ROS that induce oxidative stress in tumor cells and lead to cell death [54]. The role of antioxidants in tumor therapy is therefore a controversial issue. Some studies show that antioxidants can promote the outcome of therapy, while others show negative effects [54,55].

In summary, we were able to show antioxidant and antiproliferative but no anti-inflammatory effects of the carotenoid fucoxanthin extracted from the microalgae P. tricornutum. Fucoxanthin was able to inhibit the oxidative burst in human PMLs, scavenge radicals and increase the GSH to GSSG ratio. Additionally, the metabolic activity was decreased, and apoptosis increased by the carotenoid. This leads to the conclusion that fucoxanthin or the whole microalgae biomass, including fucoxanthin in high amounts, could be considered in nutrition in order to ameliorate the effects of diseases linked to oxidative stress. Additionally, fucoxanthin could help to support traditional cancer treatment because of its beneficial health effects. Human trials are needed in future to further support these suggestions.

Supplementary Materials: The following are available online at http://www.mdpi.com/2076-3921/8/6/183/s1, Figure S1: UHPLC-MS spectra of a commercial fucoxanthin standard (A) and fucoxanthin derived from the diatom P. tricornutum (B) showing the specific m/z-values of precursor ions (m/z = 659.6 [M+H]+; 681.5 [M+Na]+) of fucoxanthin and related daughter ions (m/z = 641.8 and 581.9). Abbreviations: m/z mass-to-charge ratio.

Author Contributions: Conceptualization, U.N., F.D., U.S.-S., T.H. and S.C.B.; methodology, U.N. and F.D.; software, F.D.; formal analysis, U.N. and F.D.; investigation, U.N., V.F.F. and F.D.; writing—original draft preparation, U.N., F.D. and S.C.B.; writing—review and editing, V.F.F., U.S.-S. and T.H.; visualization, U.N. and F.D.; supervision, U.S.-S., T.H. and S.C.B.

Funding: This work was supported by a grant to SCB and FD from the Ministry for Science, Research and Art within the Bioeconomy research Program of Baden-Württemberg (Az: 33-7533-10-5/91/1 and Az: 33-7533-10-5-93, BÖBW-105B). Furthermore, the authors acknowledge additional support from the bioeconomy graduate program BBW ForWerts.

Acknowledgments: The authors would like to thank the Max Rubner-Institute (Karlsruhe, Germany) for providing the HepG2 cell line.

Conflicts of Interest: The authors declare no conflict of interest.

References

1. Matos, Â.P. The Impact of microalgae in food science and technology. *J. Am. Oil Chem Soc.* **2017**, *94*, 1333–1350. [CrossRef]
2. Caporgno, M.P.; Mathys, A. Trends in microalgae incorporation into innovative food products with potential health benefits. *Front. Nutr.* **2018**, *5*, 58. [CrossRef] [PubMed]
3. Bowler, C.; Allen, A.E.; Badger, J.H.; Grimwood, J.; Jabbari, K.; Kuo, A.; Maheswari, U.; Martens, C.; Maumus, F.; Otillar, R.P.; et al. The *Phaeodactylum* genome reveals the evolutionary history of diatom genomes. *Nature* **2008**, *456*, 239–244. [CrossRef] [PubMed]
4. Andrianasolo, E.H.; Haramaty, L.; Vardi, A.; White, E.; Lutz, R.; Falkowski, P. Apoptosis-inducing galactolipids from a cultured marine diatom, *Phaeodactylum tricornutum*. *J. Nat. Prod.* **2008**, *71*, 1197–1201. [CrossRef] [PubMed]
5. Desbois, A.P.; Mearns-Spragg, A.; Smith, V.J. A fatty acid from the diatom *Phaeodactylum tricornutum* is antibacterial against diverse bacteria including multi-resistant *Staphylococcus aureus* (MRSA). *Mar. Biotechnol.* **2009**, *11*, 45–52. [CrossRef] [PubMed]
6. Foo, S.C.; Yusoff, F.M.; Ismail, M.; Basri, M.; Yau, S.K.; Khong, N.M.H.; Chan, K.W.; Ebrahimi, M. Antioxidant capacities of fucoxanthin-producing algae as influenced by their carotenoid and phenolic contents. *J. Biotechnol.* **2017**, *241*, 175–183. [CrossRef] [PubMed]
7. Ha, A.W.; Na, S.J.; Kim, W.K. Antioxidant effects of fucoxanthin rich powder in rats fed with high fat diet. *Nutr. Res. Pract.* **2013**, *7*, 475–480. [CrossRef] [PubMed]
8. Rico, M.; López, A.; Santana-Casiano, J.M.; Gonzàlez, A.G.; Gonzàlez-Dàvila, M. Variability of the phenolic profile in the diatom *Phaeodactylum tricornutum* growing under copper and iron stress. *Limnol. Oceanogr.* **2013**, *58*, 144–152. [CrossRef]
9. Caron, L.; Douady, D.; Quinet-Szely, M.; de Goër, S.; Berkaloff, C. Gene structure of a chlorophyll a/c-binding protein from a brown alga: Presence of an intron and phylogenetic implications. *J. Mol. Evol.* **1996**, *43*, 270–280. [CrossRef]
10. Veith, T.; Büchel, C. The monomeric photosystem I-complex of the diatom *Phaeodactylum tricornutum* binds specific fucoxanthin chlorophyll proteins (FCPs) as light-harvesting complexes. *Biochim. Biophys. Acta Bioenerg.* **2007**, *1767*, 1428–1435. [CrossRef]
11. Maeda, H.; Hosokawa, M.; Sashima, T.; Murakami-Funayama, K.; Miyashita, K. Anti-obesity and anti-diabetic effects of fucoxanthin on diet-induced obesity conditions in a murine model. *Mol. Med. Rep.* **2009**, *2*, 897–902. [CrossRef] [PubMed]
12. Heo, S.-J.; Yoon, W.-J.; Kim, K.-N.; Ahn, G.-N.; Kang, S.-M.; Kang, D.-H.; Affan, A.; Oh, C.; Jung, W.-K.; Jeon, Y.-J. Evaluation of anti-inflammatory effect of fucoxanthin isolated from brown algae in lipopolysaccharide-stimulated RAW 264.7 macrophages. *Food Chem. Toxicol.* **2010**, *48*, 2045–2051. [CrossRef] [PubMed]
13. Kang, M.-J.; Kim, S.M.; Jeong, S.-M.; Choi, H.-N.; Jang, Y.-H.; Kim, J.-I. Antioxidant effect of *Phaeodactylum tricornutum* in mice fed high-fat diet. *Food Sci. Biotechnol.* **2013**, *22*, 107–113. [CrossRef]
14. Wang, L.; Zeng, Y.; Liu, Y.; Hu, X.; Li, S.; Wang, Y.; Li, L.; Lei, Z.; Zhang, Z. Fucoxanthin induces growth arrest and apoptosis in human bladder cancer T24 cells by up-regulation of p21 and down-regulation of mortalin. *Acta Biochim. Biophys. Sin.* **2014**, *46*, 877–884. [CrossRef] [PubMed]
15. Mei, C.; Zhou, S.; Zhu, L.; Ming, J.; Zeng, F.; Xu, R. Antitumor effects of laminaria extract fucoxanthin on lung cancer. *Mar. Drugs* **2017**, *15*, 39. [CrossRef] [PubMed]
16. Kim, S.M.; Jung, Y.-J.; Kwon, O.-N.; Cha, K.H.; Um, B.-H.; Chung, D.; Pan, C.-H. A potential commercial source of fucoxanthin extracted from the microalga *Phaeodactylum tricornutum*. *Appl. Biochem. Biotechnol.* **2012**, *166*, 1843–1855. [CrossRef] [PubMed]
17. Derwenskus, F.; Metz, F.; Gille, A.; Schmid-Staiger, U.; Briviba, K.; Schließmann, U.; Hirth, T. Pressurized extraction of unsaturated fatty acids and carotenoids from wet *Chlorella vulgaris* and *Phaeodactylum tricornutum* biomass using subcritical liquids. *Glob. Bioenergy* **2019**, *11*, 335–344. [CrossRef]
18. Steinrücken, P.; Prestegard, S.K.; de Vree, J.H.; Storesund, J.E.; Pree, B.; Mjøs, S.A.; Erga, S.R. Comparing EPA production and fatty acid profiles of three *Phaeodactylum tricornutum* strains under western Norwegian climate conditions. *Algal Res.* **2018**, *30*, 11–22. [CrossRef]

19. Meiser, A.; Schmid-Staiger, U.; Trösch, W. Optimization of eicosapentaenoic acid production by *Phaeodactylum tricornutum* in the flat panel airlift (FPA) reactor. *J. Appl. Phycol.* **2004**, *16*, 215–225. [CrossRef]
20. Mirón, A.S.; Garcıa, M.C.C.; Gómez, A.C.; Camacho, F.G.; Grima, E.M.; Chisti, Y. Shear stress tolerance and biochemical characterization of *Phaeodactylum tricornutum* in quasi steady-state continuous culture in outdoor photobioreactors. *Biochem. Eng. J.* **2003**, *16*, 287–297. [CrossRef]
21. Silva Benavides, A.M.; Torzillo, G.; Kopecký, J.; Masojídek, J. Productivity and biochemical composition of *Phaeodactylum tricornutum* (Bacillariophyceae) cultures grown outdoors in tubular photobioreactors and open ponds. *Biomass Bioenergy* **2013**, *54*, 115–122. [CrossRef]
22. Bonomini, F.; Tengattini, S.; Fabiano, A.; Bianchi, R.; Rezzani, R. Atherosclerosis and oxidative stress. *Histol. Histopathol.* **2008**, *23*, 381–390. [CrossRef] [PubMed]
23. Stamp, L.K.; Khalilova, I.; Tarr, J.M.; Senthilmohan, R.; Turner, R.; Haigh, R.C.; Winyard, P.G.; Kettle, A.J. Myeloperoxidase and oxidative stress in rheumatoid arthritis. *Rheumatology* **2012**, *51*, 1796–1803. [CrossRef] [PubMed]
24. Molodecky, N.A.; Soon, I.S.; Rabi, D.M.; Ghali, W.A.; Ferris, M.; Chernoff, G.; Benchimol, E.I.; Panaccione, R.; Ghosh, S.; Barkema, H.W.; et al. Increasing incidence and prevalence of the inflammatory bowel diseases with time, based on systematic review. *Gastroenterology* **2012**, *142*, 46–54.e42. [CrossRef] [PubMed]
25. Reuter, S.; Gupta, S.C.; Chaturvedi, M.M.; Aggarwal, B.B. Oxidative stress, inflammation, and cancer: How are they linked? *Free Radic. Biol. Med.* **2010**, *49*, 1603–1616. [CrossRef] [PubMed]
26. Siegel, R.L.; Miller, K.D.; Jemal, A. Cancer statistics, 2016. *CA Cancer J. Clin.* **2016**, *66*, 7–30. [CrossRef] [PubMed]
27. Mann, J.E.; Myers, J. On pigments, growth, and photosynthesis of Phaeodactylum tricornutum. *J. Phycol.* **1968**, *4*, 349–355. [CrossRef] [PubMed]
28. Derwenskus, F.; Schmid-Staiger, U.; Bringmann, C. Verfahren zum Erhalt von Fucoxanthin und Fettsäuren aus Algenbiomasse (EN: Process for the recovery of fatty acids and fucoxanthin from algae biomass). DE-Patent Akz 102019202570.6, 26 February 2019.
29. Gille, A.; Hollenbach, R.; Trautmann, A.; Posten, C.; Briviba, K. Effect of sonication on bioaccessibility and cellular uptake of carotenoids from preparations of photoautotrophic *Phaeodactylum tricornutum*. *Food Res. Int.* **2019**, *118*, 40–48. [CrossRef] [PubMed]
30. Zhang, X.; Ibrahim, Y.M.; Chen, T.-C.; Kyle, J.E.; Norheim, R.V.; Monroe, M.E.; Smith, R.D.; Baker, E.S. Enhancing biological analyses with three dimensional field asymmetric ion mobility, low field drift tube ion mobility and mass spectrometry (μFAIMS/IMS-MS) separations. *Analyst* **2015**, *140*, 6955–6963. [CrossRef]
31. Neumann, U.; Louis, S.; Gille, A.; Derwenskus, F.; Schmid-Staiger, U.; Briviba, K.; Bischoff, S.C. Anti-inflammatory effects of *Phaeodactylum tricornutum* extracts on human blood mononuclear cells and murine macrophages. *J. Appl. Phycol.* **2018**, *30*, 2837–2846. [CrossRef]
32. El-Benna, J.; Dang, P.M.-C. Analysis of protein phosphorylation in human neutrophils. *Methods Mol. Biol.* **2007**, *412*, 85–96. [CrossRef] [PubMed]
33. Singleton, V.L.; Rossi, J.A. Colorimetry of total phenolics with phosphomolybdic-phosphotungstic acid reagents. *Am. J. Enol. Vitic.* **1965**, *16*, 144–158.
34. Benzie, I.F.; Strain, J.J. The ferric reducing ability of plasma (FRAP) as a measure of "antioxidant power": The FRAP assay. *Anal. Biochem.* **1996**, *239*, 70–76. [CrossRef] [PubMed]
35. Bachoual, R.; Talmoudi, W.; Boussetta, T.; Braut, F.; El-Benna, J. An aqueous pomegranate peel extract inhibits neutrophil myeloperoxidase in vitro and attenuates lung inflammation in mice. *Food Chem. Toxicol.* **2011**, *49*, 1224–1228. [CrossRef]
36. Ishikawa, C.; Tafuku, S.; Kadekaru, T.; Sawada, S.; Tomita, M.; Okudaira, T.; Nakazato, T.; Toda, T.; Uchihara, J.-N.; Taira, N.; et al. Anti-adult T-cell leukemia effects of brown algae fucoxanthin and its deacetylated product, fucoxanthinol. *Int. J. Cancer* **2008**, *123*, 2702–2712. [CrossRef] [PubMed]
37. Islam, M.N.; Ishita, I.J.; Jin, S.E.; Choi, R.J.; Lee, C.M.; Kim, Y.S.; Jung, H.A.; Choi, J.S. Anti-inflammatory activity of edible brown alga *Saccharina japonica* and its constituents pheophorbide a and pheophytin a in LPS-stimulated RAW 264.7 macrophage cells. *Food Chem. Toxicol.* **2013**, *55*, 541–548. [CrossRef] [PubMed]
38. Shiratori, K.; Ohgami, K.; Ilieva, I.; Jin, X.-H.; Koyama, Y.; Miyashita, K.; Yoshida, K.; Kase, S.; Ohno, S. Effects of fucoxanthin on lipopolysaccharide-induced inflammation in vitro and in vivo. *Exp. Eye Res.* **2005**, *81*, 422–428. [CrossRef]

39. Kim, K.-N.; Heo, S.-J.; Yoon, W.-J.; Kang, S.-M.; Ahn, G.; Yi, T.-H.; Jeon, Y.-J. Fucoxanthin inhibits the inflammatory response by suppressing the activation of NF-κB and MAPKs in lipopolysaccharide-induced RAW 264.7 macrophages. *Eur. J. Pharm.* **2010**, *649*, 369–375. [CrossRef]
40. Sachindra, N.M.; Sato, E.; Maeda, H.; Hosokawa, M.; Niwano, Y.; Kohno, M.; Miyashita, K. Radical scavenging and singlet oxygen quenching activity of marine carotenoid fucoxanthin and its metabolites. *J. Agric. Food Chem.* **2007**, *55*, 8516–8522. [CrossRef]
41. Müller, L.; Fröhlich, K.; Böhm, V. Comparative antioxidant activities of carotenoids measured by ferric reducing antioxidant power (FRAP), ABTS bleaching assay (αTEAC), DPPH assay and peroxyl radical scavenging assay. *Food Chem.* **2011**, *129*, 139–148. [CrossRef]
42. Lorenz, R.T.; Cysewski, G.R. Commercial potential for *Haematococcus* microalgae as a natural source of astaxanthin. *Trends Biotechnol.* **2000**, *18*, 160–167. [CrossRef]
43. Vigani, M.; Parisi, C.; Rodríguez-Cerezo, E.; Barbosa, M.J.; Sijtsma, L.; Ploeg, M.; Enzing, C. Food and feed products from micro-algae: Market opportunities and challenges for the EU. *Trends Food Sci. Technol.* **2015**, *42*, 81–92. [CrossRef]
44. Dikalov, S.I.; Harrison, D.G. Methods for detection of mitochondrial and cellular reactive oxygen species. *Antioxid. Redox Signal.* **2014**, *20*, 372–382. [CrossRef] [PubMed]
45. Kirchner, T.; Möller, S.; Klinger, M.; Solbach, W.; Laskay, T.; Behnen, M. The impact of various reactive oxygen species on the formation of neutrophil extracellular traps. *Mediat. Inflamm.* **2012**, *2012*, 849136. [CrossRef] [PubMed]
46. Zheng, J.; Piao, M.J.; Kim, K.C.; Yao, C.W.; Cha, J.W.; Hyun, J.W. Fucoxanthin enhances the level of reduced glutathione via the Nrf2-mediated pathway in human keratinocytes. *Mar. Drugs* **2014**, *12*, 4214–4230. [CrossRef] [PubMed]
47. Owen, J.B.; Butterfield, D.A. Measurement of oxidized/reduced glutathione ratio. *Methods Mol. Biol.* **2010**, *648*, 269–277. [CrossRef] [PubMed]
48. Sian, J.; Dexter, D.T.; Lees, A.J.; Daniel, S.; Agid, Y.; Javoy-Agid, F.; Jenner, P.; Marsden, C.D. Alterations in glutathione levels in Parkinson's disease and other neurodegenerative disorders affecting basal ganglia. *Ann. Neurol* **1994**, *36*, 348–355. [CrossRef] [PubMed]
49. Sechi, G.; Deledda, M.G.; Bua, G.; Satta, W.M.; Deiana, G.A.; Pes, G.M.; Rosati, G. Reduced intravenous glutathione in the treatment of early Parkinson's disease. *Prog Neuropsychopharmacol. Biol. Psychiatry* **1996**, *20*, 1159–1170. [CrossRef]
50. Kotake-Nara, E.; Sugawara, T.; Nagao, A. Antiproliferative effect of neoxanthin and fucoxanthin on cultured cells. *Fish. Sci.* **2005**, *71*, 459–461. [CrossRef]
51. Kim, K.-N.; Heo, S.-J.; Kang, S.-M.; Ahn, G.; Jeon, Y.-J. Fucoxanthin induces apoptosis in human leukemia HL-60 cells through a ROS-mediated Bcl-xL pathway. *Toxicol. Toxicol. In Vitro* **2010**, *24*, 1648–1654. [CrossRef]
52. Kumar, S.; Hosokawa, M.; Miyashita, K. Fucoxanthin: A marine carotenoid exerting anti-cancer effects by affecting multiple mechanisms. *Mar. Drugs* **2013**, *11*, 5130–5147. [CrossRef] [PubMed]
53. Kotake-Nara, E.; Terasaki, M.; Nagao, A. Characterization of apoptosis induced by fucoxanthin in human promyelocytic leukemia cells. *Biosci. Biotechnol. Biochem.* **2005**, *69*, 224–227. [CrossRef] [PubMed]
54. Mut-Salud, N.; Álvarez, P.J.; Garrido, J.M.; Carrasco, E.; Aránega, A.; Rodríguez-Serrano, F. Antioxidant intake and antitumort Therapy: Toward nutritional recommendations for optimal results. *Oxid. Med. Cell Longev.* **2016**, *2016*, 6719534. [CrossRef] [PubMed]
55. Thyagarajan, A.; Sahu, R.P. Potential contributions of antioxidants to cancer therapy: Immunomodulation and radiosensitization. *Integr. Cancer* **2018**, *17*, 210–216. [CrossRef] [PubMed]

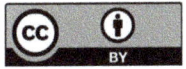

© 2019 by the authors. Licensee MDPI, Basel, Switzerland. This article is an open access article distributed under the terms and conditions of the Creative Commons Attribution (CC BY) license (http://creativecommons.org/licenses/by/4.0/).

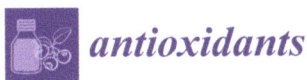

Article

Antioxidant and Photoprotection Networking in the Coastal Diatom *Skeletonema marinoi*

Arianna Smerilli [1], Sergio Balzano [1], Maira Maselli [1,2], Martina Blasio [1], Ida Orefice [1], Christian Galasso [1], Clementina Sansone [1,*] and Christophe Brunet [1]

[1] Stazione Zoologica Anton Dohrn, Istituto Nazionale di Biologia, Ecologia e Biotecnologie marine, Villa Comunale, 80121 Napoli, Italy; arianna.smerilli@gmail.com (A.S.); sergio.balzano@szn.it (S.B.); maira.maselli@bio.ku.dk (M.M.); martina.blasio@szn.it (M.B.); ida.orefice@szn.it (I.O.); christian.galasso@szn.it (C.G.); christophe.brunet@szn.it (C.B.)
[2] Department of Biology, University of Copenhagen, Strandpromenaden 5, 3000 Helsingør, Denmark
* Correspondence: clementina.sansone@szn.it

Received: 7 May 2019; Accepted: 29 May 2019; Published: 1 June 2019

Abstract: Little is known on the antioxidant activity modulation in microalgae, even less in diatoms. Antioxidant molecule concentrations and their modulation in microalgae has received little attention and the interconnection between light, photosynthesis, photoprotection, and antioxidant network in microalgae is still unclear. To fill this gap, we selected light as external forcing to drive physiological regulation and acclimation in the costal diatom *Skeletonema marinoi*. We investigated the role of light regime on the concentration of ascorbic acid, phenolic compounds and among them flavonoids and their connection with photoprotective mechanisms. We compared three high light conditions, differing in either light intensity or wave distribution, with two low light conditions, differing in photoperiod, and a prolonged darkness. The change in light distribution, from sinusoidal to square wave distribution was also investigated. Results revealed a strong link between photoprotection, mainly relied on xanthophyll cycle operation, and the antioxidant molecules and activity modulation. This study paves the way for further investigation on the antioxidant capacity of diatoms, which resulted to be strongly forced by light conditions, also in the view of their potential utilization in nutraceuticals or new functional cosmetic products.

Keywords: light; ascorbic acid; phenolic compounds; flavonoids; photoprotection

---

1. Introduction

Aerobic organisms need to deal with reactive oxygen species (ROS) which are harmful to their metabolism since high ROS concentrations can damage cellular machinery ultimately threatening cell survival; simultaneously ROS play also a role as secondary messengers. In all cells, mitochondria, NADPH oxidase (NOX) complexes and the enzyme lipoxygenase are major ROS sources. Photosynthetic eukaryotic cells possess, in addition, the chloroplasts, in which ROS are formed via energy transfer from chlorophyll or via electron transfer. Indeed, ROS intracellular concentration controls the photosystem II (PSII) activity and therefore photosynthesis and defense strategies [1]. The balance between toxicity, when ROS are in excess, and the signaling action requires cells to finely tune the ROS concentration [2–4], thanks to an efficient intracellular network composed by antioxidant molecules and enzymes. Antioxidants include molecules such as ascorbic acid (AsA), carotenoids, glutathione (GSH), tocopherols as well as phenolic compounds. AsA is a strong antioxidant component of the cell plasma [5]. AsA is also substrate of antioxidant enzymes such as peroxidases and violaxanthin de-epoxidase, thus contributing to dissipate excess energy [6]. Carotenoids occur in the chloroplast membranes interacting directly where photosynthesis-derived ROS are generated. Besides their role as photosynthetic pigments, carotenoids can efficiently quench peroxides and singlet oxygen thus preventing the formation of ROS [5,7–9]. GSH buffers the redox equilibrium of the cell by undergoing oxidation or reduction reactions, according to the redox potential of the cell. Specifically, GSH can act as an electron donor inactivating free radicals. Moreover, GSH is also a cofactor of several antioxidant enzymes [10]. Tocopherols are only produced by photoautotrophic taxa, they are lipophilic and can use resonance energy transfer to scavenge singlet oxygen, thus protecting PSII [11]. Phenolic compounds are present in all plants and derive from the shikimate-phenylpropanoids-flavonoids pathways [12]. They include a wide range of molecules with several phenol structural units. The most important phenolic compounds are flavonoids, which can donate both electrons or hydrogen atoms directly to ROS [13]. A wide range of flavonoids are present in photosynthetic microorganisms [14]. A recent study highlighted the diversity of flavonoids in phytoplankton and found that ferulic acid and apigenin are the dominant flavonoids in both cyanobacteria and eukaryotic microalgae [14]. In contrast with higher plants, their distribution and functions in microalgae are not fully clear [14,15]. Antioxidant enzymes are located in various cell compartments and include catalase (CAT), superoxide dismutase (SOD), and several peroxidases. Ascorbate peroxidase (APX) and glutathione peroxidase (GPX) accept, as substrates, AsA and GSH, respectively, in order to detoxify ROS. Furthermore, three additional enzymes, the monodehydroascorbate reductase (MDHAR), the dehydroascorbate reductase (DHAR), and the glutathione reductase (GR) contribute to regenerate the antioxidant substrates.

With the exception of carotenoids [16–18], the knowledge on antioxidant molecules and enzymes from marine microalgae is still scarce. Few studies focused on the concentration and composition of antioxidants in marine microalgae [17,19–24], and even fewer on the mechanisms for antioxidant defense in these microorganisms [24]. Indeed, both the photoprotective and antioxidant network appeared strongly controlled by light spectral composition and intensity, resulting in a complex regulation system, which allows planktonic diatoms to survive in their highly fluctuating light environment they naturally inhabit [24].

While the photoprotective mechanisms have been investigated in diatoms [25–29], only few studies investigated the role of the antioxidant network as a second defense line able to reduce the light stress [30,31]. Being light a crucial ecological axis in ruling the metabolism of photosynthetic organisms, and thus modulating the growth, the objective of this study was to investigate the impact of light intensity, photoperiod, and wave light distribution on the cellular concentrations of antioxidant molecules such as AsA and flavonoids, and total phenolic content. This knowledge can thus to be exploited to improve microalgal culturing with a productivity-driven purpose. Indeed, marine microalgae are gaining increasing attention for ecofriendly production of new antioxidant compounds. The ultimate aim of this study is to clarify the role of microalgal antioxidants in modulating light stress.

2. Materials and Methods

2.1. Skeletonema marinoi and Culture Conditions

The experiments were conducted on the diatom *Skeletonema marinoi* Sarno and Zingone (CCMP 2092); we selected *S. marinoi* since it is a cosmopolitan centric diatom broadly used in aquaculture [32] that can be cultured in different media [33] under different conditions of light intensity [34] and salinity [35].

This strain was grown at 20 °C in 4.5 L glass tanks in autoclaved seawater, pre-filtered through a 0.7 μm GF/F glass-fiber filter under water movement using an aquarium wave maker pump (Sunsun, JVP-110, Sunsun manufacturer, Zhoushan, China). A modified f/2 medium, in which the concentrations of phosphate, dissolved silica, vitamins, and trace metals are twice compared to those typically present in f/2 [36], was used.

Cells were pre-acclimated to a sinusoidal light distribution with a midday peak of 150 μmol photons m^{-2} s^{-1} and with a photoperiod equal to 12:12 dark:light, following the results obtained by [24,34,37].

The white light was composed by Red:Green:Blue (RGB) with a ratio of 10:40:50 and provided by a custom-built LED illumination system (European patent registration number: EP13196793.7), allowing to modulate the spectral composition and light intensity [38]. The three colors were provided at wavelengths of 460 nm (±36 nm, blue), 530 nm (±50 nm, green) and 626 nm (±36 nm, red).

Light intensity (Photosynthetically Active Radiation, PAR) was measured inside each tank by using a laboratory PAR 4 π sensor (QSL 2101, Biospherical Instruments Inc., San Diego, CA, USA).

2.2. Experimental Strategy

All experiments were run in triplicate and consisted in monitoring the biological responses of *S. marinoi* after the shift from pre-acclimation light condition to different light conditions, spanning from prolonged darkness to very high light climate (Table 1). The light shift started after the 12 h dark period of the previous day. The experimental conditions are presented in the Figure 1 and described in Table 1.

Table 1. Experimental strategy.

Condition	Growth Phase at T_0	Photoperiod (Light:Dark)	Light Intensity (µmol Photons m^{-2} s^{-1})	Daily Light Dose (mol Photons m^{-2} d^{-1})	Light Distribution
Sin150	Exponential	12:12	150	3.6	Sinusoidal
Stat	Stationary	12:12	150	3.6	Sinusoidal
Dark	Exponential	00:24	0	0	-
Sin10	Exponential	12:12	10	0.24	Sinusoidal
Con10	Exponential	24:00	10	1	Continuous
Sin600	Exponential	12:12	600	14.4	Sinusoidal
Quad300	Exponential	12:12	300	14.4	Square wave
Quad600	Exponential	12:12	600	28.8	Square wave

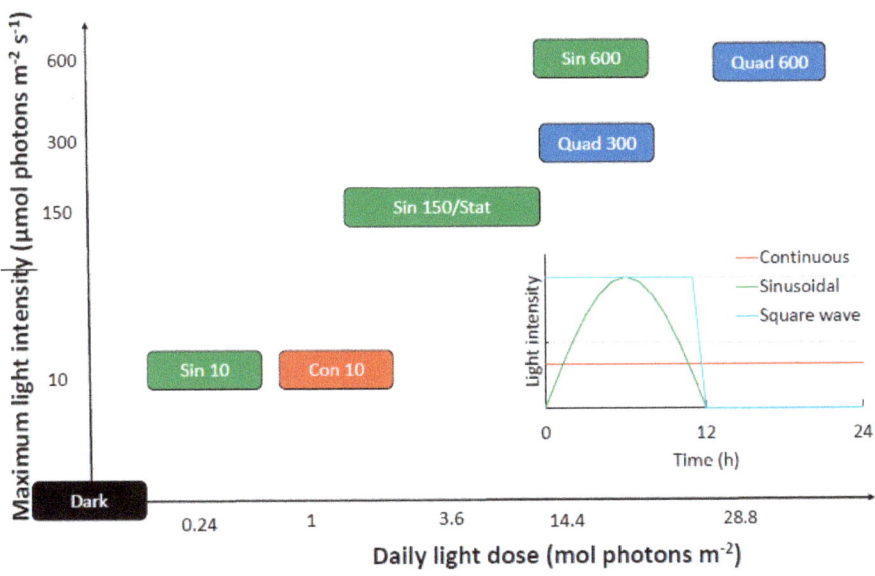

Figure 1. Details of the experimental setting used here. The different light wave distributions are explained in the inset. Treatments based on sinusoidal, quadratic or continuous light wave are shown in green, blue, and red, respectively. Refer to Table 1 for abbreviations.

The condition-oriented sampling strategy was carried out as follows. All the cultures were sampled at predawn (in the dark before the new condition operation), at 6 h (midday) and at 24 h (at the end of the dark period). Since phytoplankton cells are known to operate a rapid photoprotective mechanism when exposed to high (>200 μmol photons $m^{-2} s^{-1}$) light conditions [39] an additional sampling after 2 h from the light shift was performed in all the high light experiments (Sin 600, Quad 300 and Quad 600). Furthermore, since cultures incubated to square light wave experienced a sharp shift from 0 to 300 or 600 μmol photons $m^{-2} s^{-1}$, samples were harvested from these cultures also 10 and 30 min after the light shift in order to evaluate the short-time response of S. marinoi to cope with this unnatural and drastic enhancement of light.

2.3. Ancillary Data

2.3.1. Cell Concentration and Growth Rate

To assess cell density, 2 mL of cell suspension were collected from each tank and fixed with Lugol's iodine solution (1.5% *v/v*). Then, 1 mL of this solution was used to fill a Sedgewick Rafter counting cell chamber. Cells were then counted using a Zeiss Axioskop 2 Plus light microscope (Carl Zeiss, Göttingen, Germany).

The growth rate was estimated from cell concentration measurements using the following equation:

$$\mu \ (d^{-1}) = \ln(C_{n-1}/C_n)/(t_n - t_{n-1}),$$

where μ is the growth rate, C_{n-1} and C_n are cell concentrations (mL^{-1}) at day n − 1 (t_{n-1}) and day n (t_n).

2.3.2. Photochemical Efficiency of the Photosystem II and Non-Photochemical Quenching Measurements

To assess the photosynthetic capacities and the photophysiological state of phytoplankton cells, active chlorophyll *a* (Chl-*a*) fluorescence was measured using a DUAL-PAM fluorometer (Heinz Walz GmbH, Effeltrich, Germany). The photochemical efficiency of the PSII (F_v/F_m) was estimated by:

$$\Phi_p = (F_m - F_0)/F_m = F_v/F_m,$$

where F_v is the variable fluorescence ($F_v = F_m - F_0$).

The measurement of F_0 was done using light of low intensity (1 μmol photons $m^{-2} s^{-1}$) and low frequency (approximately 25 Hz). F_m was measured by applying a short and intense flash of actinic light which completely reduces QA. In our case, the saturation flash of bright red light (655 nm) were applied at an intensity of 2400 μmol photons $m^{-2} s^{-1}$ for a duration of 450 ms. F_v/F_m corresponds to the maximal photochemical efficiency of the PSII (or the maximal light utilization efficiency of PSII) and dark acclimation for 15 min allows the recovery of photosystems II, this leading to reliable measurements of F_0 [38].

Estimation of the non-photochemical quenching is calculated by the Stern–Volmer expression [40]:

$$NPQ = (F_m - F'_m)/F'_m = F_m/F'_m - 1.$$

The estimation of NPQ consisted of measuring F_0 and F_m on 15 min dark-acclimated samples and then measuring F_m' and F_0' every minute on the same sample illuminated by an actinic light (setup at 399 μmol photons $m^{-2} s^{-1}$) for 10 min.

2.3.3. Electron Transport Rate-Light Curves Determination

The electron transport rate (ETR) vs. irradiance (E) curves were determined on 15-min dark-acclimated samples by applying a series of 10 increasing intensity actinic lights (composed by 2/3 of blue and 1/3 of red light, lasting 1.5 min each, ranging from 1 to 1222 μmol photons $m^{-2} s^{-1}$). The photochemical efficiency of the PSII was measured on the 15-min dark-acclimated sample, while the light utilization efficiency of the PSII ($\Delta\Phi$) was measured after each actinic light level.

The relative ETR, taking into account the part of incident light energy effectively absorbed by the photosystem, was calculated as follows:

$$relETR = F'_v/F'_m \cdot E \cdot 0.5 \cdot a *,$$

where E is irradiance, and $a *$ is the cell specific absorption coefficient expressed in m^2 $cell^{-1}$ [24]. A factor of 0.5 was applied since it is assumed that half of the incident light is absorbed by the PSI and half by the PSII. The relative ETR is expressed in nmol e^- h^{-1} $cell^{-1}$.

Determination of $relETR_{max}$ was retrieved according to the equation of Eilers and Peeters (1988) [41].

2.4. Pigment Analysis

Pigment analysis was conducted by High Performance Liquid Chromatography (HPLC) as described by Smerilli et al. [24]. An aliquot of algal culture (10 mL) was filtered on GF/F glass-fiber filter (25 mm, Whatman, Maidstone, UK) and immediately stored in liquid nitrogen until further analysis. Pigments were extracted by mechanical grounding for 3 min in 2 mL of absolute methanol. The homogenate was then filtered onto Whatman 25-mm GF/F filters and the volume of the extract accurately measured. Prior to injection into the HPLC, 250 µL of 1 M ammonium acetate were added to 500 µL of the pigment extract and incubated for 5 min in darkness at 4 °C. This extract was then injected in the 50 µL loop of the Hewlett Packard series 1100 HPLC (Hewlett-Packard, Wilmington, NC, USA). The reversed-phase column (2.6 mm diameter C8 Kinetex column; 50 × 4.6 mm; Phenomenex®, Torrance, CA, USA) corresponded to an apolar stationary phase composed of silica beads possessing aliphatic chains of eight carbon atoms (C8). The temperature of the column was steadily maintained at 20 °C and the flow rate of the mobile phase was set up at 1.7 mL min^{-1}.

The mobile phase was composed of two solvents mixtures: A, methanol:0.5 N aqueous ammonium acetate (70:30, v/v) and B, absolute methanol. During the 12-min elution, the gradient between the solvents was programmed: 75% A (0 min), 50% A (1 min), 0% A (8 min), 0% A (11 min), 75% A (12 min).

Pigments were detected at 440 nm using a Hewlett Packard photodiode array detector model DAD series 1100 which gives the 400–700 nm spectrum for each detected pigment. A fluorometer (Hewlett Packard standard FLD cell series 1100) with excitation at 410 nm and emission at 665 nm allowed the detection of fluorescent molecules (chlorophylls and their degraded products). Pigments were identified based on their retention time and quantified based on pure standards from the D.H.I. Water and Environment (Hørsholm, Denmark) as described previously [38].

2.5. Antioxidant Molecules and Antioxidant Activity Analysis

2.5.1. Ascorbic Acid Content Determination

To assess the ascorbic acid (AsA) content in cells, the procedure modified from [42] was the following. A 150 mL volume of culture was centrifuged at 3600 g for 15 min at 4 °C (DR15P centrifuge, B. Braun Biotech International, Melsungen, Germany), the pellet was weighed, flash frozen in liquid nitrogen, and stored at −20 °C. Pellets were resuspended in 5% trichloroacetic acid (TCA) and sonicated for 1 min with a microtip at 20% output on ice (S-250A Branson Ultrasonic). Cell debris were precipitated by centrifugation at 5000× g for 5 min at 4 °C. The supernatant was then used for spectrophotometric analysis after mixing it with a reagent. The reagent consisted of a 0.5% solution of 2,2'-dipyridyl mixed with an 8.3 mM ferric ammonium sulfate solution in 15% (v/v) o-phosphoric acid in a ratio 4 to 1. Supernatant and reagent were mixed (1:5) immediately before use. After 1 h the absorbance was read at 520 nm and AsA concentration was calculated thanks to factor calibration retrieved from calibration curves using AsA standards. AsA concentration is reported in fg AsA $cell^{-1}$.

2.5.2. Preparation of the Methanolic Extracts

For the determination of 2,2′-azino-bis (3-ethylbenzothiazoline-6-sulphonic acid) (ABTS) radical scavenging activity, total phenolic content (TPC) and total flavonoid content (TFC), the pellets were prepared as follows. Cells were re-suspended in methanol and sonicated for 1 min with a microtip at 20% output on ice (S-250A Branson Ultrasonic). The suspension was left for 30 min at room temperature in the dark, and then was centrifuged at 3600× g for 10 min at 4 °C. Supernatant was collected and the pellet was re-suspended in an equal volume of methanol and left other 30 min at room temperature in the dark. The suspension was centrifuged again in the same conditions, and the two supernatants were combined.

2.5.3. Total Phenolic Content

Polyphenols in plant extracts react with specific redox reagents (Folin-Ciocalteu reagent) to form a blue complex that can be quantified by visible-light spectrophotometry. Total phenolic content (TPC) was estimated by the Folin–Ciocalteu method [43] as described by Li and collaborators [44].

Briefly, 200 µL of the sample was mixed with 1 mL of Folin-Ciocalteu's phenol reagent, pre-diluted in distilled water 1:10 v/v. After 4 min, 800 µL 75 g/L Na_2CO_3 were added to the mixture, shacked vigorously and stored at room temperature for 2 h. The absorbance was read at 765 nm. Gallic acid was used for the standard calibration curve. The results were expressed in fg of gallic acid equivalents (GAEq) cell^{-1}.

2.5.4. Total Flavonoid Content

The total flavonoid content was estimated by aluminum chloride colorimetric method [45]. Briefly, 600 µL of sample were pre-diluted 1:2 v/v in methanol 80% v/v and mixed with an equal volume of $AlCl_3$ 2%. The mix was shaken and incubated at room temperature for 1 h. The absorbance was measured at 410 nm and quercetin was used for the standard calibration curve. The results were expressed in fg of quercetin equivalents (QEq) cell^{-1}.

2.5.5. ABTS Radical Scavenging Activity

The antioxidant activity was assessed by the 2,2′-azino-bis (3-ethylbenzothiazoline-6-sulphonic acid) (ABTS) radical scavenging activity assay. The scavenging activity of ABTS radical was measured following [16]. The ABTS free radical was generated by mixing 7 mM ABTS diammonium salt with 2.45 mM potassium persulfate and stored overnight at room temperature. The solution was diluted with methanol till the absorbance at 734 nm reached 0.70 ± 0.01 units. Then one part of sample was mixed with three parts of ABTS radical solution. The mix was shaken and left 1 h at room temperature in the dark. The absorbance was read at 734 nm. Ascorbic acid was used for the standard calibration curve. The results were expressed in fg of ascorbic acid equivalents (AEq) cell^{-1}.

2.6. Statistical Analysis

Calculations of mean, standard deviation, variance, coefficient of variation (CV), Student's t-test for mean comparison, Spearman rank correlation, analysis of variance (ANOVA) and Tukey test for multiple comparisons were performed using the PAST software package, version 3.10 [46].

3. Results

3.1. Growth Rate and Photosynthesis

After 24 h from the light shifts, in all the experimental conditions the growth rate of *S. marinoi* decreased (Table 2), in contrast with what observed in the control condition, revealing a physiological stress induced by the variations of light environment. The highest decrease in cell abundance was observed for cultures shifted to square wave light distribution at 600 µmol photons m^{-2} s^{-1} and to continuous light (Table 2).

Table 2. Cell concentration and growth rate at time T$_0$ and after 24 h from the start of the experiment.

Condition	Cell Concentration (10^5 Cells mL^{-1})		Growth Rate (µ, s^{-1})	
	0 h	24 h	0 h	24 h
Sin150	2.9 ± 0.4	6.7 ± 0.5	1.2 ± 0.1	1.2 ± 0.3
Stat	5.3 ± 0.7	4.0 ± 0.4	−0.4 ± 0.3	-
Dark	4.6 ± 0.5	4.0 ± 0.4	1.0 ± 0.2	−0.1 ± 0.1
Sin10	4.4 ± 0.6	4.8 ± 0.4	1.0 ± 0.2	0.1 ± 0.1
Con10	6.8 ± 0.5	0.8 ± 0.4	1.0 ± 0.1	−1.5 ± 0.6
Sin600	7.2 ± 0.4	8.1 ± 2.1	1.1 ± 0.1	0.1 ± 0.2
Quad300	4.7 ± 1.0	1.8 ± 2.0	0.5 ± 0.2	−1.5 ± 1.4
Quad600	5.9 ± 1.7	1.5 ± 1.0	0.8 ± 0.2	−1.5 ± 0.4

Photosynthetic electron transport rate (ETR) did not vary significantly over time under Sin 150, dark conditions, and Sin 10. Significant increases were observed under continuous light (Con 10), stationary conditions (Sin 150 Stat), and for cultures incubated under high light conditions (Table 3). The photochemical efficiency of photosystem II (Fv/Fm, Table 3) decreased significantly after 6 h for cultures exposed to square-wave light distribution type. Fv/Fm restored after 24 h in Quad 600, whereas it did not reach its initial value in Quad 300 probably because of photoinhibition. Fv/Fm decreased over time in Sin 10, Con 10 and Sin 600 treatments, whereas it did not change significantly for the control and the dark treatments.

Table 3. Electron photosynthetic rate (ETR, nmol e$^-$ h^{-1} cell^{-1}), Fv/Fm, Chlorophyll-*a* concentration (Chl-*a*, fg cell^{-1}), and Fucoxanthin concentration (Fuco, fg cell^{-1}) measured under the different light conditions.

	Sampling Time (h)	Sin150	Dark	Sin10	Con10	Sin600	Quad300	Quad600
ETR	0	22.6 ± 6.2	11.55 ± 3.01	23.21 ± 5.70	82.01 ± 26.81	15.92 ± 2.28	30.14 ± 14.60	20.56 ± 5.31
	0.17							
	0.5						33.60 ± 5.20	19.79 ± 1.00
	2					26.18 ± 6.25	42.03 ± 15.53	21.39 ± 1.00
	6	25.1 ± 3.7	8.58 ± 1.68	23.82 ± 4.63	47.85 ± 7.46	16.20 ± 3.03	26.71 ± 0.72	26.72 ± 1.02
	24	19.2 ± 7.9	8.33 ± 3.74	15.39 ± 3.52	22.56 ± 3.03	23.92 ± 3.97	32.87 ± 0.23	35.35 ± 1.00
Fv/Fm	0	0.80 ± 0.06	0.82 ± 0.08	0.97 ± 0.04	0.92 ± 0.04	0.78 ± 0.03	0.78 ± 0.00	0.79 ± 0.03
	0.17						0.82 ± 0.11	0.81 ± 0.08
	0.5						0.81 ± 0.06	0.81 ± 0.10
	2					0.77 ± 0.06	0.82 ± 0.05	0.82 ± 0.04
	6	0.79 ± 0.04	0.94 ± 0.04	0.93 ± 0.08	0.79 ± 0.04	0.74 ± 0.08	0.56 ± 0.03	0.65 ± 0.05
	24	0.74 ± 0.01	0.72 ± 0.09	0.78 ± 0.05	0.68 ± 0.05	0.88 ± 0.01	0.63 ± 0.00	0.75 ± 0.01
Chl-*a*	0	93.7 ± 13.9	49.50 ± 1.35	55.70 ± 2.74	23.80 ± 1.30	87.50 ± 2.40	237.80 ± 8.40	10.39 ± 4.41
	0.17						242.70 ± 3.96	17.40 ± 3.73
	0.5						242.70 ± 5.30	20.07 ± 8.53
	2					96.50 ± 1.99	150.60 ± 6.04	17.30 ± 7.37
	6	126.5 ± 22.0	80.70 ± 1.13	27.00 ± 0.98	17.40 ± 0.77	104.00 ± 3.16	221.70 ± 2.30	20.67 ± 2.14
	24	102.00 ± 5.74	78.30 ± 2.16	21.50 ± 2.53	22.80 ± 11.80	98.30 ± 3.74	636.40 ± 61.30	26.75 ± 8.94
Fuco	0	32.0 ± 5.0	22.5 ± 10.7	18.1 ± 8.8	20.2 ± 4.7	39.3 ± 10.0	95.10 ± 18.00	44.2 ± 12.0
	0.17						97.9 ± 8.4	64.3 ± 6.5
	0.5						109.9 ± 5.7	66.7 ± 26.8
	2					35.4 ± 7.6	60.6 ± 16.0	78.8 ± 25.3
	6	26.4 ± 10.2	27.60 ± 0.70	28.1 ± 9.2	36.4 ± 1.2	33.1 ± 5.3	79.6 ± 16.0	57.7 ± 16.3
	24	35.6 ± 15.0	28.6 ± 11.0	52.3 ± 8.4	101.60 ± 2.58	37.2 ± 9.8	287.60 ± 29.93	89.5 ± 59.0

3.2. Photosynthetic Pigments

The cellular concentration of Chl-*a* varied differently depending on the light climate cells were exposed to. Decreases were observed in the Sin 150 Stat (6 h), whereas sharp increases occurred in the dark treatment (6 h) and in the Con 10 (24 h). In the Quad 300 the concentration of Chl-*a* decreased

(24 ± 1 to 15.1 ± 6.0 fg cell^{-1}) after 2 h and then increased again in the following 4 h (22.2 ± 2.1 fg cell^{-1}). The cellular concentration of fucoxanthin (fuco) increased in the cultures incubated under low light conditions (Con 10 and Sin 10) and did not change significantly in the other cultures except in Quad 300, where it decreased after 2 h and then increased again during the following 22 h (Table 3). Under control condition (Sin 150), the increase in Chl-*a* content per cell at midday was attributed to cell cycle progression, and its decrease at 24 h was the result of cell division occurring during night (Table 3). Conversely, under Sin 600 or Quad 600 and 300, cell pigment content did not change significantly with time, probably because of the arrest of cell cycle progression or related to the two antagonist effects of high light regulation (lowering Chl-*a* concentration) and cell cycle progression (increasing it).

Prolonged darkness induced an increase of Chl-*a* with time revealing an acclimation strategy in the reaction centers of photosystems (Table 3). Under Sin 10, after 6 h Chl-*a* decreased significantly while Fuco tended to increase.

Under Con 10, both Fuco and Chl-*a* were strongly enhanced the second day of experiment (Table 3).

3.3. Photoprotection: NPQ and Xanthophyll Cycle

Major changes in NPQ as well as the pigments related to the xanthophyll cycle were mostly observed in the cultures exposed to high light. Indeed, the NPQ was found to be more variable in cultures incubated under Sin 600 and square light wave conditions compared to the other treatments (Figure 2). Under continuous light (Con 10) the cellular concentration of Dt increased and the NPQ decreased over time. While the increase in Dt (Figure 2A–C) mostly occurred in the last 18 h, the NPQ decreased during the first 6 h (Figure 2D–F). Cells incubated under sinusoidal conditions in both exponential (Sin 150) and stationary (Sin 150 stat) phases did not exhibit significant infradiel variations in Dt and NPQ (Figure 2B,D). Under Sin 600, NPQ increased rapidly in the first 2 h ($p < 0.05$), coming back to the pre-dawn values at midday (Figure 2F). At 24 h NPQ was significantly higher ($p < 0.001$) with respect to the previous predawn day value (Figure 2F). Under Quad 300, NPQ slightly increased after 10 min and later on decreased progressively reaching the lowest value after 6 h ($p < 0.05$, Figure 2C). Conversely, Dt progressively increased reaching its maximal concentration at 6 h ($p < 0.05$, Figure 2C) and the DES significantly increased after 30 min (data not shown). Under Quad 600, the cellular concentration of Dt increased after 2 h and then decreased again; the NPQ was fairly constant within the first 2 h while it decreased significantly after 6 h ($p < 0.05$, Figure 2F).

The cellular concentrations of Dd and β-car did not change significantly over time in most cases (Figure 3). A small increase in both Dd and β-car was only observed in the Con 10 treatment after 24 h since the beginning of the experiments (Figure 3A,D). NPQ and the concentration of the photoprotective pigment Dt were thus not correlated (Table 4), as previously observed under sinusoidal light distribution [24,47].

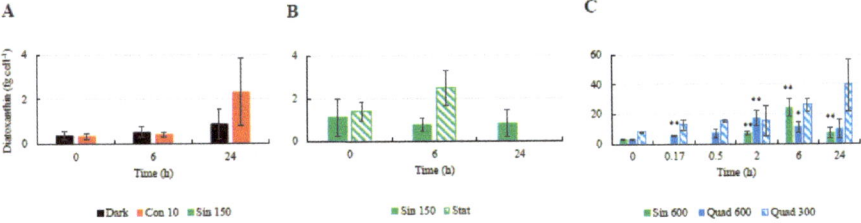

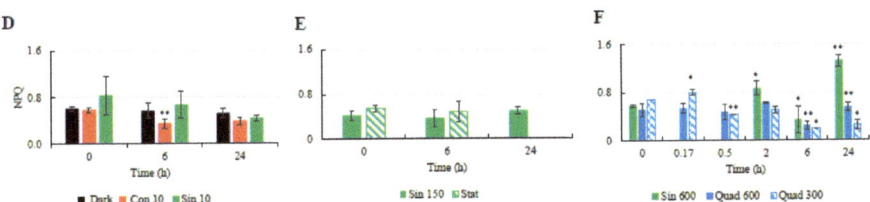

Figure 2. Temporal changes in the cellular concentrations of diatoxanthin ((**A**): low light climates, (**B**): moderate light, (**C**): high light climates) and non-photochemical quenching (NPQ; (**D**): low light climates, (**E**): moderate light, (**F**): high light climates) in the different culturing treatments of *Skeletonema marinoi* CCMP 2092. Refer to Table 1 for abbreviations. "*" means significantly different from time 0 ($p < 0.05$); "**" means significantly different from time 0 ($p < 0.01$).

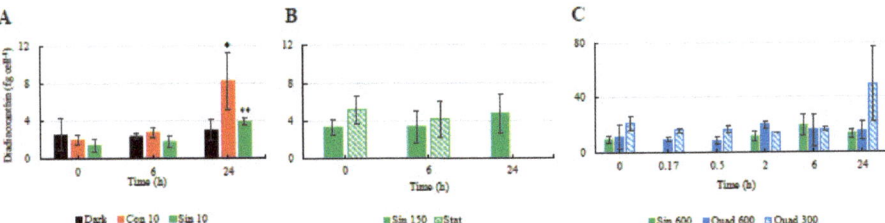

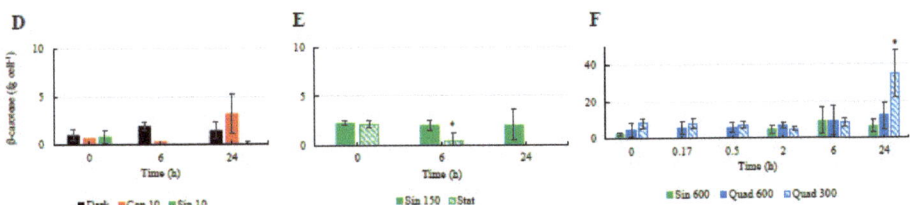

Figure 3. Temporal changes in the cellular concentrations of diadinoxanthin ((**A**): low light climates, (**B**): moderate light, (**C**): high light climates) and β-carotene ((**D**): low light climates, (**E**): moderate light, (**F**): high light climates) in the different culturing treatments of *S. marinoi* CCMP 2092. Refer to Table 1 for abbreviations. "*" means significantly different from time 0 ($p < 0.05$); "**" means significantly different from time 0 ($p < 0.01$).

Table 4. Spearman correlation matrix between the antioxidant capacity, antioxidant molecules, and the photoprotection-related parameters evaluated under control (Sin150) and stationary phase (Stat) conditions [1,2].

	Sin150	Stat	Sin150	Stat	Sin150	Stat	Sin150	Stat	Sin150	Stat	Sin150	Stat
	ABTS		AsA		Phenolics		Flavonoids		Dd		Dt	
AsA	0.83	0.83										
Phenolics	0.87	0.95	0.81	0.80								
Flavonoids	0.84	n.s	0.60	n.s	0.76	n.s						
Dd	0.64	n.s	0.53	n.s	0.58	n.s	0.62	n.s				
Dt	0.60	0.70	0.63	n.s	0.61	0.62	0.66	n.s	n.s	n.s		
β-car	0.54	n.s	0.47	n.s	0.51	n.s	0.54	n.s	n.s	n.s	0.84	−0.58
Light	0.75	n.s	0.68	n.s	0.72	n.s	0.75	0.61	n.s	n.s	0.57	n.s
NPQ	n.s	n.s	n.s	n.s	n.s	n.s	n.s	−0.67	n.s	n.s	n.s	n.s

[1] Abbreviations and units used for the correlation are as follows: Ascorbic acid (AsA in fg/cell); Phenolics (in fg GAEq/cell); Flavonoids (in fg QEq/cell); ABTS test (in fg AEQ/cell); Diatoxanthin (Dt in fg/cell); Diadinoxanthin (Dd in fg/cell); β-carotene (β-car in fg/cell); Light (in μmol photons m^{-2} s^{-1}). [2] n.s. = non-significant (p-value > 0.01).

3.4. Antioxidant Molecules and Activity

Similarly to the NPQ and the xanthophyll-cycle related pigments, most changes in the cellular concentrations of antioxidant molecules occurred in the cultures incubated under high light (Figures 4 and 5). Under the control condition (Sin 150), the cellular concentration of ascorbic acid (AsA) increased at midday (Figure 4). The phenolic content followed the same trend, with higher values found at midday compared to pre-dawn (Figure 5A–C). As AsA and phenolic content, flavonoids increased at midday compared to pre-dawn (Figure 5D–F). In contrast when cells entered stationary phase, these daily variations disappeared and the flavonoids, phenolics, and AsA concentrations stabilized on higher values with respect of those recorded in the exponential phase (Figures 4 and 5).

Consistent with this observation, the ABTS test reflected the trend observed for the antioxidant molecules, following infradiel variations, with an enhancement at midday, and further increase during the stationary phase (Figure 6).

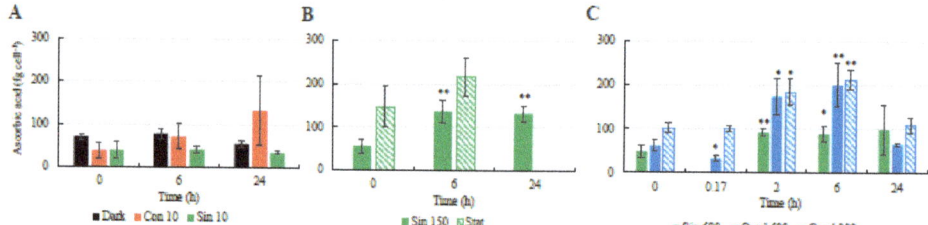

Figure 4. Temporal changes in the cellular concentrations of ascorbic acid ((**A**): low light climates, (**B**): moderate light, (**C**): high light climates) in the different culturing treatments of *S. marinoi* CCMP 2002. Refer to Table 1 for abbreviations. "*" means significantly different from time 0 ($p < 0.05$); "**" means significantly different from time 0 ($p < 0.01$).

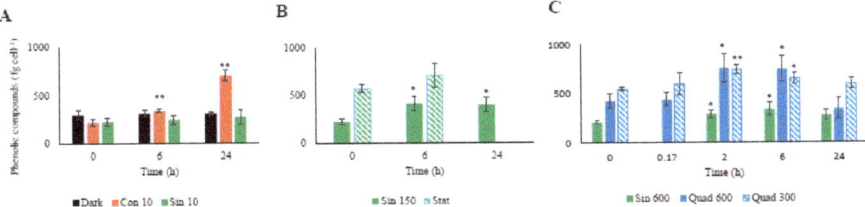

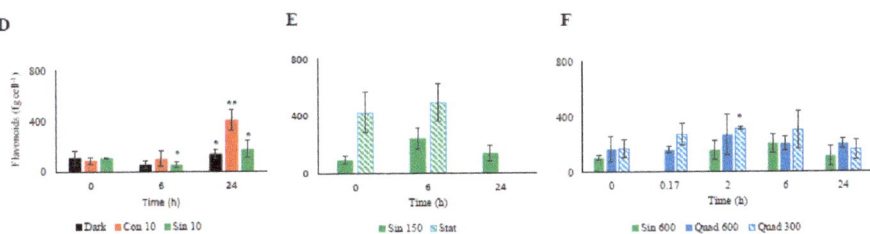

Figure 5. Temporal changes in the cellular concentrations of phenolic compounds ((**A**): low light climates, (**B**): moderate light, (**C**): high light climates) and flavonoids ((**D**): low light climates, (**E**): moderate light, (**F**): high light climates) in the different culturing treatments of *S. marinoi* CCMP 2002. Refer to Table 1 for abbreviations. "*" means significantly different from time 0 ($p < 0.05$); "**" means significantly different from time 0 ($p < 0.01$).

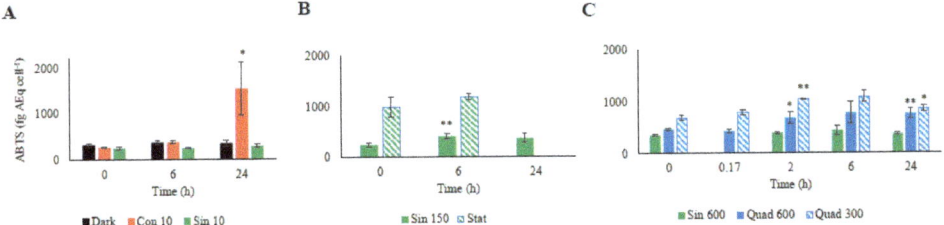

Figure 6. Radical scavenging activity of the different culturing treatment based on the assay of 2,2'-azino-bis (3 ethylbenzthiazoline-6-sulfonic acid, ABTS; (**A**): low light climates, (**B**): moderate light, (**C**): high light climates). Data are indicated in fg of ascorbic acid equivalent per cell (fg AEq cell^{-1}). Refer to Table 1 for abbreviations. "*" means significantly different from time 0 ($p < 0.05$); "**" means significantly different from time 0 ($p < 0.01$).

Antioxidant activity (ABTS) and antioxidant compounds (AsA, phenolics, and flavonoids content) were significantly correlated with all the parameters related to photoprotection (Dt and its two precursors Dd and β-car) except NPQ as well as light intensity (Table 4). The situation changed a little when cells entered into the stationary phase, in which light was no longer the only parameter inducing antioxidant response (lack of correlation, Table 4). ABTS activity was linked to phenolic content, AsA, and Dt, these three parameters being linked between them (Table 4). In this condition, a negative correlation between Dt and β-car was noticed on the opposite to the exponentially grown cells, revealing that Dt might be enhanced from β-car pool that was not fully replenished.

Under Sin 600, AsA conserved the infradiel variation previously observed (Figure 4C). AsA concentration doubled already at 2 h, keeping its concentration fairly constant towards the end of the experiments. The total phenolic content and flavonoids concentration followed a trend similar to AsA in Sin 600, although the increase was observed after 6 h since the beginning of the experiments (Figure 5C,F). Under Quad 600 the infradiel trend of AsA previously observed was still present (Figure 4C). Intriguingly, AsA concentration was halved in 10 min revealing its very fast consumption, then AsA was recycled and newly synthesized, reaching the highest values at 2 and 6 h ($p < 0.05$ and $p < 0.01$, respectively, Figure 4C). The increase between the time 0 and 2–6 h was greater than the increase observed in the control condition, being of circa three times against 2.4 in Sin 150 and 1.8 in Sin 600 (Figure 4B,C).

The ABTS test paralleled the increase of the antioxidants' concentration, remaining high at 6 h (Figure 6). After one day since the light shift, the antioxidant capacity was still higher than T_0 ($p < 0.01$), while the antioxidant molecules decreased or were stable with respect to the previous day (Figures 4–6).

Under both square light wave conditions AsA content (Figure 4C) did not vary within the first minutes of the experiment, increasing at 2 and 6 h ($p < 0.05$) and restoring the starting values after 24 h. The increase in AsA found in Sin 600 was lower than the one observed in Quad 300 and Quad 600 (Figure 4C). The phenolic content in both Quad 300 and Quad 600 peaked at 2 h ($p < 0.05$), then decreased restoring the initial values at 24 h while flavonoids did not show any significant variation (Figure 5C,F). The ABTS followed the same trend of AsA, increasing at 2 h and keeping high values at 6 h ($p < 0.05$, Figure 6).

During the shift to Sin 600, the ABTS activity was correlated with light distribution as well as with phenolic content and the pigments Dt and β-car (Table 5). On the difference to the Sin 150 condition, AsA and flavonoids seemed to do not be involved in ABTS activity (lack of correlation, Table 5), conversely to what was observed in Sin 150. When cells coped with high light square wave distribution, the correlations changed again. Under Quad 600, ABTS activity was only related to flavonoids content (Table 5) while phenolic content was linked to Dt. Under Quad 300, i.e., a square wave distribution with a daily light dose similar to Sin 600, the ABTS activity was related to AsA, with the latter negatively correlated to NPQ (Table 5).

Under prolonged darkness, phenolic compounds, flavonoids, AsA, and ABTS did not vary significantly over time (Figures 4–6). Under continuous light the cellular concentration of AsA did not change over time while that of both phenolic compounds and flavonoids doubled and quadrupled, respectively, after 24 h (Figure 4). The increase of ABTS by five fold after 24 h in the Con 10 treatment was coupled to the antioxidant molecules increase (Figures 5 and 6).

Changes in the cellular concentration of antioxidants, as well as ABTS over time were not significant for both Sin 10 and dark treatments (Figure 5A–D and Figure 6A). In continuous dark, ABTS scavenging activity was significantly related to the Dt and β-car while none of the antioxidant molecules was correlated to ABTS (Table 6). Conversely, under Con 10, the unique parameter significantly involved in the ABTS activity was the flavonoids concentration. Under Sin 10, ABTS activity was correlated to phenolic compounds (but not flavonoids, Table 6). These results highlighted the diversity of the responses of the cells when copying with different low light treatments.

Table 5. Spearman correlation matrix between the antioxidant capacity, antioxidant molecules, and the photoprotection-related parameters evaluated under light conditions [1].

	ABTS			AsA			Phenolics			Flavonoids			Dd			Dt	
	Sin600	Quad300	Quad600	Quad300	Sin600	Quad300	Quad600	Sin600	Quad300	Quad600	Sin600	Quad600	Quad300	Sin600	Quad600	Quad300
AsA	n.s	0.82	n.s			n.s	n.s	n.s	n.s	n.s	n.s	n.s	n.s	n.s	n.s	n.s
Phenolics	0.59	n.s	n.s	0.67	0.64	n.s	n.s	n.s	n.s	n.s	n.s	n.s	n.s	n.s	n.s	n.s
Flavonoids	n.s	0.74	n.s	n.s	n.s	n.s	0.81	n.s	n.s	n.s	0.71	0.81	0.89	n.s	n.s	n.s
Dd	n.s	n.s	n.s	n.s	n.s	n.s	n.s	n.s	n.s	n.s	n.s	n.s	n.s	n.s	n.s	n.s
Dt	0.56	n.s	n.s	n.s	n.s	n.s	0.63	0.61	n.s	n.s	n.s	n.s	n.s	n.s	n.s	n.s
β-car	0.76	n.s	n.s	n.s	n.s	n.s	n.s	n.s	n.s	n.s	n.s	n.s	n.s	0.56	n.s	n.s
Light	0.61	n.s	0.79	n.s	n.s	0.93	n.s	n.s	n.s	n.s	n.s	0.74	n.s	0.76	0.76	n.s
NPQ	n.s	n.s	n.s	n.s	n.s									n.s	n.s	n.s

[1] Abbreviations and measurement units as in Table 4.

Table 6. Spearman correlation matrix between the antioxidant capacity, antioxidant molecules, and the photoprotection-related parameters evaluated under low light and dark conditions [1].

	ABTS			AsA			Phenolics			Flavonoids			Dd			Dt		
	Dark	Con10	Sin10	Dark	Con10	Sin10	Dark	Con10	Sin10	Dark	Con10	Sin10	Dark	Con10	Sin10	Dark	Con10	Sin10
AsA	n.s	n.s	n.s															
Phenolics	n.s	n.s	0.82	n.s	n.s	n.s												
Flavonoids	n.s	0.90	n.s	n.s	n.s	n.s	0.90	n.s										
Dd	n.s	n.s	n.s	n.s	n.s	n.s	n.s	n.s	n.s	n.s	n.s	n.s						
Dt	0.61	n.s	n.s	n.s	n.s	n.s	n.s	n.s	n.s	n.s	n.s	0.81	0.80	0.82	n.s			
β-car	0.70	n.s	n.s	n.s	0.82	n.s	n.s	n.s	n.s	n.s	n.s	n.s	0.56	n.s	n.s	0.68	n.s	n.s
Light	n.s	0.87	n.s	n.s	n.s	n.s	0.87	n.s	n.s	0.87	n.s	n.s	n.s	n.s	n.s	n.s	n.s	n.s
NPQ	n.s	n.s	−0.96	n.s	n.s	n.s	n.s	n.s	−0.89	n.s	n.s	n.s	n.s	n.s	n.s	−0.78	n.s	n.s

[1] Abbreviations and measurement units as in Table 4.

4. Discussion

Current results highlighted that *Skeletonema marinoi* turned out to be rich in phenolic compounds, which are the most widespread antioxidant substances in photosynthetic organisms [48,49]. Phenolic compounds are able to act directly against radical species as well as indirectly via the inhibition of pro-oxidant enzymes such as lipoxygenase or through metal chelation, preventing the occurrence of the Haber–Weiss and the Fenton reactions, which are important sources of radical species [50]. Although some studies reported that phenolic compounds are the main contributors to microalgal antioxidant capacity [17,24,48,51], the microalgal phenolic content is studied little [14,17,20]. The most abundant phenolic compounds in phytoplankton are phloroglucinol, *p*-coumaric acid as well as flavonoids such as ferulic acid and apigenin [14]. Among them, few studies explored their modulation in response to environmental forcing changes [44,49,52,53]. As reported previously [17,24], the content of phenolic compounds in microalgae is higher than in macroalgae and many higher plants. Assuming a dry weight per cell equivalent to 55 pg as in *Skeletonema costatum* [54], we estimate an average phenolic content ≈ 5.5 mg GAE g^{-1} DW, with values up to 12.7 mg GAE g^{-1} DW in some conditions. These values are in the range of previous estimations on the same species object of the present study [24] and in the higher range of results from different studies [17,44,48,51]. Yet, another study [20] reported high phenolic content (8–17.5 mg GAE g^{-1} DW) in four microalgae from different taxa: *Nannochloropsis oceanica* (Eustigmatophyceae), *Chaetoceros calcitrans* (diatom), *Skeletonema costatum* (diatom), and *Chroococcus turgidus* (cyanophyte).

Among the phenolic compounds family, recent findings demonstrated diatoms' ability to produce flavonoids [49], which display relevant antioxidant activity and act as signaling molecules able to up-regulate the defense strategies [13,49]. In most of the light conditions tested in our study, flavonoids' concentration generally shows the same trend observed for the phenolic compounds. Flavonoids are located in different organelles, including chloroplasts where they play a key photoprotective role [55–57]; in particular, they can scavenge radical species and stabilize membranes containing non-bilayer lipids, such as monogalactosyldiacylglycerol (MGDG) [58].

Our study shows that flavonoids are strictly related to ABTS scavenging activity under unnatural light stress, such as continuous (0:24 h, light: dark) and very high light (600 μmol photons m^{-2} s^{-1}; Quad 600), conversely to AsA. This might confirm the powerful capacity of flavonoids to act as defense against stress as photoprotector [59]. Their concentration ranges from circa 50 to 400 fg quercetin equivalent (QEq) $cell^{-1}$, corresponding to ≈ 1 to 8 mg quercetin equivalent (QEq) g^{-1} DW. Interestingly, these values correspond to concentrations reported in a wide range of vegetables, fruits or higher plants [60–62].

AsA concentration in *S. marinoi* is also high, with values spanning from 10 to 300 fg AsA $cell^{-1}$ (≈1.8–5.5 mg AsA g^{-1} DW) in the range of the values previously reported for the same species [24], as well as other phytoplankters [32,63,64]. The latter study highlighted the high variability of AsA concentration among different groups and between exponential and stationary growth phases, with concentrations up to 16 mg AsA g^{-1} DW. Our results highlight the huge potential of *S. marinoi*, the diatom model used in this study, as alternative source of antioxidant molecules. This study also shows the relevance of light driven-modulation on the intracellular concentrations of these molecules.

Current results highlight a substantial infradiel variability in the cellular concentrations of antioxidants. The increase in antioxidants observed at midday confirms the role of light in controlling antioxidant synthesis; antioxidants counteract the detrimental effect of the ROS which are produced as consequence of light exposure, as already observed in higher plants [65,66]. In the absence of light or under an extremely low sinusoidal light, infradiel variations of protective or antioxidant responses disappear, highlighting a direct light stimulus control, excluding an internal circadian clock, of these variations. A circadian clock synchronized with predictable daily environmental cyclic variations generally represents an evolutionary adaptation able to increase the fitness of the organism [67]. Instead, under the highly fluctuating light environment naturally experienced by diatoms, which frequently move along the water column, the presence of a rigid scheme ruling cell physiology could be a disadvantage. A better strategy might consist of promptly modifying the metabolism following the external stimuli, resulting in a great plasticity, which is a known feature attributed to diatoms.

In contrast with what was reported under sinusoidal light distribution, square wave distribution does not induce cyclical infradiel variability. The sinusoidal high light distribution, although slowing microalgal growth, is well tolerated, thanks to the activation and functioning of the antioxidant-photoprotective network. By contrast, square wave distribution with high light intensity strongly affects cell performance impairing the normal functioning of the defense processes network.

Light climate changes experienced by cells induce an uncoupling of the regulative responses (photoprotection vs. AsA, phenol and flavonoid contents) compared to the synergy of these photoresponses observed under pre-acclimation light (Sin 150). Sinusoidal high light exposition leads ABTS scavenging activity to be related to phenolic content as well as Dt and β-car while a non-significant role of flavonoids or AsA content is observed. Parallel responses of Dt and phenolic compounds' concentrations have been already reported [24], along with no significant relationship between Dt and NPQ ([24,37,47]; this study) confirming an alternative role of this pigment, which is likely to have an additional antioxidant function. Under sinusoidal light distribution, with either moderate or high intensity, significant contribution of Dt in ROS scavenging activity is detected. Intriguingly, the relationship between Dt and ABTS is always accompanied by the significant correlation between β-car and ABTS (except when cells enter the stationary phase) that might reveal a similar role of these two pigments in ROS scavenging. The discrepancy between NPQ and Dt is related to an earlier NPQ response compared to Dt as observed under Sin 600, with the highest NPQ recorded after 2 h and subsequently decreasing. This uncoupling between NPQ and Dt confirms the role of NPQ as first defense strategy against light-related stress and that of Dt as a less quick ROS quencher [47].

In Quad 600 the significant role of flavonoids into the ABTS scavenging activity, by contrast to the other phenolic compounds, agree with the fact that flavonoids are known to have strong antioxidant activity [68–70], together with a relevant role in photoprotection [58] that relies on their enhanced concentration in chloroplasts, sites of light-driven ROS production [71,72].

The peculiar response of AsA under Quad 600, with a decrease recorded after 10 min of light exposure, might be due to its fast consumption to counteract the oxidative process induced by abrupt and strong high light exposure.

By contrast in lower light square wave distribution (Quad 300) AsA seems to control ABTS scavenging activity since they are both significantly correlated.

Under low light conditions, different bioactive compounds families with respect to the light climate modulate ABTS scavenging activity.

Under prolonged darkness the increased concentration of Dt is induced by the chlororespiration-dependent trans-thylakoid ΔpH [39,73,74], and significantly linked to ABTS scavenging activity. Under very low light conditions (Sin 10), ABTS only significantly relies on phenolic content, as it was also observed—together with Dt—in Sin 600. This very low light intensity does not determine any increase in Dt, probably because of the absence of chlororespiratory pathway development as observed in prolonged darkness.

By contrast, the continuous low light causes a strong impairment of the normal cell functioning inducing high cell mortality. Under this condition, such as under Quad 600 ABTS scavenging activity is only related to flavonoids content.

Not only light distribution and/or intensity, but also culture age changes dramatically the photoresponses of the cells. All the antioxidant molecules as well as Dt increase during cell senescence. The accumulation AsA has been already observed in the senescent diatom S. marinoi [64]. The infradiel variations observed during the active growth phase were disrupted during the stationary phase, vouching for the drastic changes to which the cells were subjected [75]. Conversely to exponentially grown cells, NPQ remains high at midday together with the antioxidant capacity and molecule concentration. The integrated defense strategy development suggests the high level of ROS produced in senescent cultures. In higher plants, the early event of cell senescence is the inactivation of the enzyme Rubisco [76,77] not paralleled by a loss of the thylakoid proteins, which happens at a later time [77]. Therefore, the potential exposure to increasing light induces the development of the first defense mechanism represented by NPQ and, subsequently, the antioxidant network is involved in the scavenging of the ROS, which are produced by the accumulation of electrons from the photosynthetic process.

5. Conclusions

In conclusion, phenols do account for scavenging activity in the case of natural gradual light variations (moderate, high, or extremely low light), while flavonoids are the family of compounds "selected" in the case of un-natural and very stressful change of light (Con 10, Quad 600).

This study provides evidence of the interconnection between xanthophyll-cycle-relied photoprotection and synthesis of antioxidant molecules. This study highlights the great potential of diatoms as alternative source of natural antioxidant molecules such as carotenoids, phenolic compounds, flavonoids, and ascorbic acid—as well as on the role of light manipulation as an effective tool for enhancing antioxidant molecules synthesis in diatoms.

Author Contributions: C.B. supervised the work. A.S., M.M., I.O. and C.B. carried out the experiments and analyzed the samples. A.S., S.B., M.M., M.B., C.G., C.S., C.B. contributed to data interpretation, analyzed the results and drafted the manuscript. All authors approved the submitted version and agreed to be personally accountable for the authors' own contributions.

Funding: This research received no external funding. Arianna Smerilli was funded by a PhD grant from the Stazione Zoologica Anton Dohrn.

Acknowledgments: The authors thank Federico Corato for the light system device realization. We acknowledge the three reviewers for their comments on the previous version of the manuscript.

Conflicts of Interest: The authors declare no conflict of interest

References

1. Foyer, C.H.; Shigeoka, S. Understanding Oxidative Stress and Antioxidant Functions to Enhance Photosynthesis. *Plant Physiol.* **2011**, *155*, 93–100. [CrossRef] [PubMed]
2. Mittler, R. Oxidative stress, antioxidants and stress tolerance. *Trends Plant Sci.* **2002**, *7*, 405–410. [CrossRef]
3. Foyer, C.H.; Noctor, G. Oxidant and antioxidant signalling in plants: A re-evaluation of the concept of oxidative stress in a physiological context. *Plant Cell Environ.* **2005**, *28*, 1056–1071. [CrossRef]
4. Foyer, C.H.; Noctor, G. Redox homeostasis and antioxidant signaling: A metabolic interface between stress perception and physiological responses. *Plant Cell Environ.* **2005**, *17*, 1866–1875. [CrossRef] [PubMed]
5. Snoeijs, P.; Sylvander, P.; Häubner, N. Oxidative stress in aquatic primary producers as a driving force for ecosystem responses to large-scale environmental changes. In *Oxidative Stress in Aquatic Ecosystems*; Abele, D., Vázquez-Medina, J.P., Zenteno-Savín, T., Eds.; Wiley-Blackwell: Oxford, UK, 2012; pp. 72–88.
6. Smirnoff, N.; Wheeler, G.L. Ascorbic acid in plants: Biosynthesis and function. *Crit. Rev. Biochem. Mol. Biol.* **2000**, *35*, 291–314. [CrossRef] [PubMed]
7. Stahl, W.; Sies, H. Antioxidant activity of carotenoids. *Mol. Asp. Med.* **2003**, *24*, 345–351. [CrossRef]
8. Boon, C.S.; McClements, D.J.; Weiss, J.; Decker, E.A. Factors influencing the chemical stability of carotenoids in foods. *Crit. Rev. Food Sci. Nutr.* **2010**, *50*, 515–532. [CrossRef]
9. Kuczynska, P.; Jemiola-Rzeminska, M.; Strzalka, K. Photosynthetic pigments in diatoms. *Mar. Drugs* **2015**, *13*, 5847–5881. [CrossRef]
10. Marí, M.; Morales, A.; Colell, A.; García-Ruiz, C.; Fernández-Checa, J.C. Mitochondrial glutathione, a key survival antioxidant. *Antioxid Redox Signal.* **2009**, *11*, 2685–2700. [CrossRef]
11. Krieger-Liszkay, A. Singlet oxygen production in photosynthesis. *J. Exp. Bot.* **2006**, *56*, 337–346. [CrossRef]
12. Cheynier, V.; Comte, G.; Davies, K.M.; Lattanzio, V.; Martens, S. Plant phenolics: Recent advances on their biosynthesis, genetics, and ecophysiology. *Plant Physiol. Biochem.* **2013**, *72*, 1–20. [CrossRef]
13. Pietta, P.G. Flavonoids as antioxidants. *J. Nat. Prod.* **2000**, *63*, 1035–1042. [CrossRef]
14. Goiris, K.; Muylaert, K.; Voorspoels, S.; Noten, B.; De Paepe, D.; Baart, G.J.E.; De Cooman, L. Detection of flavonoids in microalgae from different evolutionary lineages. *J. Phycol.* **2014**, *50*, 483–492. [CrossRef]

15. Klejdus, B.; Lojková, L.; Plaza, M.; Snóblová, M.; Sterbová, D. Hyphenated technique for the extraction and determination of isoflavones in algae: Ultrasound-assisted supercritical fluid extraction followed by fast chromatography with tandem mass spectrometry. *J. Chromatogr. A* **2010**, *1217*, 7956–7965. [CrossRef]
16. Xia, S.; Wang, K.; Wan, L.; Li, A.; Hu, Q.; Zhang, C. Production, characterization, and antioxidant activity of fucoxanthin from the marine diatom *Odontella aurita*. *Mar. Drugs* **2013**, *11*, 2667–2681. [CrossRef]
17. Foo, S.C.; Yusoff, F.M.; Ismail, M.; Basri, M.; Yau, S.K.; Khong, N.M.H.; Chan, K.W.; Ebrahimi, M. Antioxidant capacities of fucoxanthin-producing algae as influenced by their carotenoid and phenolic contents. *J. Biotechnol.* **2017**, *241*, 175–183. [CrossRef]
18. Galasso, C.; Corinaldesi, C.; Sansone, C. Carotenoids from Marine Organisms: Biological Functions and Industrial Applications. *Antioxidants* **2017**, *6*, 96. [CrossRef]
19. Rico, M.; López, A.; Santana-Casiano, J.M.; Gonzàlez, A.G.; Gonzàlez-Dàvila, M. Variability of the phenolic profile in the diatom *Phaeodactylum tricornutum* growing under copper and iron stress. *Limnol. Oceanogr.* **2013**, *58*, 144–152. [CrossRef]
20. Sushanth, V.R.; Rajashekhar, M. Antioxidant and antimicrobial activities in the four species of marine microalgae isolated from Arabian Sea of Karnataka Coast. *Indian J. Geo-Mar. Sci.* **2015**, *44*, 69–75.
21. Gastineau, R.; Turcotte, F.; Pouvreau, J.-B.; Morançais, M.; Fleurence, J.; Windarto, E.; Prasetiya, F.; Arsad, S.; Jaouen, P.; Babin, M.; et al. Marennine, Promising Blue Pigments from a Widespread Haslea Diatom Species Complex. *Mar. Drugs* **2014**, *12*, 3161–3189. [CrossRef]
22. López, A.; Rico, M.; Santana-Casiano, J.M.; González, A.G.; González-Dávila, M. Phenolic profile of *Dunaliella tertiolecta* growing under high levels of copper and iron. *Environ. Sci. Pollut. Res.* **2015**, *22*, 14820–14828. [CrossRef]
23. Jerez-Martel, I.; García-Poza, S.; Rodríguez-Martel, G.; Rico, M.; Afonso-Olivares, C.; Gómez-Pinchetti, J.L. Phenolic Profile and Antioxidant Activity of Crude Extracts from Microalgae and Cyanobacteria Strains. *J. Food Qual.* **2017**, *2017*, 2924508. [CrossRef]
24. Smerilli, A.; Orefice, I.; Corato, F.; Gavalás Olea, A.; Ruban, A.V.; Brunet, C. Photoprotective and antioxidant responses to light spectrum and intensity variations in the coastal diatom S keletonema marinoi. *Environ. Microbiol.* **2017**, *19*, 611–627. [CrossRef]
25. Lavaud, J.; Rousseau, B.; Etienne, A.-L. General features of photoprotection by energy dissipation in planktonic diatoms (Bacillariophyceae). *J. Phycol.* **2004**, *40*, 130–137. [CrossRef]
26. Ruban, A.V.; Lavaud, J.; Rousseau, B.; Guglielmi, G.; Horton, P.; Etienne, A.-L. The super-excess energy dissipation in diatom algae: Comparative analysis with higher plants. *Photosynth. Res.* **2004**, *82*, 165–175. [CrossRef]
27. Lavaud, J. Fast regulation of photosynthesis in diatoms: Mechanisms, evolution and ecophysiology. *Funct. Plant Sci. Biotechnol.* **2007**, *1*, 267–287.
28. Derks, A.; Schaven, K.; Bruce, D. Diverse mechanisms for photoprotection in photosynthesis. Dynamic regulation of photosystem II excitation in response to rapid environmental change. *BBA Bioenerg.* **2015**, *1847*, 468–485. [CrossRef]
29. Goss, R.; Lepetit, B. Biodiversity of NPQ. *J. Plant Physiol.* **2015**, *172*, 13–32. [CrossRef]
30. Waring, J.; Klenell, M.; Bechtold, U.; Underwood, G.J.C.; Baker, N.R. Light-induced responses of oxygen photoreduction, reactive oxygen species production and scavenging in two diatom species. *J. Phycol.* **2010**, *46*, 1206–1217. [CrossRef]
31. Cartaxana, P.; Domingues, N.; Cruz, S.; Jesus, B.; Laviale, M.; Serodio, J.; Marques da Silva, J. Photoinhibition in benthic diatom assemblages under light stress. *Aquat. Microb. Ecol.* **2013**, *70*, 87–92. [CrossRef]
32. Brown, M.R.; Jeffrey, S.W.; Volkman, J.K.; Dunstan, G. Nutritional properties of microalgae for mariculture. *Aquaculture* **1997**, *151*, 315–331. [CrossRef]
33. Kourtchenko, O.; Rajala, T.; Godhe, A. Growth of a common planktonic diatom quantified using solid medium culturing. *Sci. Rep.* **2018**, *8*, 9757. [CrossRef]
34. Chandrasekaran, R.; Barra, L.; Carillo, S.; Caruso, T.; Corsaro, M.M.; Dal Piaz, F.; Graziani, G.; Corato, F.; Pepe, D.; Manfredonia, A.; et al. Light modulation of biomass and macromolecular composition of the diatom *Skeletonema marinoi*. *J. Biotechnol.* **2014**, *192*, 114–122. [CrossRef]
35. Balzano, S.; Sarno, D.; Kooistra, W. Effects of salinity on the growth rate and morphology of ten *Skeletonema* strains. *J. Plankton Res.* **2011**, *33*, 937–945. [CrossRef]

36. Orefice, I.; Musella, M.; Smerilli, A.; Sansone, C.; Chandrasekaran, R.; Corato, F.; Brunet, C. Role of nutrient concentrations and water movement on diatom's productivity in culture. *Sci. Rep.* **2019**, *9*, 1479. [CrossRef]
37. Orefice, I.; Chandrasekaran, R.; Smerilli, A.; Corato, F.; Caruso, T.; Casillo, A.; Corsaro, M.M.; Dal Piaz, F.; Ruban, A.V.; Brunet, C. Light-induced changes in the photosynthetic physiology and biochemistry in the diatom *Skeletonema marinoi*. *Algal Res.* **2016**, *17*, 1–13. [CrossRef]
38. Brunet, C.; Chandrasekaran, R.; Barra, L.; Giovagnetti, V.; Corato, F.; Ruban, A. V Spectral radiation dependent photoprotective mechanism in the diatom *Pseudo-nitzschia multistriata*. *PLoS ONE* **2014**, *9*, e87015. [CrossRef]
39. Brunet, C.; Johnsen, G.; Lavaud, J.; Roy, S. Pigments and photoacclimation processes. In *Phytoplankton Pigments. Characterization, Chemotaxonomy and Applications in Oceanography*; Roy, S., Llewellyn, C.A., Egeland, E.S., Johnsen, G., Eds.; Cambridge University Press: Cambridge, UK, 2011; pp. 445–471.
40. Bilger, W.; Rimke, S.; Schreiber, U.; Lange, O.L. Inhibition of Energy-Transfer to Photosystem II in Lichens by Dehydration: Different Properties of Reversibility with Green and Blue-green Phycobionts. *J. Plant Physiol.* **1989**, *134*, 261–268. [CrossRef]
41. Eilers, P.H.C.; Peeters, J.C.H. A model for the relationship between light intensity and the rate of photosynthesis in phytoplankton. *Ecol. Model.* **1988**, *42*, 199–215. [CrossRef]
42. Running, J.A.; Severson, D.K.; Schneider, K.J. Extracellular production of L-ascorbic acid by *Chlorella protothecoides*, *Prototheca* species and mutants of *P. moriformis* during aerobic culturing at low pH. *J. Ind. Microbiol. Biotechnol.* **2002**, *29*, 93–98. [CrossRef]
43. Singleton, V.L.; Rossi, J.A. Colorimetry of total phenolics with phosphomolybdic-phosphotungstic acid reagents. *Am. J. Enol. Vitic.* **1965**, *16*, 144–158.
44. Li, H.-B.; Cheng, K.-W.; Wong, C.-C.; Fan, K.-W.; Chen, F.; Jiang, Y. Evaluation of antioxidant capacity and total phenolic content of different fractions of selected microalgae. *Food Chem.* **2007**, *102*, 771–776. [CrossRef]
45. Lamaison, J.L.C.; Carnet, A. Teneurs en Principaux Flavonoides des Fleurs de Crataegus monogyna Jacq et de Crataegus laevigata (Poiret D. C) en Fonction de la Vegetation. *Pharm. Acta Helv.* **1990**, *65*, 315–320.
46. Hammer, Ø.; Harper, D.A.T.; Ryan, P.D. PAST: Paleontological Statistics Software Package for education and data analysis. *Palaeontol. Electron.* **2001**, *4*, 1–9.
47. Giovagnetti, V.; Flori, S.; Tramontano, F.; Lavaud, J.; Brunet, C. The velocity of light intensity increase modulates the photoprotective response in coastal diatoms. *PLoS ONE* **2014**, *9*, e103782. [CrossRef]
48. Goiris, K.; Muylaert, K.; Fraeye, I.; Foubert, I.; De Brabanter, J.; De Cooman, L. Antioxidant potential of microalgae in relation to their phenolic and carotenoid content. *J. Appl. Phycol.* **2012**, *24*, 1477–1486. [CrossRef]
49. Goiris, K.; Van Colen, W.; Wilches, I.; León-Tamariz, F.; De Cooman, L.; Muylaert, K. Impact of nutrient stress on antioxidant production in three species of microalgae. *Algal Res.* **2015**, *7*, 51–57. [CrossRef]
50. Quideau, S.; Deffieux, D.; Douat-Casassus, C.; Pouysegu, L. Plant polyphenols: Chemical properties, biological activities, and synthesis. *Angew. Chem. Int. Ed. Engl.* **2011**, *50*, 586–621. [CrossRef]
51. Hajimahmoodi, M.; Faramarzi, M.A.; Mohammadi, N.; Soltani, N.; Oveisi, M.R.; Nafissi-Varcheh, N. Evaluation of antioxidant properties and total phenolic contents of some strains of microalgae. *J. Appl. Phycol.* **2010**, *22*, 43–50. [CrossRef]
52. Duval, B.; Shetty, K.; Thomas, W.H. Phenolic compounds and antioxidant properties in the snow alga Chlamydomonas nivalis after exposure to UV light. *J. Appl. Phycol.* **2000**, *11*, 559–566. [CrossRef]
53. Kováčik, J.; Klejdus, B.; Bačkor, M. Physiological Responses of *Scenedesmus quadricauda* (Chlorophyceae) to UV-A and UV-C Light. *Photochem. Photobiol.* **2010**, *86*, 612–616. [CrossRef]
54. FAO Micro-algae. In *Manual on the Production and Use of Live Food for Aquaculture*; Lavens, P.; Sorgeloos, P. (Eds.) FAO: Rome, Italy, 1996; Volume 361.
55. Agati, G.; Tattini, M. Multiple functional roles of flavonoids in photoprotection. *New Phytol.* **2010**, *186*, 786–793. [CrossRef]
56. Saewan, N.; Jimtaisong, A. Photoprotection of natural flavonoids. *J. Appl. Pharm. Sci.* **2013**, *3*, 129–141.
57. Zhou, R.; Su, W.H.; Zhang, G.F.; Zhang, Y.N.; Guo, X.R. Relationship between flavonoids and photoprotection in shade-developed *Erigeron breviscapus* transferred to sunlight. *Photosynthetica* **2016**, *54*, 201–209. [CrossRef]
58. Agati, G.; Brunetti, C.; Di Ferdinando, M.; Ferrini, F.; Pollastri, S.; Tattini, M. Functional roles of flavonoids in photoprotection: New evidence, lessons from the past. *Plant Physiol. Biochem.* **2013**, *72*, 35–45. [CrossRef]
59. Winkel-Shirley, B. Biosynthesis of flavonoids and effects of stress. *Curr. Opin. Plant Biol.* **2002**, *5*, 218–223. [CrossRef]

60. Ghasemzadeh, A.; Jaafar, H.Z.E.; Rahmat, A. Identification and Concentration of Some Flavonoid Components in Malaysian Young Ginger (*Zingiber officinale* Roscoe) Varieties by a High Performance Liquid Chromatography Method. *Molecules* **2010**, *15*, 6231–6243. [CrossRef]
61. Chandra, S.; Khan, S.; Avula, B.; Lata, H.; Yang, M.H.; ElSohly, M.A.; Khan, I.A. Assessment of Total Phenolic and Flavonoid Content, Antioxidant Properties, and Yield of Aeroponically and Conventionally Grown Leafy Vegetables and Fruit Crops: A Comparative Study. *Evid. Based Complement. Altern. Med.* **2014**, *2014*, 253875. [CrossRef]
62. Kamtekar, S.; Keer, V.; Patil, V. Estimation of Phenolic content, Flavonoid content, Antioxidant and Alpha amylase Inhibitory Activity of Marketed Polyherbal Formulation. *J. Appl. Pharm. Sci.* **2014**, *4*, 61–065.
63. Abalde, J.; Fabregas, J.; Herrero, C. β-Carotene, vitamin C and vitamin E content of the marine microalga *Dunaliella tertiolecta* cultured with different nitrogen sources. *Bioresour. Technol.* **1991**, *38*, 121–125. [CrossRef]
64. Brown, M.R.; Miller, K.A. The ascorbic acid content of eleven species of microalgae used in mariculture. *J. Appl. Phycol.* **1992**, *4*, 205–215. [CrossRef]
65. Massot, C.; Stevens, R.; Génard, M.; Longuenesse, J.-J.; Gautier, H. Light affects ascorbate content and ascorbate-related gene expression in tomato leaves more than in fruits. *Planta* **2012**, *235*, 153–163. [CrossRef]
66. Wang, J.; Zhang, Z.; Huang, R. Regulation of ascorbic acid synthesis in plants. *Plant Signal. Behav.* **2013**, *8*, e24536. [CrossRef]
67. Vaze, K.M.; Sharma, V.K. On the adaptive significance of circadian clocks for their owners. *Chronobiol. Int.* **2013**, *30*, 413–433. [CrossRef]
68. Mierziak, J.; Kostyn, K.; Kulma, A.; Mierziak, J.; Kostyn, K.; Kulma, A. Flavonoids as Important Molecules of Plant Interactions with the Environment. *Molecules* **2014**, *19*, 16240–16265. [CrossRef]
69. Panche, A.N.; Diwan, A.D.; Chandra, S.R. Flavonoids: An overview. *J. Nutr. Sci.* **2016**, *5*, e47. [CrossRef]
70. Treml, J.; Šmejkal, K. Flavonoids as Potent Scavengers of Hydroxyl Radicals. *Compr. Rev. Food Sci. Food Saf.* **2016**, *15*, 720–738. [CrossRef]
71. Saunders, J.A.; McClure, J.W. The distribution of flavonoids in chloroplasts of twenty five species of vascular plants. *Phytochemistry* **1976**, *15*, 809–810. [CrossRef]
72. Agati, G.; Azzarello, E.; Pollastri, S.; Tattini, M. Flavonoids as antioxidants in plants: Location and functional significance. *Plant Sci.* **2012**, *196*, 67–76. [CrossRef]
73. Jakob, T.; Goss, R.; Wilhelm, C. Unusual pH-dependence of diadinoxanthin de-epoxidase activation causes chlororespiratory induced accumulation of diatoxanthin in the diatom *Phaeodactylum tricornutum*. *J. Plant Physiol.* **2001**, *158*, 383–390. [CrossRef]
74. Cruz, S.; Goss, R.; Wilhelm, C.; Leegood, R.; Horton, P.; Jakob, T. Impact of chlororespiration on non-photochemical quenching of chlorophyll fluorescence and on the regulation of the diadinoxanthin cycle in the diatom *Thalassiosira pseudonana*. *J. Exp. Bot.* **2010**, *62*, 509–519. [CrossRef]
75. Vidoudez, C.; Pohnert, G. Comparative metabolomics of the diatom *Skeletonema marinoi* in different growth phases. *Metabolomics* **2012**, *8*, 654–669. [CrossRef]
76. Grover, A. How do senescing leaves lose photosynthetic activity? *Curr. Sci.* **1993**, *64*, 226–234.
77. Mae, T.; Thomas, H.; Gay, A.P.; Makino, A.; Hidema, J. Leaf development in *Lolium temulentum*: Photosynthesis and photosynthetic proteins in leaves senescing under different irradiances. *Plant Cell Physiol.* **1993**, *34*, 391–399.

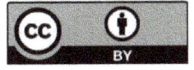

© 2019 by the authors. Licensee MDPI, Basel, Switzerland. This article is an open access article distributed under the terms and conditions of the Creative Commons Attribution (CC BY) license (http://creativecommons.org/licenses/by/4.0/).

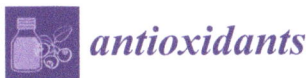 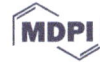

Article

Red Light Control of β-Carotene Isomerisation to 9-cis β-Carotene and Carotenoid Accumulation in *Dunaliella salina*

Yanan Xu and Patricia J. Harvey *

Faculty of Engineering and Science, University of Greenwich, Central Avenue, Chatham Maritime, Kent ME4 4TB, UK; y.xu@greenwich.ac.uk
* Correspondence: p.j.harvey@greenwich.ac.uk

Received: 14 May 2019; Accepted: 26 May 2019; Published: 27 May 2019

Abstract: *Dunaliella salina* is a rich source of *9-cis* β-carotene, which has been identified as an important biomolecule in the treatment of retinal dystrophies and other diseases. We previously showed that chlorophyll absorption of red light photons in *D. salina* is coupled with oxygen reduction and phytoene desaturation, and that it increases the pool size of β-carotene. Here, we show for the first time that growth under red light also controls the conversion of extant *all-trans* β-carotene to *9-cis* β-carotene by β-carotene isomerases. Cells illuminated with red light from a light emitting diode (LED) during cultivation contained a higher *9-cis* β-carotene content compared to cells illuminated with white or blue LED light. The *9-cis/all-trans* β-carotene ratio in red light treated cultures reached >2.5 within 48 h, and was independent of light intensity. Illumination using red light filters that eliminated blue wavelength light also increased the *9-cis/all-trans* β-carotene ratio. With norflurazon, a phytoene desaturase inhibitor which blocked downstream biosynthesis of β-carotene, extant *all-trans* β-carotene was converted to *9-cis* β-carotene during growth with red light and the *9-cis/all-trans* β-carotene ratio was ~2. With blue light under the same conditions, *9-cis* β-carotene was likely destroyed at a greater rate than *all-trans* β-carotene (*9-cis/all-trans* ratio 0.5). Red light perception by the red light photoreceptor, phytochrome, may increase the pool size of anti-oxidant, specifically *9-cis* β-carotene, both by upregulating phytoene synthase to increase the rate of biosynthesis of β-carotene and to reduce the rate of formation of reactive oxygen species (ROS), and by upregulating β-carotene isomerases to convert extant *all-trans* β-carotene to *9-cis* β-carotene.

Keywords: *9-cis* β-carotene; *all-trans* β-carotene; *Dunaliella salina*; red LED; blue LED; growth; light intensity; carotenoids; isomerisation

1. Introduction

Carotenoids are synthesized by photosynthetic organisms for light-harvesting and for photo-protection of the pigment-protein light-harvesting complexes and photosynthetic reaction centres in the thylakoid membrane [1–4]. *Dunaliella salina*, a halotolerant chlorophyte, is one of the richest sources of natural carotenoids, and accumulates up to 10% of the dry biomass as β-carotene under conditions that are sub-optimal for growth, i.e., high light intensity, sub-optimal temperatures, nutrient limitation and high salt concentrations [5–8]. Two pools of β-carotene have been identified, which may be distinguished on the basis of geometric isomer configuration, *cis* or *trans* (Z/E), and enzyme complement. Thylakoid β-carotene consists principally of *all-trans* β-carotene (*all-trans* βC), and may be constitutively expressed; the 'accumulated' β-carotene, which is found in globules of lipid and proline-rich, β-carotene globule protein (the βC-plastoglobuli) in the inter-thylakoid spaces of the chloroplast, appears in high concentration of both *cis/trans* (Z/E) configurations, ratio ~1 [5,9–11].

The occurrence of such high concentrations of *9-cis* βC in *D. salina* is of great pharmaceutical interest. *9-cis* βC has a higher antioxidant activity than *all-trans* βC, and may also be more efficient than *all-trans* βC in vivo [12,13]. *9-cis* βC has been proposed in treatments for retinal dystrophies, chronic plaque psoriasis and atherosclerosis and as an anti-ageing therapy [14–18]. Importantly, a synthetic pure preparation of *9-cis* βC has recently been shown to inhibit photoreceptor degeneration of eye cups from mice with a retinoid cycle genetic defect [19].

However, the mechanism and regulation of the biosynthesis of *9-cis* βC in *D. salina* is unclear. Using different inhibitors of β-carotene biosynthesis, Shaish et al. [20] found that all the intermediates between phytoene and β-carotene in cultures maintained under low light intensity and N-starvation contained similar ratios of *9-cis/all-trans* stereoisomers. They concluded that the isomerisation step must occur at or before phytoene, and that no further isomerisation was likely to occur during the further transformation of phytoene to β-carotene. On the other hand, in cultures maintained under light stress, *9-cis/all-trans* βC isomerases were identified in high concentrations in plastidic globules, and were shown in vitro to catalyse conversion of *all-trans* βC to *9-cis* βC, whilst the expression of the corresponding genes was enhanced under stress conditions [21]. The *9-cis/all-trans* βC ratio has been shown to increase four-fold and the β-carotene content two-fold when the culture temperature decreased from 30 °C to 10 °C [22], and to increase with increased light intensity [21,23,24], but to be independent of light wavelength within the photosynthetically active range [7]. There have also been reports of a higher *9-cis/all-trans* βC ratio in *D. salina* cultivated under low light intensities [25,26].

Recently, we showed that growth of *D. salina* under high intensity red light was associated with carotenoid accumulation and a high rate of oxygen uptake [1]. We proposed a mechanism for carotenoid synthesis under red light, which involved absorption of red light photons by chlorophyll to reduce plastoquinone in photosystem II, coupled with phytoene desaturation by a plastoquinol:oxygen oxidoreductase, with oxygen as electron acceptor. Partitioning of electrons between photosynthesis and carotenoid biosynthesis would depend on both red photon flux intensity and phytoene synthase upregulation by the red light photoreceptor, phytochrome.

In this paper, the effects of red, white and blue light on the β-carotene isomeric composition in *D. salina* were investigated. Isomerisation between *all-trans* and *9-cis* βC in *D. salina* was regulated by light wavelength but not light intensity, with red light shifting the equilibrium in the direction of *9-cis* βC production. In blue light, *9-cis* βC was more rapidly destroyed than *all-trans* βC.

2. Materials and Methods

2.1. Strains and Cultivation

D. salina strain CCAP 19/41 (PLY DF15) was isolated from a salt pond in Israel and obtained from the Marine Biological Association (MBA, Plymouth, UK). Algae were cultured in Modified Johnsons Medium [27] in an ALGEM Environmental Modeling Labscale Photobioreactor (Algenuity, Bedfordshire, UK) and growth was monitored as described previously [1]. For initial experiments described by Figure 1, *D. salina* cells were grown under 12/12 light/dark (L/D) with 200 μmol photons $m^{-2}\ s^{-1}$ supplied by white light emitting diode (LED) light (Figure A1a) to exponential growth phase, then dark-adapted for 36 h. After dark adaptation, they were transferred to continuous white, blue or red LED light at light intensities of 200, 500, or 1000 μmol photons $m^{-2}\ s^{-1}$ for 48 h. Samples were taken at 0, 24 and 48 h for carotenoids analysis. For experiments with norflurazon described by Figure 5, cultures were grown for 24 h under white LED light then norflurazon as added to cultures to a working concentration of 5 μM and maintained for a further 48 h under red, blue or a mix of red and blue LED light at 200 μmol $m^{-2}\ s^{-1}$ or kept in the dark. Red filters (Lee filter 26 Bright red, 27 Medium red, and 787 Marius red (Figure A1b–d)) when used, were purchased from Lee Filters Andover (Hampshire, UK) and placed over the LED lights. The cultures were shaken for 10 min at 100 rpm every hour before taking samples to monitor cell growth in order to minimise sheer stress to the cells which have no cell wall.

2.2. Carotenoids Analysis

The composition of pigments was analysed by High-Performance Liquid Chromatography with Diode-Array Detection (HPLC-DAD) (Agilent Technologies 1200 series, Agilent, Santa Clara, United States). Biomass was harvested and extracted for HPLC analysis as described previously [1], and analysed at least in triplicate. A carotene standard for *all-trans* βC was obtained from Sigma-Aldrich Inc. (Merck KGaA, Darmstadt, Germany); a carotene standard for *9-cis* βC was obtained from Dynamic Extractions (Tredegar, Gwent, UK). The *all-trans* and *9-cis* βC contents were quantified from their absorption at 450 nm.

2.3. Statistical Analysis

Each experiment was carried out at least in triplicate. The collected data were analyzed in R by one way analysis of variance (ANOVA) with posterior Dunnett's test and Turkey multiple pairwise-comparisons. A $p < 0.05$ value was considered significant.

3. Results

9-cis βC and *all-trans* βC were the major carotenoids that accumulated in *D. salina* biomass after 48 h exposure to red or blue LED light, but the relative pool sizes of each depended on the concentration of red and blue photons of light received. Under blue light, the contents of both *9-cis-* and *all-trans* βC per cell increased with time (Figure 1a,b), and the ratio of *cis/trans* βC isomers remained approximately the same at all light intensities (Figure 1c). The concentration of *9-cis* βC was ~half as much as *all-trans* βC. Under red light, by contrast, the concentration of *9-cis* βC and total pool of carotenoids increased massively compared to that in blue in all light intensities and the content of *9-cis* βC was ~twice as much as *all-trans* βC (Figure 1a,b). With increasing light intensity, the relative pool sizes of the isomers changed; that of *all-trans* βC decreased and that of *9-cis* βC increased. Furthermore *9-cis* βC increased with time to >60% of total β-carotene under red light (Figure 1d). HPLC profiles of the carotenoid extracts showed *9-cis* βC and *all-trans* βC were the major carotenoids that accumulated in *D. salina* biomass, and that the ratios of the two isomers were different under different wavelengths (Figure 1e).

To test the effect of blue light exposure on carotene isomers that had accumulated in red light and vice versa, dark-adapted cultures of *D. salina* were cultivated in red or blue LED high intensity light for 24 h (T0), and then cultivated for a further 24 h in red, blue, or a mixture of red and blue LED light (1:1) with the same light intensity, or the dark. As before, red-shifted cells maintained in red light produced the greatest amount of carotenoids with ~twice as much as *9-cis* βC as *all-trans* βC (Figure 2). On the other hand, *9-cis* βC decreased when red-shifted cells were transferred to blue light (Figure 2), to the same level as for blue-shifted cells maintained continuously in blue (Figure 3); the pool size of carotenoids for both conditions was about the same and the concentration of *9-cis* βC was ~half as much as *all-trans* βC. Conversely, blue-shifted cells when transferred to red LED produced more carotenoids (28% greater content), principally as *9-cis* βC (Figure 3).

Since red light increased the net content of *9-cis* βC, the effects of red light/dark cycles of increasing red light duration during cultivation were tested. Increasing red light duration increased the total amount of β-carotene, in particular the amount of *9-cis* βC (Figure 4). With a red light/dark cycle of 10 min/110 min, the ratio of *9-cis/all-trans* βC was 1.1, but in a red light/dark cycle of 30 min/30 min, this increased to 2.2, similar to that in continuous red (2.3). However, in continuous red light, the total pool size β-carotene was nearly 25% greater.

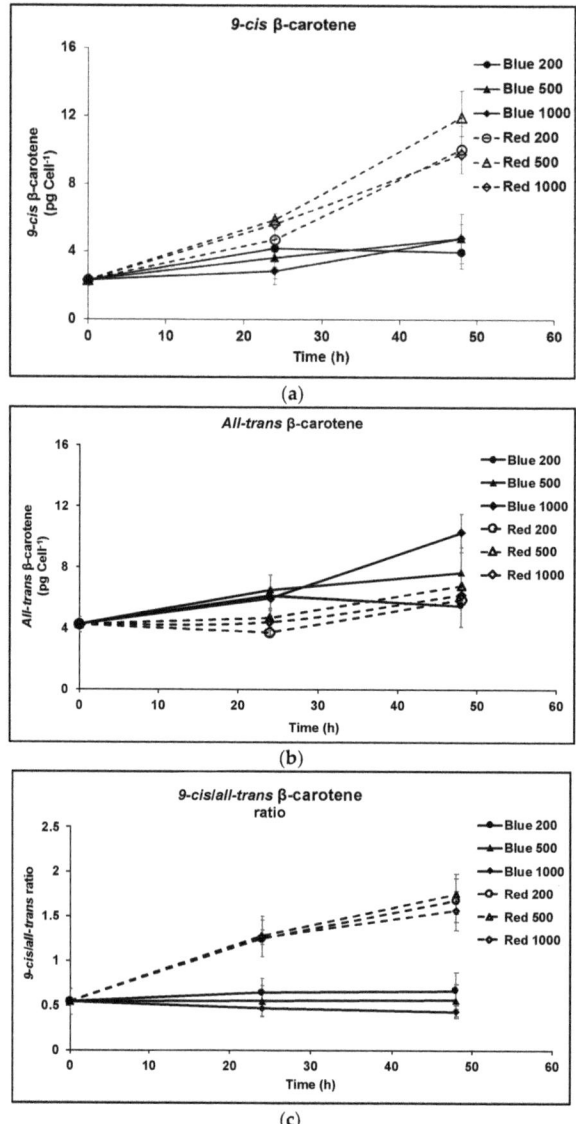

Figure 1. Cont.

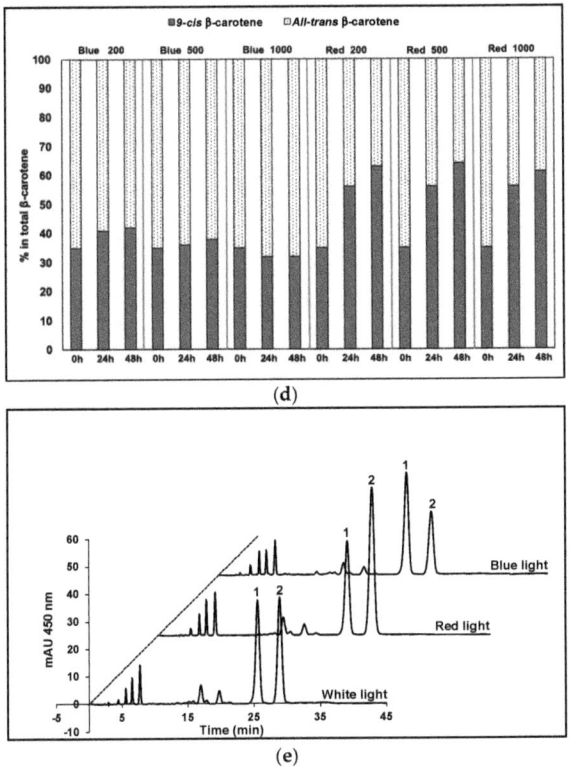

Figure 1. Cultivation of *D. salina* under continuous blue or red LED light at three different light intensities of 200, 500 and 1000 µmol m^{-2} s^{-1} for 48 h. (**a**) Cellular content of *9-cis* βC, (**b**) cellular content of *all-trans* βC; (**c**) *9-cis/all-trans* βC ratio. (**d**) Percentage of *9-cis* and *all-trans* βC in total βC. (**e**) HPLC profiles at 450 nm of carotenoid extracts from *D. salina* cultivated under continuous white light, red light or blue light, each at 1000 µmol m^{-2} s^{-1} for 48 h. Peak 1: *all-trans* β-carotene; peak 2: *9-cis* β-carotene. Biomass was collected at 48 h illumination and carotenoids extracted for HPLC analysis. Each culture condition was set up at least in triplicate. mAU: milli-absorbance unit.

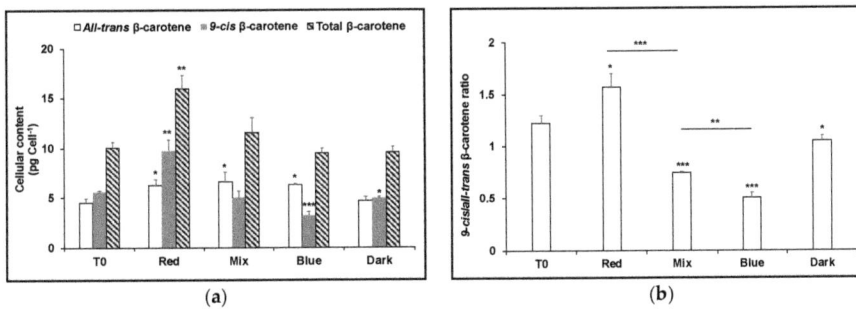

Figure 2. (**a**) Cellular content of *9-cis* βC and *all-trans* βC and (**b**) *9-cis/all-trans* βC ratio in *D. salina* cultures exposed to continuous red LED light at 1000 µmol m^{-2} s^{-1} for 24 h followed by 24 h under either red light, a mix of 1:1 red and blue light, blue light at the same light intensity of 1000 µmol m^{-2} s^{-1} or dark. Each culture condition was set up at least in triplicate. Results were analysed by one way analysis of variance (ANOVA) with posterior Dunnett's test compared to T0 and Tukey multiple pairwise-comparisons. Asterisks represent different levels of significance (*** $0 < p \leq 0.001$, ** $0.001 < p \leq 0.01$, * $0.01 < p \leq 0.05$).

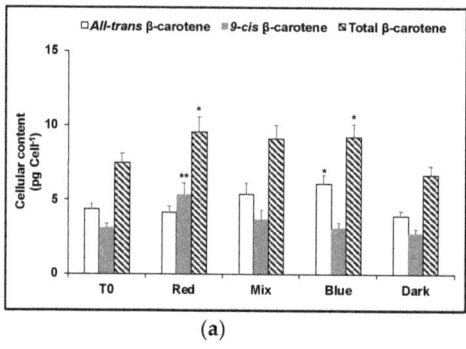
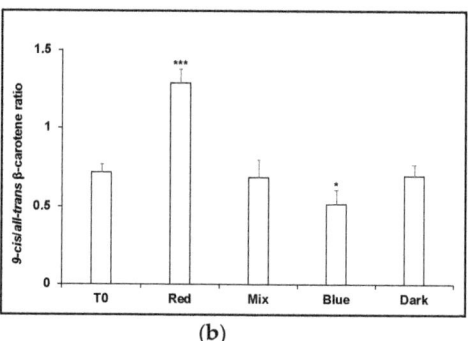

Figure 3. (a) Cellular content of *9-cis* βC and *all-trans* βC and (b) *9-cis/all-trans* βC ratio in *D. salina* cultures exposed to continuous blue LED light at 1000 µmol m^{-2} s^{-1} for 24 h followed by 24 h under either red light, a mix of 1:1 red and blue light, blue light at the same light intensity of 1000 µmol m^{-2} s^{-1} or dark. Each culture condition was set up at least in triplicate. Results were analysed by one way ANOVA with posterior Dunnett's test compared to T0 and Tukey multiple pairwise-comparisons. Asterisks represent different levels of significance (*** $0 < p \leq 0.001$, ** $0.001 < p \leq 0.01$, * $0.01 < p \leq 0.05$).

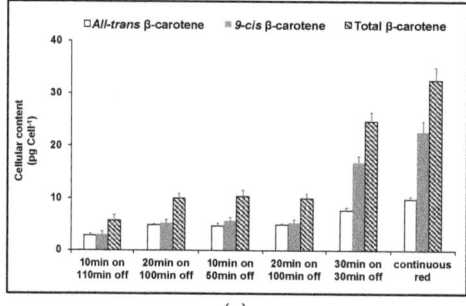
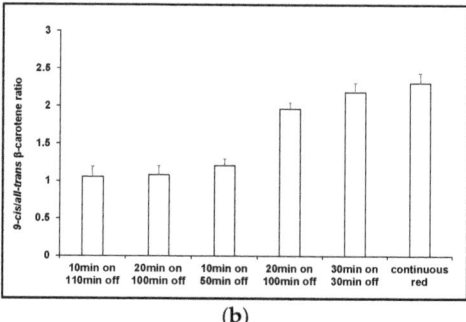
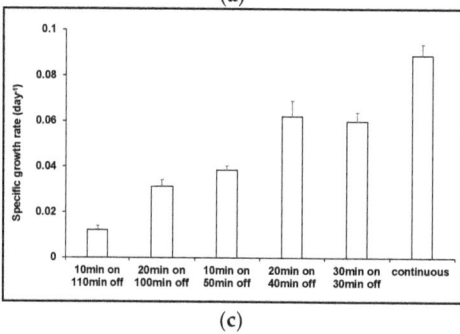

Figure 4. Effect of cultivating *D. salina* under different red light/dark cycles. (a) Cellular content of *9-cis* βC, *all-trans* βC and total βC and (b) *9-cis/all-trans* βC ratio and (c) specific growth rate of *D. salina* cultures grown under different light/dark cycles of red LED light supplied at 500 µmol m^{-2} s^{-1}. Cultures of *D. salina* were grown to a cell density of ~0.2 million cells mL^{-1} under white LED light and then transferred into red LED light growth cycles of different duration. Carotenoids were analysed after 6 days growth.

The accumulation of carotenoids under red light has previously been shown to involve upregulation of phytoene synthase to increase the pool size of phytoene in *D. salina* cultures [1]. In order to test the effect of blue and red light on the β-carotene isomer composition, but without interference of de novo synthesis of β-carotene from phytoene, norflurazon, a phytoene desaturase inhibitor, was applied to the *D. salina* cultures (Figure 5). After 48 h without light, the total pool size of carotenoids was the same as that at the outset of the experiment (T0) before light treatment i.e., norflurazon blocked any further downstream synthesis of β-carotene. Under these conditions, the β-carotene isomer composition, *9-cis/all-trans* βC, was 1.1, the same as that recorded for growth in a red light/dark cycle of 10 min/110 min. Both red and blue light treatments lowered the total pool size of total β-carotene, blue more than red: ~31–32% total β-carotene was destroyed under red light and under the 1:1 red/blue light mix, and ~41% under blue light. Carotenoids absorb photons in the range 400–550 nm, exactly overlapping the emission spectrum of the blue LED (440–500 nm) therefore the greater loss in blue light compared to red was to be anticipated. Furthermore, although both *all-trans* βC and *9-cis* βC were destroyed under blue light, the loss of *9-cis* βC was very much greater: only ~40% of the content of *9-cis* βC recorded in dark-treated cultures remained, compared to 78% for *all-trans* βC. Since *9-cis* βC has a higher antioxidant activity than *all-trans* βC, this result might also be anticipated. Somewhat surprisingly, however, loss of *9-cis* βC under red light compared to blue was much smaller and the ratio of *9-cis/all-trans* βC was 3-fold greater than under blue light. Since the emission spectrum of the red LED (625–680 nm) emits photons that are not absorbed by β-carotene, these data imply isomerisation of extant *all-trans* βC to *9-cis* βC to increase the content of *9-cis* βC at the expense of *all-trans* βC during growth.

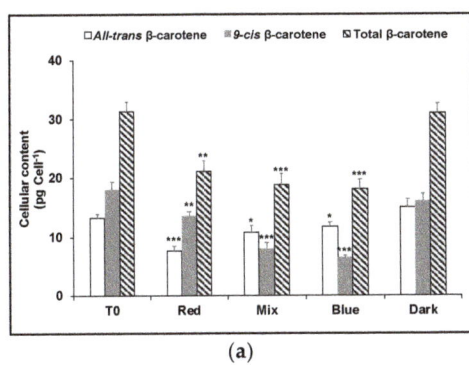
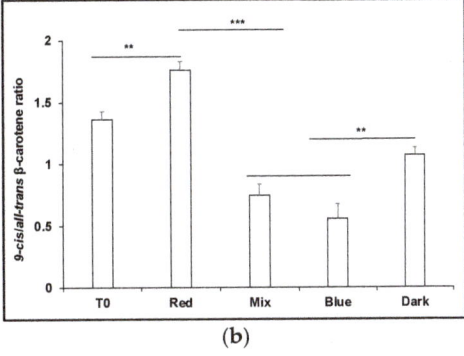

Figure 5. Production of carotenes in *D. salina* cultures treated with 5 μM norflurazon. (**a**) cellular content of *9-cis* βC, *all-trans* βC and total βC and (**b**) *9-cis/all-trans* βC ratio. Cultures were grown for 24 h under white LED light then treated with norflurazon and maintained for a further 48 h under red, blue or a mix of red and blue LED light at 200 μmol photons m^{-2} s^{-1} or kept in the dark. T0: time point after growth for 24h under white LED light only, before addition of norflurazon. Results were analysed by one way ANOVA with posterior Dunnett's test compared to T0 and Tukey multiple pairwise-comparisons. Asterisks represent different levels of significance (*** $0 < p \leq 0.001$, ** $0.001 < p \leq 0.01$, * $0.01 < p \leq 0.05$).

A similarly greater loss of *all-trans* βC compared to *9-cis* βC in red light was obtained using Lee Bright Red, Medium Red or 787 Marius Red filters: these transmitted only a fraction (8.6%, 3.6% and 1.0%) of the light intensity applied with a red LED (1000 μmol m^{-2} s^{-1}), but importantly excluded light wavelengths below 550 nm (Figure A1b–d). Each increased the total β-carotene pool size and the *9-cis/all-trans* βC ratio was higher (Figure 6). With the 787 Marius Red filter, cells received only approximately 10–17 μmol m^{-2} s^{-1} light intensity of the red wavelength but this was still sufficient to increase the ratio of *9-cis/all-trans* βC ratio, the amount of *9-cis* βC per cell and total β-carotene to values approaching those found using white light at 1000 μmol m^{-2} s^{-1}.

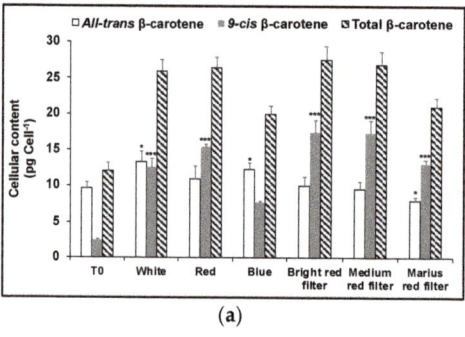
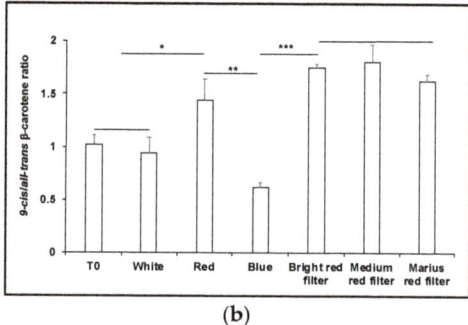

Figure 6. Cultivation of *D. salina* using red light filters. *D. salina* was cultivated under white light to early orange phase (cell density of ~0.5 × 10^6 cells mL^{-1}; carotenoid: chlorophyll ratio ~3), and then cultures were diluted with fresh medium to a cell density of ~0.2 × 10^6 cells mL^{-1} (no nutrient stress) (T0) and then further cultivated for 48 h under white, red or blue LED light at 1000 µmol m^{-2} s^{-1} or under white LED light at 1000 µmol m^{-2} s^{-1} covered with one of three different red filters (Lee filter 26 Bright red; Lee filter 27 Medium red; or Lee filter 787 Marius red). (**a**) Cellular content of *9-cis*, *all-trans* and total β-carotene. (**b**) *9-cis/all-trans* β-carotene ratio. Results were analysed by one way ANOVA and Tukey multiple pairwise-comparisons. Asterisks represent different levels of significance (*** 0 < p ≤ 0.001, ** 0.001 < p ≤ 0.01, * 0.01 < p ≤ 0.05).

The co-regulation by light and temperature on the β-carotene production and isomeric composition in *D. salina* is shown in Figure 7. Cultivation at 15 °C compared to 25 °C increased the *9-cis/all-trans* βC ratio, especially under red light, but decreased the pool size of β-carotene measured over the same time frame (48 h).

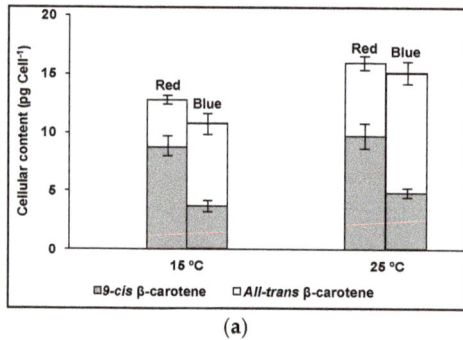
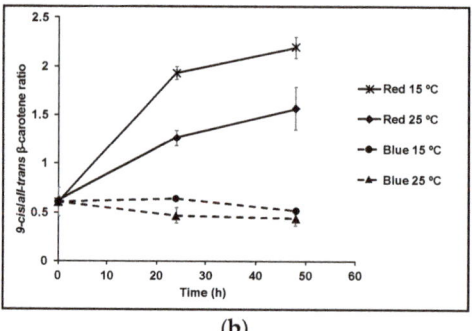

Figure 7. *D. salina* cultivated under red or blue light at either 15 °C or 25 °C. (**a**) Cellular content of *9-cis* βC and *all-trans* βC (**b**) *9-cis/all-trans* βC ratio. Cells were cultured under a light:dark 12h:12h white light growth regime to mid-log phase of the growth cycle (0.1–0.2 × 10^6 cells mL^{-1}) then transferred to the dark for 24 h before treatment for 48 h at either 15 °C or 25 °C under continuous blue or red LED light at 1000 µmol m^{-2} s^{-1}. Each culture condition was set up at least in triplicate.

Finally, the effects of blue and red light on the destruction of *all-trans* βC were evaluated. No reaction of *all-trans* βC solutions was detected under red light in nitrogen (Figure 8a). Under red light in air, (Figure 8b), 40% destruction of *all-trans* βC was recorded, whereas in blue light (Figure 8c), *all-trans* βC was fully destroyed within the same time frame. These data show that blue light is more damaging to *all-trans* βC than red light.

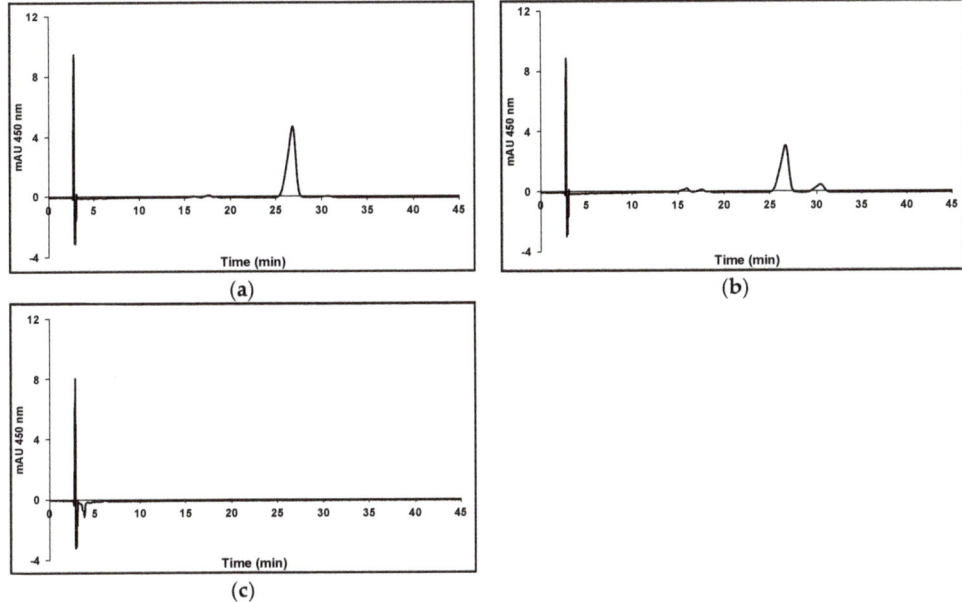

Figure 8. Effect of red or blue LED light on the photo-destruction of *all-trans* βC. *All-trans* βC was dissolved in chloroform to a final concentration of 2.4 µM and vials were thoroughly flushed with either nitrogen or air, sealed and incubated for 24 h at 25 °C under different LED lights at 200 µmol m^{-2} s^{-1}. (a) Red light under nitrogen; (b) Red light in air; (c) Blue light in air.

4. Discussion

In the present work, we found that under high intensity red LED light (up to 1000 µmol m^{-2} s^{-1}) but in conditions of nutrient sufficiency, *D. salina* accumulated carotenoids rapidly within 48 h. Surprisingly, the major accumulated isomer was *9-cis* βC, ~twice as much as *all-trans* βC. In vitro, *9-cis* βC is a better scavenger of free radicals than *all-trans* βC [12], and reportedly degrades more rapidly compared to *all-trans* βC under both light and dark conditions [28]. Furthermore, chlorophyll absorbs photons in the range of the emission spectrum of the red LED used here (625–680 nm) and therefore in *D. salina* cultures in high intensity red light, a high rate of photo-oxidation of *9-cis* βC might have been anticipated. Carotenoids are known antioxidants synthesized by many microalgae to prevent photoinhibition caused by photo-oxidation of photosynthetic reaction centres. Photooxidative damage occurs when species such as singlet oxygen ($^1O_2$) are formed under saturating light conditions as a result of transfer of energy from chlorophyll in the triplet excited state (^{3}Chl*) to the ground state of O_2. $^1O_2$ react readily with fatty acids to form lipid peroxides and will set up a chain of oxygen activation events that may eventually lead to a hyperoxidant state and cell death [29]. Carotenoids protect the photosystems in the following ways: (i) by reacting with lipid peroxidation products and terminating free radical chain reactions as a result of the presence of the polyene chain; (ii) by scavenging $^1O_2$ and dissipating the energy as heat; and (iii) by reacting with triplet excited chlorophyll ^{3}Chl* to prevent formation of $^1O_2$ or by dissipation of excess excitation energy through the xanthophyll cycle [3,30,31].

The simplest explanation to resolve the seeming anomaly, namely accumulation of the more readily degraded *9-cis* βC under high intensity red light conditions that should be associated with high rates of photo-oxidation, invokes the activity of β-carotene isomerases, the gene transcripts of which are increased in light stress [21]. Davidi et al. [11] showed that all the enzymes in the biosynthetic pathway from phytoene to β-carotene were present in the plastidic lipid globules and included enriched concentrations β-carotene isomerases; two of these, *9-cis*-βC-ISO1 and *9-cis*-βC-ISO2, were shown to be responsible for the catalytic conversion of *all-trans* βC to *9-cis* βC. Based on the data presented here we propose that the expression of gene transcripts of β-carotene isomerases may be triggered by specific light sensing, possibly through phytochrome.

In red light compared to blue, the apparent loss of *9-cis* βC with norflurazon was surprisingly small and the ratio of *9-cis/all-trans* βC was 3-fold greater than in blue light (Figure 5). Accumulation of *9-cis* βC by phytoene synthase (PSY) gene activation, whose expression has been shown to be greatly increased 6–48 h following stress [11] was precluded by the presence of norflurazon, which blocked phytoene desaturation and consequent carotene synthesis. Under these conditions, the relative increase in pool size of *9-cis* βC in red light implies a much higher rate of *9-cis* βC formation from extant *all-trans* βC, caused by increased isomerase activity, than the rate of *9-cis* βC destruction (see Figure 5). Carotenes absorb photons in the range 400–550 nm, exactly overlapping the emission spectrum of the blue LED (440–500 nm). However blue light catalysed a much more rapid rate of destruction of carotenes than red light (Figure 8). In blue LED light, *9-cis* βC would be destroyed more rapidly than could be replenished by adjustment of the *9-cis/all-trans* βC equilibrium position because increased β-carotene isomerase activity from red-light activated gene expression for β-carotene isomerases is not possible in blue light (see Figure 5).

Red light stimulation of the expression of gene transcripts of β-carotene isomerases by a phytochrome to increase the rate of accumulation of *9-cis* βC by β-carotene isomerases is also supported by the increase in pool size of *9-cis* βC under low intensity red light (Figure 6). Each of the Lee red light filters increased the total β-carotene pool size and the *9-cis/all-trans* βC ratio was higher despite the much lower light intensity of the red wavelength compared to the red LED light. The effects of low temperature on *9-cis* βC-accumulation in *D. salina* are also noteworthy, since enzyme catalysis typically shows a Q_{10} (temperature coefficient) ~2, yet in the present work, formation of *9-cis* βC in low temperature compared to high was increased under red light, and had little effect in blue. In higher plants, the activated phytochrome B, a red light photoreceptor, is considered to function as the thermal sensor to sense environmental temperature [32]. Mutants with no phytochromes showed a constitutive warm temperature transcriptome even at low temperatures [33]. Red light sensing to increase the concentration of β-carotene isomerases and catalyse conversion of *all-trans* βC at low temperatures, as well as high, may play a significant role in photoprotection in *D. salina*.

We recently proposed that red light enhanced the production of carotenoids in a mechanism dependent on both photon flux density as well as upregulation of phytoene synthase by the red light photoreceptor phytochrome and that chlorophyll absorption of red light photons and subsequent plastoquinone reduction in photosystem II was coupled with oxygen reduction and phytoene desaturation by plastoquinol:oxygen oxidoreductase [1]. According to the findings in the previous work [1], the partitioning electron flux between photosynthesis and carotenoid biosynthesis could be augmented by addition of the regulation of the pool size of *9-cis* βC, as seen in the Scheme 1.

Red light sensing by phytochrome to increase the pool size of phytoene by phytoene synthase has been reported in higher plants [34]. Red light control of carotenoid biosynthesis coupled with the accumulation of the more readily oxidized *9-cis* βC as a consequence of isomerisation from *all-trans* βC reserves would therefore rapidly increase the pool size of anti-oxidant to reduce the rate of formation of ROS under stress (See Scheme 1).

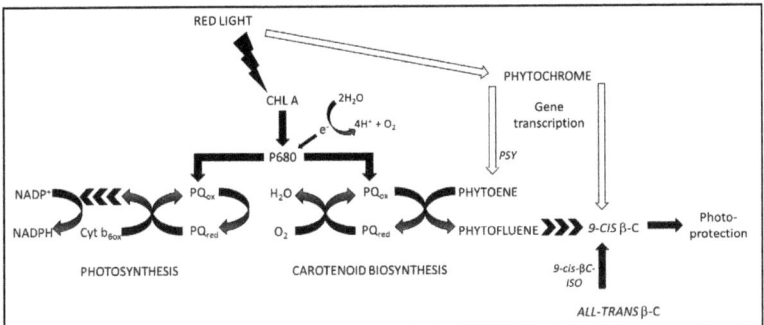

Scheme 1. Regulation of the pool size of *9-cis* βC. Red photon flux intensity controls the partitioning of electrons either for carotenoid biosynthesis or for photosynthesis, via energy absorption by chlorophyll and the PQ pool [1]. Red photon flux also controls phytochrome regulation of the production of gene transcripts for phytoene synthase and β-carotene isomerases. CHL A: chlorophyll a; P680: chlorophyll a, primary electron donor of Photosystem II; PQ_{ox}: plastoquinone, oxidised form; PQ_{red}: plastoquinone, reduced form; Cyt b_{6ox}: cytochrome b6f complex, oxidised form; $NADP^+$: NADP oxidised form; NADPH: NADP reduced form; PSY: phytoene synthase; 9-cis-βC-ISO: 9-cis βC isomerase.

5. Conclusions

Red light availability regulates the isomerisation of *all-trans* β-carotene to *9-cis* β-carotene and upregulates carotenoid biosynthesis in the halotolerant microalga *Dunaliella salina*. In red light *9-cis* βC accumulated, caused by increase in the rate of isomerisation of *all-trans* βC to *9-cis* βC relative to the rate of its destruction. Red light may have industrial value as an energy-efficient light source for production of natural *9-cis* βC from *D. salina*.

Author Contributions: Y.X. and P.J.H. conceived the work, analysed the data, and wrote the article; Y.X. conducted experiments and curated data; P.J.H. agrees to serve as the author responsible for contact and ensures communication.

Funding: This work was supported by EU KBBE.2013.3.2-02 programme (D-Factory: 368 613870) and by the Interreg 2 Seas programme 2014-2020 co-funded by the European Regional Development Fund under subsidy contract No ValgOrize 2S05017.

Conflicts of Interest: The authors declare no conflict of interest.

Appendix A

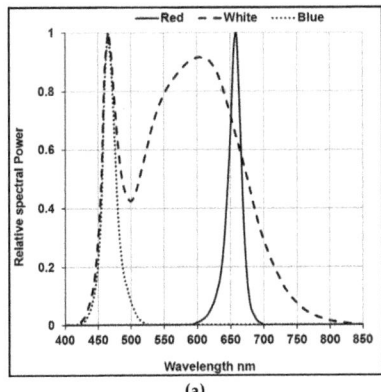
(a)

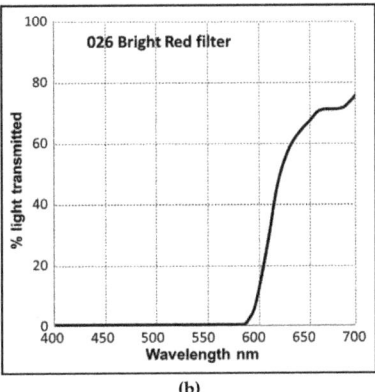
(b)

Figure A1. *Cont.*

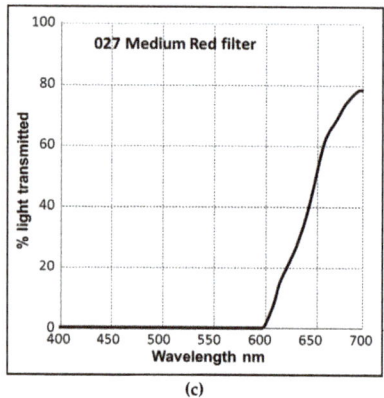
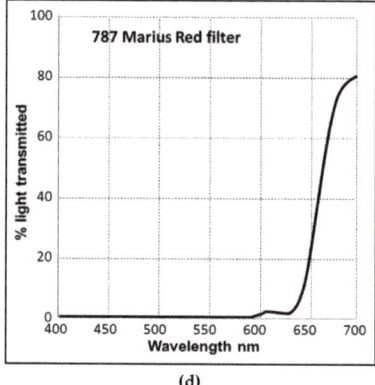

Figure A1. (a) Typical relative spectral power distribution of white, blue and red LED lights in the Algem bioreactor; (**b–d**) The light transmission (Y%) for each wavelength (nm) of filters that were used to transmit red light. (**b**) Lee Filters 026 Bright red (Transmission 8.6%), (**c**) 027 Medium Red (Transmission 3.6%), (**d**) 787 Marius Red (Transmission 1.0%).

References

1. Xu, Y.; Harvey, P.J. Carotenoid production by *Dunaliella salina* under red light. *Antioxidants* **2019**, *8*, 123. [CrossRef] [PubMed]
2. Khoo, H.E.; Nagendra, P.K.; Kong, K.W.; Jiang, Y.; Ismail, A. Carotenoids and their isomers: Color pigments in fruits and vegetables. *Molecules* **2011**, *16*, 1710–1738. [CrossRef] [PubMed]
3. Hashimoto, H.; Sugai, Y.; Uragami, C.; Gardiner, A.T.; Cogdell, R.J. Natural and artificial light-harvesting systems utilizing the functions of carotenoids. *J. Photochem. Photobiol. C: Photochem. Rev.* **2015**, *25*, 46–70. [CrossRef]
4. Rodriguez-Concepcion, M.; Avalos, J.; Bonet, M.L.; Boronat, A.; Gomez-Gomez, L.; Hornero-Mendez, D.; Limon, M.C.; Meléndez-Martínez, A.J.; Olmedilla-Alonso, B.; Palou, A.; et al. A global perspective on carotenoids: Metabolism, biotechnology, and benefits for nutrition and health. *Prog. Lipid Res.* **2018**, *70*, 62–93. [CrossRef]
5. Ben-Amotz, A.; Katz, A.; Avron, M. Accumulation of β-carotene in halotolerant algae: Purification and characterization of β-carotene-rich globules from *Dunaliella Bardawil* (Chlorophyceae). *J. Phycol.* **1982**, *18*, 529–537. [CrossRef]
6. Ben-Amotz, A. Analysis of carotenoids with emphasis on 9-cis β-carotene in vegetables and fruits commonly consumed in Israel. *Food Chem.* **1998**, *62*, 515–520. [CrossRef]
7. Ben-Amotz, A.; Shaish, A.; Avron, M. Mode of action of the massively accumulated β-carotene of *Dunaliella bardawil* in protecting the alga against damage by excess irradiation. *Plant Physiol.* **1989**, *91*, 1040–1043. [CrossRef]
8. Lamers, P.P.; Janssen, M.; De Vos, R.C.H.; Bino, R.J.; Wijffels, R.H. Exploring and exploiting carotenoid accumulation in *Dunaliella salina* for cell-factory applications. *Trends Biotechnol.* **2008**, *26*, 631–638. [CrossRef]
9. Jiménez, C.; Pick, U. Differential stereoisomer compositions of β, β-carotene in thylakoids and in pigment globules in *Dunaliella*. *J. Plant Physiol.* **1994**, *143*, 257–263. [CrossRef]
10. Davidi, L.; Shimoni, E.; Khozin-Goldberg, I.; Zamir, A.; Pick, U. Origin of β-carotene-rich plastoglobuli in *Dunaliella bardawil*. *Plant Physiol.* **2014**, *164*, 2139–2156. [CrossRef]
11. Davidi, L.; Levin, Y.; Ben-Dor, S.; Pick, U. Proteome analysis of cytoplasmatic and plastidic β-carotene lipid droplets in *Dunaliella bardawil*. *Plant Physiol.* **2015**, *167*, 60–79. [CrossRef]
12. Levin, G.; Mokady, S. Antioxidant activity of 9-cis compared to all-trans β-carotene in vitro. *Free Radic. Biol. Med.* **1994**, *17*, 77–82. [CrossRef]
13. Jaime, L.; Mendiola, J.A.; Ibáñez, E.; Martin-Alvarez, P.J.; Cifuentes, A.; Reglero, G.; Señoráns, F.J. Beta-carotene isomer composition of sub- and supercritical carbon dioxide extracts. Antioxidant activity measurement. *J. Agric. Food Chem.* **2007**, *55*, 10585–10590. [CrossRef]
14. Greenberger, S.; Harats, D.; Salameh, F.; Lubish, T.; Harari, A.; Trau, H.; Shaish, A. *9-cis*-rich β-carotene powder of the alga *Dunaliella* reduces the severity of chronic plaque psoriasis: A randomized, double-blind, placebo-controlled clinical trial. *J. Am. Coll. Nutr.* **2012**, *31*, 320–326. [CrossRef]

15. Harari, A.; Abecassis, R.; Relevi, N.; Levi, Z.; Ben-Amotz, A.; Kamari, Y.; Harats, D.; Shaish, A. Prevention of atherosclerosis progression by 9-cis-β-carotene rich alga *Dunaliella* in apoE-deficient mice. *Biomed. Res. Int.* **2013**, *2013*. [CrossRef]
16. Rotenstreich, Y.; Belkin, M.; Sadetzki, S.; Chetrit, A.; Ferman-Attar, G.; Sher, I.; Harari, A.; Shaish, A.; Harats, D. Treatment with 9-cis β-carotene-rich powder in patients with retinitis pigmentosa: A randomized crossover trial. *JAMA Ophthalmol.* **2013**, *131*, 985–992. [CrossRef]
17. Zolberg Relevy, N.; Bechor, S.; Harari, A.; Ben-Amotz, A.; Kamari, Y.; Harats, D.; Shaish, A. The inhibition of macrophage foam cell formation by 9-cis β-carotene is driven by BCMO1 activity. *PLoS ONE* **2015**, *10*, e0115272. [CrossRef] [PubMed]
18. Weinrich, T.; Xu, Y.; Wosu, C.; Harvey, P.J.; Jeffery, G. Mitochondrial Function, Mobility and Lifespan Are Improved in Drosophila melanogaster by Extracts of 9-cis-β-Carotene from *Dunaliella salina*. *Marine Drugs* **2019**, *17*, 279. [CrossRef]
19. Sher, I.; Tzameret, A.; Peri-Chen, S.; Edelshtain, V.; Ioffe, M.; Sayer, A.; Buzhansky, L.; Gazit, E.; Rotenstreich, Y. Synthetic 9-cis-beta-carotene inhibits photoreceptor degeneration in cultures of eye cups from rpe65rd12 mouse model of retinoid cycle defect. *Sci. Rep.* **2018**, *8*, 6130. [CrossRef] [PubMed]
20. Shaish, A.; Avron, M.; Ben-Amotz, A. Effect of inhibitors on the formation of stereoisomers in the biosynthesis of β-carotene in *Dunaliella bardawil*. *Plant Cell Physiol.* **1990**, *31*, 689–696.
21. Davidi, L.; Pick, U. Novel *9-cis/all-trans* β-carotene isomerases from plastidic oil bodies in *Dunaliella bardawil* catalyze the conversion of *all-trans* to *9-cis* β-carotene. *Plant Cell Rep.* **2017**, *36*, 807–814. [CrossRef]
22. Ben-Amotz, A. Effect of low temperature on the stereoisomer composition of β-carotene in the halotolerant alga *Dunaliella bardawil* (chlorophyta). *J. Phycol.* **1996**, *32*, 272–275. [CrossRef]
23. Ben-Amotz, A.; Lers, A.; Avron, M. Stereoisomers of β-carotene and phytoene in the alga *Dunaliella bardawil*. *Plant Physiol.* **1988**, *86*, 1286–1291. [CrossRef]
24. Ben-Amotz, A.; Avron, M. The wavelength dependence of massive carotene synthesis in *Dunaliella bardawil* (Chlorophyceae). *J. Phycol.* **1989**, *25*, 175–178. [CrossRef]
25. Orset, S.C.; Young, A.J. Exposure to low irradiances favors the synthesis of 9-cis beta, beta-carotene in *Dunaliella salina* (Teod.). *Plant Physiol.* **2000**, *122*, 609–618. [CrossRef]
26. Gómez, P.I.; González, M.A. The effect of temperature and irradiance on the growth and carotenogenic capacity of seven strains of *Dunaliella salina* (Chlorophyta) cultivated under laboratory conditions. *Biol. Res.* **2005**, *38*, 151–162. [CrossRef]
27. Borowitzka, M.A. Algal growth media and sources of algal cultures. In *Micro-algal Biotechnology*, 1st ed.; Borowitzka, M.A., Borowitzka, L.J., Eds.; Cambridge University Press: Cambridge, UK, 1988; pp. 456–465.
28. Jimenez, C.; Pick, U. Differential reactivity of β-carotene isomers from *Dunaliella bardawil* toward oxygen radicals. *Plant Physiol.* **1993**, *101*, 385–390. [CrossRef] [PubMed]
29. Hansberg, W.; Aguirre, J. Hyperoxidant states cause microbial cell differentiation by cell isolation from dioxygen. *J. Theor. Biol.* **1990**, *142*, 201–221. [CrossRef]
30. Yokthongwattana, K.; Jin, E.; Melis, A. Chloroplast acclimation, photodamage and repair reactions of Photosystem-II in the model green alga, *Dunaliella salina*. In *The Alga Dunaliella Biodiversity, Physiology, Genomics and Biotechnology*, 1st ed.; Ben-Amotz, A., Polle, E.W., Subba Rao, D.V., Eds.; CRC Press: Enfield, NH, USA, 2009; pp. 273–299.
31. Erickson, E.; Wakao, S.; Niyogi, K.K. Light stress and photoprotection in *Chlamydomonas reinhardtii*. *Plant J.* **2015**, *82*, 449–465. [CrossRef] [PubMed]
32. Legris, M.; Burgie, E.S.; Rojas, C.C.R.; Neme, M.; Wigge, P.A.; Vierstra, R.D.; Casal, J.J. Phytochrome B integrates light and temperature signals in *Arabidopsis*. *Science* **2016**, *354*, 897–900. [CrossRef] [PubMed]
33. Viczián, A.; Klose, C.; Ádám, É.; Nagy, F. New insights of red light-induced development. *Plant Cell Environ.* **2017**, *40*, 2457–2468. [CrossRef] [PubMed]
34. Welsch, R.; Beyer, P.; Hugueney, P.; Kleinig, H.; von Lintig, J. Regulation and activation of phytoene synthase, a key enzyme in carotenoid biosynthesis, during photomorphogenesis. *Planta* **2000**, *211*, 846–854. [CrossRef] [PubMed]

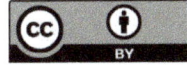

© 2019 by the authors. Licensee MDPI, Basel, Switzerland. This article is an open access article distributed under the terms and conditions of the Creative Commons Attribution (CC BY) license (http://creativecommons.org/licenses/by/4.0/).

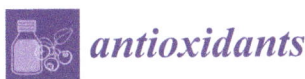

Article

Optimization of Microwave-Assisted Extraction of Polysaccharides from *Ulva pertusa* and Evaluation of Their Antioxidant Activity

Bao Le [1], Kirill S. Golokhvast [2], Seung Hwan Yang [1,*] and Sangmi Sun [1,*]

1. Department of Biotechnology, Chonnam National University, Yeosu 59726, Korea; lebaobiotech@gmail.com
2. Educational Scientific Center of Nanotechnology, Engineering School, Far Eastern Federal University, 37 Pushkinskaya Street, 690950 Vladivostok, Russia; droopy@mail.ru
* Correspondence: ymichigan@jnu.ac.kr (S.H.Y.); smsun@chonnam.ac.kr (S.S.); Tel.: +82-61-659-7306 (S.H.Y.); +82-61-659-7302 (S.S.)

Received: 22 April 2019; Accepted: 11 May 2019; Published: 14 May 2019

Abstract: The use of green marine seaweed *Ulva* spp. as foods, feed supplements, and functional ingredients has gained increasing interest. Microwave-assisted extraction technology was employed to improve the extraction yield and composition of *Ulva pertusa* polysaccharides. The antioxidant activity of ulvan was also evaluated. The impacts of four independent variables, i.e., extraction time (X_1, 30 to 60 min), power (X_2, 500 to 700 W), water-to-raw-material ratio (X_3, 40 to 70), and pH (X_4, 5 to 7) were evaluated. The chemical structure of different polysaccharides fractions was investigated via FT-IR and the determination of their antioxidant activities. A response surface methodology based on a Box–Behnken design (BBD) was used to optimize the extraction conditions as follows: extraction time of 43.63 min, power level of 600 W, water-to-raw-material ratio of 55.45, pH of 6.57, and maximum yield of 41.91%, with a desired value of 0.381. Ulvan exerted a strong antioxidant effect against 1,1-diphenyl-2-picrylhydrazyl (DPPH) and 2,2′-azino-bis(3-ethylbenzothiazoline-6-sulphonic acid) (ABTS) and showed reducing power in vitro. Ulvan protected RAW 264.7 cells against H_2O_2-induced oxidative stress by upregulating the expression and enhancing the activity of oxidative enzymes such as superoxide dismutase (SOD) and superoxide dismutase (CAT). The results suggest that the polysaccharides from *U. pertusa* might be promising bioactive compounds for commercial use.

Keywords: antioxidant activities; Box–Behnken design; microwave-assisted extraction; polysaccharide; *Ulva pertusa*; seaweed

1. Introduction

The genus *Ulva* (Chlorophyta) is a cosmopolitan, abundant, and fast-growing green macroalgae forming natural beds in shallow waters throughout the world [1]. *Ulva* is widely distributed, grows rapidly, and causes "green tides" in response to elevated levels of nitrogenous and phosphorus materials in coastal areas [2]. *Ulva* spp. are a relatively rich source of different bioactive compounds, in particular, polyphenols and dietary fiber [3].

Ulva contains a polysaccharide present in high amounts in the cell wall (38% to 54% in dry weight) and commonly known as ulvan [4], which belongs to a group of sulfated hetero-polysaccharides comprising glucose, glucuronic acid, rhamnose, xylose, and galactose [5]. Ulvan has been demonstrated to play an important role as an antitumor [6] and antihyperlipidemic [7] substance in living organisms and induces a defense mechanism in crops [8]. It is also one of the important antioxidant compounds, whose antioxidant properties are mainly attributed to its scavenging activity against superoxide and hydroxyl radicals, its chelating ability, singlet and triplet oxygen quenching activity, and reducing power [9]. However, the understanding of the structural characteristics of polysaccharides extracted from *Ulva pertusa* is limited, which affects their application.

Hot water or aqueous organic solvents are the most common and conventional methods for extracting water-soluble polysaccharides from *Ulva* sp. [7]. However, such methods are time-consuming and have a low extraction efficiency owing to the complex polymers of the algae cell wall [10]. Therefore, additional methods are being used to improve the extraction process, such as microwaving [11], ultrasonication [5], and enzymatic reduction [12]. Microwave-assisted extraction (MAE) methods have demonstrated better performances with the advantages of a short operation time, simplicity, low cost, and high efficiency [13]. MAE is a "green" extraction process based on the use of electromagnetic waves with high frequencies. The high temperature produced by molecular motions increases the solubility of the extracted compounds and the solvent diffusion rate, thereby enhancing their quality and yield [14]. Although this extraction method has been proved efficient in fucoidan and carrageenan isolation from brown and red seaweed [15,16], only a few studies have been carried out on green seaweed such as *Ulva meridional*, *Ulva ohnoi*, and *Monostroma latissimum* [11].

The main aim of this study was to optimize the operational parameters (power, time, water-to-raw-material ratio, and pH) of MAE to obtain the maximum yield of ulvan extracted from *U. pertusa*. Furthermore, the antioxidant activity of ulvan was evaluated in hydrogen peroxide (H_2O_2)-treated RAW 264.7 cells through in vitro assays.

2. Materials and Methods

2.1. Seaweeds and Chemicals

U. pertusa gametophytes were collected from June to July 2018 in Dolsan, Yeosu, Korea (34°40′ N, 127°46′ E), put into sterilized plastic bags containing seawater, placed in an ice box, and transferred to the laboratory immediately. The vegetative materials were rinsed several times to clear their surface, oven-dried at 40 °C, and maintained at −80 °C until use. All chemicals and reagents applied were of analytical grade.

2.2. Microwave Extraction of Ulvan

The dried *U. pertusa* thallus (100 g) was ground in a high-speed disintegrator to make a fine powder. The powder was pretreated with 80% ethanol (400 mL) in a water bath at 85 °C for 2 h to remove pigments and low-molecular-weight compounds. After incubation, the precipitate was collected through centrifugation at 4000× g for 10 min and was then dried in an oven at 50 °C. The pretreated sample (1 g) was extracted using MAE based on specific extraction time, amount of microwave power, water-to-raw-material ratio, and pH (Table 1). The aqueous extract was separated from the insoluble residue through centrifugation (6000× g, 20 min). The solution was precipitated with the addition of ethanol to a final concentration of 85% and maintained at 4 °C overnight. The crude polysaccharide was separated through centrifugation (6000× g for 20 min) and air-dried for 12 h. Ulvan was weighed and stored at −20 °C until analyzed. The total content of the polysaccharides was measured using a phenol–sulfuric acid method [17]. The yield of ulvan (%) was calculated as follows:

Yield of ulvan (%) = polysaccharides content of the extract (g)/weight of the pretreated sample (g)　　(1)

2.3. Single-Factor MAE Experiments

The influence of the process parameters including extraction time, microwave power, water-to-raw-material ratio, and pH on the extraction yield and identify the independent variables as well as on the optimum ranges of the Box–Behnken Design (BBD) was determined using a series of single-factor experiments. The effects of each factor were evaluated by determining the ulvan yield.

Table 1. Box–Behnken (BBD) matrix of the four variables, levels for response surface methodology (RSM), experimental data, and predicted values of ulvan extraction.

Run	Variable Levels				Ulvan Yield (%)	
	X_1 (Time, min)	X_2 (Power, W)	X_3 (Water-To-Raw-Material, mL/g)	X_4 (pH)	Predicted	Observed
1	45	500	70	6	32.72	32.22
2	45	700	55	5	31.61	31.26
3	45	600	70	7	32.30	31.38
4	30	600	70	6	32.18	32.48
5	30	600	40	6	29.93	29.46
6	45	600	55	6	40.84	40.84
7	45	500	55	5	35.22	35.47
8	60	600	70	6	27.36	28.46
9	60	600	40	6	30.45	30.78
10	45	500	55	7	34.78	35.75
11	60	600	55	5	25.88	25.71
12	30	600	55	5	30.51	29.79
13	45	500	40	6	36.29	35.89
14	60	600	55	7	32.92	33.11
15	45	600	40	5	28.15	28.97
16	45	700	70	6	37.27	37.14
17	30	600	55	7	32.60	32.24
18	30	500	55	6	32.94	33.45
19	45	700	55	7	41.18	41.56
20	60	500	55	6	32.46	31.63
21	45	600	70	5	31.85	32.01
22	30	700	55	6	36.01	36.74
23	45	600	55	6	40.84	40.84
24	45	600	55	6	40.84	40.83
25	45	700	40	6	34.53	34.51
26	45	600	40	7	36.83	36.56
27	60	700	55	6	32.18	31.56

2.4. Experimental Design

A response surface methodology (RSM) was used to optimize the effects of the independent variables on the extraction yield of ulvan polysaccharide. Four processing variables, i.e., time (X_1), power (X_2), water-to-raw-material ratio (X_3), and pH (X_4) were chosen on the basis of the results of single-factor experiments and were then investigated using BBD (Table 1). The yield was taken as the response to the design experiments. The selected variables were coded using the following equation:

$$x_i = (X_i - X_o)/\Delta X, \tag{2}$$

where x_i is a variable, X_o and X_i are the actual values for the ith independent variable at the center point, and ΔX is the value of the step change.

A second-order regression analysis of the data was defined using the response function (Y) including the linear, quadratic, and interactive components and the proposed model, as follows:

$$Y = \beta_o + \sum \beta_i x_i + \sum \beta_{ii} x_i^2 + \sum \beta_{ij} x_i x_j \tag{3}$$

where Y is a dependent variable, β_o is a constant coefficient, and β_i, β_{ii}, and β_{ij} are the regression coefficients for the intercept, linear, quadratic, and two-factor interaction variables, respectively.

2.5. FT-IR Spectrometric Analysis

The ulvan extract was ground with potassium bromide (KBr) powder before measurement. IR spectra were acquired on an FT-IR spectrophotometer (VERTEX 70, Bruker, Germany) in the frequency range of 4000–400 cm^{-1}.

2.6. Determination of the Antioxidant Activity of Ulvan Extracts in Vitro

2.6.1. DPPH Radical-Scavenging Activity

The free scavenging activity on 1,1-diphenyl-2-picrylhydrazyl (DPPH) was investigated using the method mentioned by Bondet et al. [18]. The reaction mixtures consisted of 2 mL of ulvan extracted under optimal conditions (0 to 0.8 mg/mL) and 2 mL DPPH (0.05 mM in ethanol). The reaction tubes were incubated in darkness at 25 °C for 30 min. The absorbance of the mixture was measured at 517 nm using ascorbic acid as a positive control. The scavenging DPPH activity was calculated according to Equation (4):

$$\text{Scavenging activity (\%)} = (1 - (A_1 - A_2)/A_0) \times 100 \tag{4}$$

where A_0, A_1, A_2 are the absorbance of the DPPH solution used as a negative control, of the sample with the DPPH solution, and of the sample without the DPPH solution, respectively.

2.6.2. ABTS Radical-Scavenging Activity

The assay was carried out using the procedure described by Hromadkova et al. [19]. The working solution was prepared by mixing 25 mL of a 7 mM 2,2′-azino-bis(3-ethylbenzothiazoline-6-sulphonic acid) (ABTS) solution and 12.5 mL of 2.4 mM potassium persulfate. The mixture was kept in the dark at room temperature for 12 to 16 h prior to use. The ABTS solution was adjusted to an absorbance of 0.7. For the assays, 0.1 mL of extract was allowed to react with 1 mL of the ABTS solution, and the absorbance was recorded at 734 nm after 7 min using a spectrophotometer. The scavenging ABTS activity was calculated according to Equation (5):

$$\text{Scavenging activity (\%)} = (1 - (A_1 - A_2)/A_0) \times 100 \tag{5}$$

where A_0, A_1, A_2 are the absorbance of the ABTS solution used as a negative control, of the sample with the ABTS solution, and of the sample without the ABTS solution, respectively.

2.6.3. Determination of the Reducing Power

The reducing power was evaluated using a method by Dahmoun et al. [20]. The reaction mixture consisted of 2.5 mL of a 0.2 M phosphate solution, 2.5 mL of 1% (w/v) potassium ferricyanide, and 2.4 mL of varying concentrations of the ulvan extracts. After the mixture was incubated at 50 °C for 20 min, 2.5 mL of 10% (w/v) trichloroacetic acid was added, and the mixture was centrifuged at 900× g for 10 min. The supernatant (5 mL) was mixed with 5 mL of distilled water and 1 mL of 0.1% (w/v) ferric chloride. The absorbance of the resulting solution was measured for 2 min at 700 nm.

2.7. In Vitro Antioxidant Activity

The RAW 264.7 murine macrophage cell line was cultured in Dulbecco's modified Eagle's medium (DMEM) (Wellgen, Daegu, Korea) containing 4.5 g/L glucose, 4 mM L-glutamine, 25 mM HEPES, 1 mM sodium pyruvate, 15 mg/L phenol red, 3.7 g/L sodium bicarbonate, 10% fetal bovine serum (FBS), 100 units/mL penicillin, and 50 ug/mL streptomycin in a humidified atmosphere at 37°C, 5% CO_2. RAW 264.7 cells were split and seeded in 96-well cell culture plates (2.0×10^4 cells/well) and incubated in the same culture conditions overnight. The medium was replaced with fresh DMEM medium containing various concentration of ulvan or 600 μM hydrogen peroxide (H_2O_2) for 24 h. After incubation, the cell viability was determined using the 3-[4,5-dimethylthiazol-2-yl]-2,5 diphenyl tetrazolium bromide (MTT) (Sigma Aldrich, St. Louis, MO, USA) assay [21].

Oxidative damage of the cells was induced using hydrogen peroxide [22]. RAW 264.7 cells (2.0×10^4 cells/well) were seeded in 96-well cell culture plates and incubated overnight. The cells were then washed with 0.1 PBS (pH 7.2) and pretreated with fresh DEME medium containing various concentrations of ulvan for 2 h. To stimulate oxidative stress, the cells were then incubated with 600 μM H_2O_2 for 24 h under the same conditions. Ascorbic acid was used as a positive control. After incubation, the cells were collected, suspended in 0.1 M cold PBS buffer, and lysed using ultrasonic decomposition in an ice-water bath. The cell-free supernatant was used for analysis of superoxide dismutase (SOD; cat. no. STA-340, Cell Biolabs Inc., San Diego, CA, USA) and catalase (CAT; cat. no. STA-340, Cell Biolabs Inc., San Diego, CA, USA) activities using commercial kits following the manufacturers' instructions.

To determine the expression levels of antioxidant-related genes, total RNA from the treated RAW 264.7 cells was purified by using the Trizol reagent (Invitrogen, USA) according to the manufacturer's protocol. Total RNA (1 µg) was reverse-transcribed into cDNA using the ImProm-II™ Reverse Transcription System (Promega, USA), and the target cDNA was amplified using the following primers: β-actin, forward 5'-AAG ACC TCT ATG CCA ACA CAG T-3', reverse 5'-CAT CGT ACT CCT GCT TGC TGA T-3'; glutathione S-transferases (GST), forward 5'-TGA GAG GAA CCA AGT GTT TGA G-3', reverse 5'-CAG GGG GAC TTT AGC TTT AGA A-3'; catalase (CAT), forward 5'-GGG ATT CCC GAT GGT-3', reverse 5'-GCC AAA CCT TGG TCA G-3'; MnSOD, forward 5'-TCC CAGACC TGC CTT ACG A-3', reverse 5'-TCG GTG GCG TTG AGA TTG-3'; GPx, forward 5'-CTC GGT TTC CCG TGC AAT CAG-3', reverse 5'-GTG CAG CCA GTA ATC ACC AAG-3' [23].

2.8. Statistical Analysis

The experimental design and graphical and statistical analysis for the RSM were conducted using Minitab 17 (Minitab Inc., State College, Pennsylvania). All trials were conducted in triplicate. Data differences between two groups were analyzed using the Student's t test ($p < 0.05$) by the SPSS 16.0 software (SPSS, Inc., Chicago, IL, USA).

3. Results

3.1. Effect of Process Parameters on Microwave Extraction Efficiency

As shown in Figure 1a, the yield of the polysaccharides increased significantly with increasing extraction times ranging from 15 to 45 min; the highest extraction yield was obtained at 45 min. To study the effect of microwave powers on the yield of the polysaccharides, the extraction processes were carried out at 300, 400, 500, 600, 700, and 800 W for 45 min. The results shown in Figure 1b indicate that the maximum ulvan yield (35.14%) occurred when the power was 600 W. The yield of ulvan affected by the different ratios between water and raw materials is shown in Figure 1c, whereas the other extraction variables were as follows: 600 W power, pH of 6, and extraction time of 45 min. The extraction yields increased as the water-to-raw-material ratio ascended slightly from 25 to 85 mL/g and reached the maximum value (25.23%) when the ratio was 70 mL/g. To evaluate the pH effects on the yield, the extraction process was conducted at different pH values, and the results are shown in Figure 1d. As shown in the figure, the polysaccharide yield increased with an increase in the pH level and significantly decreased when the pH was higher than 7.

3.2. Optimization of the Procedure Using RSM

In the present study, the ulvan extraction yield was investigated according to BBD (27 batch experiments), and the corresponding results are shown in Table 1. The experimental data were then investigated using a multiple regression analysis and an analysis of variance, and the adequacy and fitness of the models are summarized in Table 2. As the results demonstrated, the fitness of the model was highly significant ($p < 0.0001$). According to the multiple regression analysis, the independent variables were related on the basis of a mathematical model describing the ulvan extraction yield (Y) and following a second-order polynomial equation:

$$Y = 40.84 - 1.076X_1 + 0.697X_2 - 0.207X_3 + 2.283X_4 - 0.84X_1X_2 - 1.335X_1X_3 + 1.238X_1X_4 \\ + 1.575X_2X_3 + 2.505X_2X_4 - 2.055X_3X_4 - 6.333X_1^2 - 1.111X_2^2 - 4.526X_3^2 - 4.032X_4^2 \quad (6)$$

where X_1, X_2, X_3, and X_4 are the time, power, water-to-raw-material ratio, and pH, respectively.

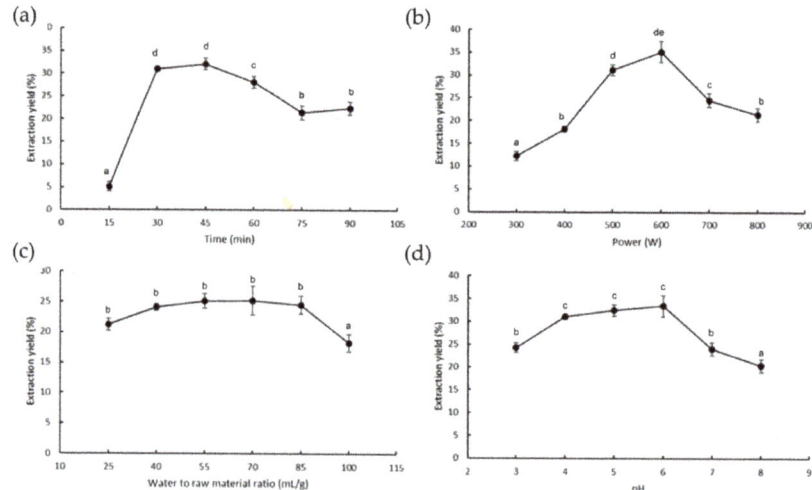

Figure 1. Effect of different times (**a**), powers (**b**), water-to-raw material ratios (**c**), and pH (**d**) on the extraction yield of ulvan. Different letters show statistically significant differences among the groups ($p < 0.05$).

Table 2. ANOVA of the RSM model for the prediction of ulvan yield.

	Source	Sum of Squares	DF	Mean Square	F Value	p-Value
	Model	433.962	14	30.997	49.48	<0.0001 **
	X_1	13.889	1	13.889	22.17	0.001 *
Linear effects	X_2	5.824	1	5.824	9.30	0.010 *
	X_3	0.513	1	0.513	0.82	0.384
	X_4	62.518	1	62.518	99.79	<0.0001 **
	$X_1 \cdot X_2$	2.822	1	2.822	4.51	0.055
	$X_1 \cdot X_3$	7.129	1	7.129	11.38	0.006 *
Interaction effects	$X_1 \cdot X_4$	6.126	1	6.126	9.78	0.009 *
	$X_2 \cdot X_3$	9.923	1	9.923	15.84	0.002 *
	$X_2 \cdot X_4$	25.100	1	25.100	40.06	<0.0001 **
	$X_3 \cdot X_4$	16.892	1	16.892	26.96	<0.0001 **
	X_1^2	128.979	1	213.870	341.38	<0.0001 **
	X_2^2	6.76	1	6.586	10.51	0.007 *
	X_3^2	60.754	1	109.264	174.41	<0.0001 **
	X_4^2	86.726	1	86.726	138.43	<0.0001 **
	Residual	7.518	12	0.626		
Quadratic effects	Lack of fit	7.518	10	0.752		
	Pure error	0.000	2	0.000		
	Cor. Total	441.480	26			
	R^2	98.30				
	Adj. R^2	96.31				
	Pred. R^2	90.19				
	C.V.%	1.37				

* Significant coefficient ($p < 0.05$). ** Highly significant coefficient ($p < 0.01$).

Among the four independent variables studied, only the power and pH exerted a positive linear effect on ulvan extraction. However, the quadratic effects of all parameters negatively affected the extraction process (Table 2). In this study, ulvan yield was significantly influenced by nitrate, time, power, water-to-raw-material ratio, and pH.

The coefficient of determination ($R^2 = 0.9830$) and the adjusted determination coefficient (adj. $R^2 = 0.9631$) for the model exhibited a high correlation between the experimental and theoretical values [24]. In this study, the coefficient of variation (C.V., 1.15%) was no greater than 10%, indicating a high precision and strong reliability of the experimental values. A smaller C.V. is a better expression of low variance than the percentage of the mean [25].

The optimal extraction conditions used to obtain the maximum ulvan extraction yield were determined according to Derringer's desired function methodology [26], with extraction time of 43.63 min, power level of 600 W, water-to-raw-material ratio of 55.45, pH of 6.57, and maximum yield of 41.91%, with a desired value of 0.381. The verification experiments were carried out under the optimized conditions, and the mean values (42.12 ± 0.674%, n = 3) demonstrated the validity of the optimized conditions.

Response surface plots were generated to understand the significant interaction between the variables. Figures 2a and 3a, which show the polysaccharide extraction yield as a function of extraction time and power, showed that the extraction yield increased rapidly with the increase of the extraction time from 30 to 45 min, while it only slowly increased with the increase of power from 500 to 600 W. Time affected the yield more than power. The interaction effects of different extraction times and water-to-raw-material ratios are illustrated in Figures 2b and 3b. Ulvan yield increased linearly at first with the increase of time from 30 to 45 min and of the water-to-raw-material ratio from 40 to 55 but then decreased for further increases of these variables. Figures 2c and 3c show the relationship between extraction time and pH. The yield initially increased quickly reaching its maximum as both time and pH increased and decreased thereafter. Moreover, the interaction between power and water-to-raw-material ratio (Figures 2d and 3d, and power and pH (Figures 2e and 3e) on the yield were shown to be both positive and significant. In Figures 2f and 3f, the yield improved significantly with the increase of pH from 6 to 6.5. However, the interaction between pH and water-to-raw-material ratio on the yield was characterized by a negative coefficient in the fitting equation. In summary, extraction time and pH were the major factors causing significant effects on the yield of polysaccharides.

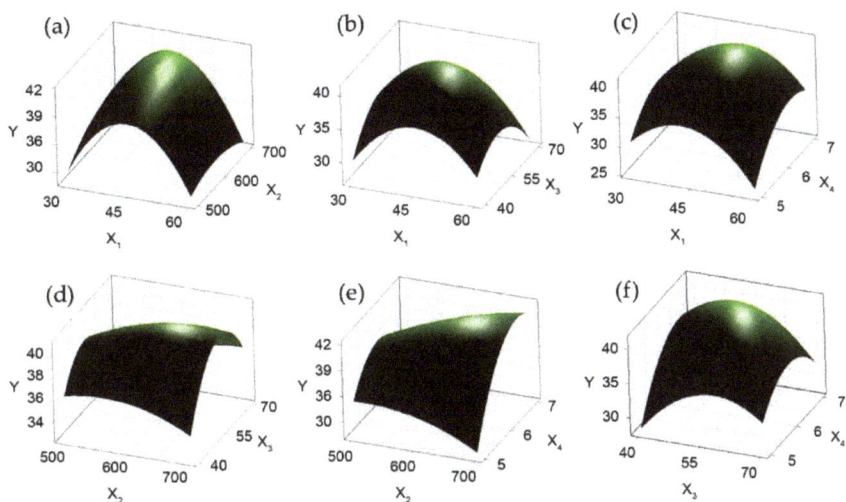

Figure 2. Response surface (3D) showing the effects of variables on the yield of ulvan. Effects of (**a**) extraction time (X_1) and power (X_2), (**b**) extraction time and water-to-raw-material ratio (X_3), (**c**) extraction time and pH (X_4), (**d**) power and water-to-raw-material ratio, (**e**) power and pH, (**f**) water-to-raw-material ratio and pH on ulvan yield (Y, %).

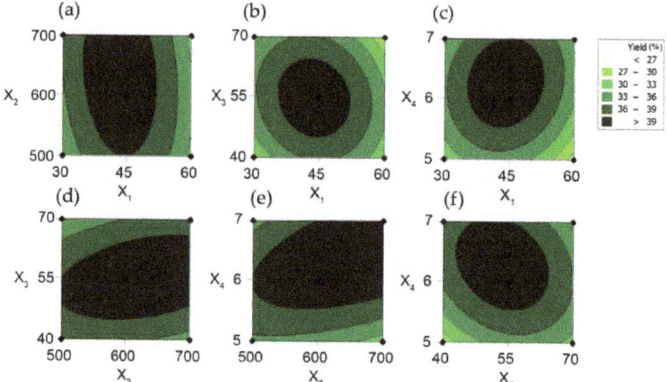

Figure 3. Contour plots showing the effects of the above-mentioned variables on the yield of ulvan. Effects of (**a**) extraction time (X_1) and power (X_2), (**b**) extraction time and water-to-raw-material ratio (X_3), (**c**) extraction time and pH (X_4), (**d**) power and water-to-raw-material ratio, (**e**) power and pH, (**f**) water-to-raw-material ratio and pH on ulvan yield (Y, %).

3.3. FT-IR Spectral Analysis

The FT-IR spectrum of the ulvan extract is shown in Figure 4a. The high absorptions at 874 and 1623 cm^{-1} were attributed to the bending vibration of sulfate in axial position in C–O–S [27]. The specific intense peaks at 3353, 2926, and 1034 cm^{-1} were due to O–H, C–H, C–O stretching vibrations, respectively. The absorption at 1623 cm^{-1} was indicative of C=O [28]. The signal at approximately 1414 cm^{-1} may suggest the presence of uronic acid [16]. In addition, the spectra of ulvan extract obtained by MAE were quite similar to those obtained after autoclaving [27]. Overall, these results showed that the ulvan extract exhibited the typical absorption peaks of a polysaccharide.

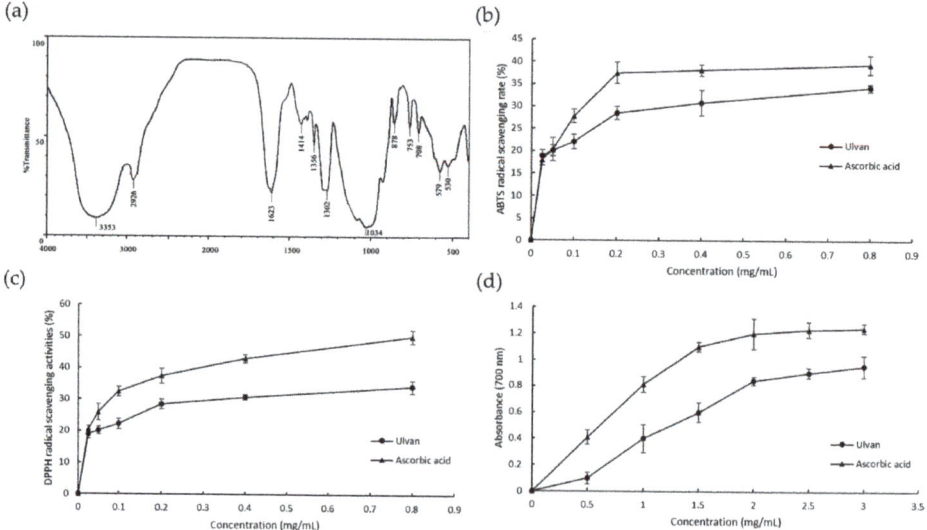

Figure 4. FT-IR spectra and antioxidant activity of the polysaccharide extracts from *Ulva pertusa* by the microwave-assisted extraction (MAE) method (mean ± SD, $n = 3$). (**a**) FT-IR spectra, (**b**) ABTS free radical scavenging assay, (**c**) DPPH free radical scavenging assay and (**d**) Reducing power assay. ABTS: 2,2′-azino-bis(3-ethylbenzothiazoline-6-sulphonic acid), DPPH: 1,1-diphenyl-2-picrylhydrazyl.

3.4. In Vitro Antioxidant Activities of Ulvan

In this study, the scavenging capabilities of different ulvan extracts for ABTS radicals were measured and are shown in Figure 4b. The scavenging capability of ulvan for ABTS radicals was 20.15% at 0.5 mg/L, with a 1.5-fold increase in activity at 0.8 mg/mL. As shown in Figure 4c, ulvan showed a dose-dependent DPPH scavenging effect weaker than that of ascorbic acid at each concentration. The scavenging capability of the polysaccharide increased from 5.61% to 46.51% as the concentration of the polysaccharide increased from 0.025 to 0.800 mg/mL. The reducing power of ulvan is depicted in Figure 4d. The reducing power of ulvan increased with increasing concentrations (0.5–3 mg/mL).

3.5. Effect of Ulvan on RAW 264.7 Macrophage Cell Viability and SOD and CAT Activities

The toxicity of ulvan in RAW 264.7 macrophage cells was evaluated in Figure 5A. An MTT assay demonstrated that ulvan did not significantly affect cell viability at concentrations below 200 µg/mL compared with untreated cells. At the concentration of 400 µg/mL of ulvan, cell viability reduced significantly ($p < 0.05$) (Figure 5A). Ulvan at concentration from 50 to 200 µg/mL showed no cytotoxic effects, thus concentrations in this range were selected for further study.

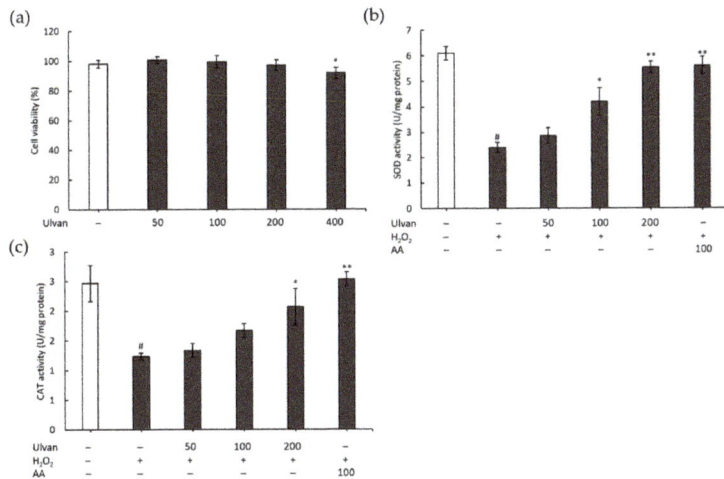

Figure 5. Effects of ulvan (µg/mL) on cell viability (**a**) and production of superoxide dismutase (SOD) (**b**) and catalase (CAT) (**c**) in RAW 264.7 cells. The results are presented as means ± SD ($n = 3$); * $p < 0.05$ and ** $p < 0.01$ vs H2O2 treatment; # $p < 0.05$ compared with control group. AA, ascorbic acid at concentration of 100 µg/mL.

The induction of SOD and CAT was determined to evaluate the antioxidant activity of ulvan in RAW 264.7 cells stimulated by H_2O_2. As shown in Figure 5B, compared with the control group, treatment with 600 µM of H_2O_2 significantly decreased SOD activity ($p < 0.05$). SOD activity was significantly increased after treatment with 100 and 200 µg/mL of ulvan. At 200 µg/mL of ulvan, SOD activity was close to that measured in cells treated with ascorbic acid (positive control) at 100 µg/mL. In addition, CAT activity showed a similar trend to that of SOD activity in cells treated with H_2O_2. However, CAT activity increased upon ulvan treatment at 200 µg/mL. We found that the reduction of SOD and CAT activities in RAW 264.7 cells stimulated by H_2O_2 could be prevented by a high concentration of ulvan (≥200 µg/mL).

3.6. Effects of Ulvan on the Expression of Antioxidant Genes

We examined whether ulvan affected the transcriptional profiles of genes associated with the antioxidant system, such as *GST*, *CAT*, *MnSOD*, and *GPx*, in RAW 264.7 cells (Figure 6). The results showed the downregulation of mRNA expression for these genes compared with the control group ($p < 0.05$) upon treatment with H_2O_2. In contrast, ulvan significantly increased the expression of *GST*, *CAT*, *MnSOD*, and *GPx* compared in the presence of H_2O_2 in macrophage RAW 264.7 cells in a dose-dependent manner.

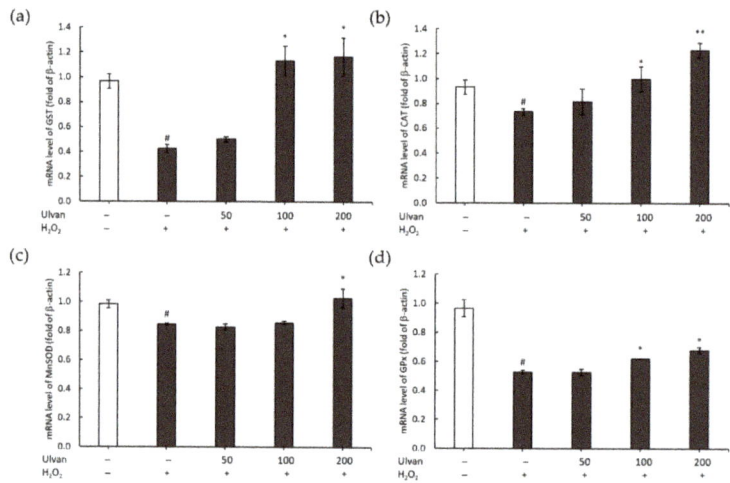

Figure 6. Effects of ulvan (μg/mL) on the expression of the antioxidant genes *GST* (**a**), *CAT* (**b**), *MnSOD* (**c**), *GPx* (**d**) in 264.7 cells treated with H_2O_2. The results are presented as means ± SD ($n = 3$); * $p < 0.05$ and ** $p < 0.01$ vs H_2O_2 treatment; # $p < 0.05$ compared with the control group.

4. Discussion

In this study, we developed an extraction process that allows to obtain high yields of polysaccharides from *U. pertusa* while maintaining their antioxidant effects, as confirmed through functional and molecular experiments. To our knowledge, this is the first study to describe the mechanism of the antioxidant activity of ulvan on RAW 264.7 cells.

A single-factor experimental analysis was applied to select the appropriate conditions and enhance ulvan extraction yields. The microwave power controls the extraction temperature, which is the main parameter influencing water physicochemical properties, thereby increasing the solubility of lowly polar compounds in water [29]. Therefore, four extraction parameters including extraction time, microwave power, water-to-raw-material ratio, and pH were investigated separately. After 45 min of extraction, the extraction efficiency decreased slightly owing to the degradation of the polysaccharides [30]. The diffusion coefficient and solubility of the polysaccharides increases at high temperatures [31] which were achieved using the microwave power control. Moreover, high power causes the disruption of the vegetable cell, which allows the target compounds to dissolve more quickly. However, the structure of the target compound is degraded at high values of microwave power [19]. The degradation of polysaccharides by temperature was reported in different materials such as the roots of valerian [19], *Polygonatum sibiricum* [32], and *Eucommia ulmoides* Oliver leaves [33]. As the water-to-raw-materials ratio continued to increase, the yield tended to decrease. Many studies have reported that a high water-to-raw-material ratio is beneficial for the enhancement of the solvent diffusivity and polysaccharide desorption [26]. However, excess water can absorb the energy in the extraction process, resulting in a lower ulvan extraction yield [34]. The optimal water-to-raw-material ratio to ensure homogeneous and effective heating was determined to be from 40 to 70 mL/g. A possible reason for this phenomenon is that the increase in pH enhances the dissociation of the acidic groups of the polysaccharide, thereby leading to an increase in the polysaccharide solubility in water [35], whereas a decrease of the solubility of the polysaccharide occurs in alkaline solutions [36]. On the basis of the result of single-factor experiments, time, power, water-to-raw-material ratio, and pH were further optimized by RSM using the BBD method to increase the extraction yield of ulvan.

ABTS and DPPH radical scavenging activity and reducing power were determined as reference indicators to evaluate the potential antioxidant activities of the polysaccharide [37]. The antioxidant activity of ulvan depend on many factors, such as the sulfate group, the contribution of the monosaccharides with a variable content of hydroxy and carboxyl groups, as well as the hydrogen donation capability [37]. Ulvan reducing power was weaker than that of ascorbic acid at all concentrations tested. However, it was relatively higher than at the absorption of no more than 0.15 reducing power of *Laminaria japonica* at 3 mg/mL [38]. The antioxidant activity of polysaccharides has been confirmed in other species including *Ulva linza* and *Ulva intestinalis* [39,40]. The antioxidant activity of polysaccharides depends on the degree of substitutions, monosaccharides, and glycosidic linkages [41]. These relations are not always described by linear regression. Wang, Hu, Nie, Yu, and Xie [41] found that DPPH radical scavenging ability of polysaccharides from *Pleurotus eryngii* was improved by an increasing degree of sulfation. Another study also revealed a unlinear regression between the polysaccharides from pumpkin (*Cucurbita moschata*) and the scavenging effects [42]. Lo et al. [43] investigated the relationship between the antioxidant properties of polysaccharides and monosaccharides or glycosyl linkages, using four conventional antioxidant models (conjugated diene, reducing power, DPPH scavenging activity, and ferrous ions chelation) by multiple linear regression analysis (MLRA).

Macrophages are usually employed to evaluate the response to oxidative stress for host defense. Hydrogen peroxide (H_2O_2) is commonly used for inducing oxidative stress-mediated cell injury in various kinds of cells [44,45]. We confirmed that 600 µM H_2O_2 was sufficient to induce oxidative injury in RAW 264.7 macrophages. The present study was designed to investigate whether treatment with ulvan decreased the cytotoxicity caused by H_2O_2 in RAW 264.7 cells and, thus, if ulvan could be proposed as an antioxidant agent. In order to evaluate the protective mechanism of ulvan against H_2O_2 stress in RAW 264.7 cells, we analyzed SOD and CAT enzymatic activities and the mRNA expression of *GST*, *CAT*, *MnSOD*, and *GPx*. In our study, SOD and CAT activities were found to be significantly increased after 24 h of ulvan treatment in RAW 264.7 cells. These results are in line with those of Yan et al. [46], who reported that polysaccharides from green tea could decrease H_2O_2-induced cell death and increase the levels of SOD and CAT in human ARPE-19 cells. Although many studies have shown a strong protective effect of polysaccharides from green and other seaweed [47] and have suggested a correlation between the antioxidant activity of polysaccharides and the expression of antioxidant gene, they did not provide any experimental evidence proving these observations. In this study, the expression of antioxidant genes was also found to increase in a dose-dependent manner. These results indicate that ulvan may upregulate antioxidant enzymes and enhance their enzymatic activity.

5. Conclusions

This study provides an efficient extraction process leading to a high yield of polysaccharides from *U. pertusa* according to an RSM model. An analysis of variance showed that the optimal extraction conditions leading to a yield of 41.91% were 43.63 min with 600 W of power, water-to-raw-material ratio of 55.45, and pH of 6.57. Ulvan extracted from *U. pertusa* showed a strong in vitro antioxidant capacity by increasing the activity of anti-oxidant enzymes. Ulvan provided a protective effect against cytotoxicity induced by H_2O_2 in macrophage cells. This effect was related to the upregulation of SOD and CAT.

Ulvan can be useful as a potential supplement food and reduce the problems in utilizing waste algae from "green bloom". Further studies are needed to understand the relationship between the chemical properties of ulvan and its antioxidant activity.

Author Contributions: Conceptualization, S.S.; Methodology, B.L.; Software, B.L. and K.S.G.; Formal analysis, K.S.G.; Investigation, S.S.; Data curation, K.S.G.; writing—original draft preparation, B.L.; Writing—review and editing, S.H.Y.; Supervision, S.H.Y. and S.S.; Project administration, S.S.; Funding acquisition, S.S.

Funding: This research was supported by the Basic Science Research Program through the National Research Foundation of Korea (NRF) funded by the Ministry of Education(NRF-2017R1D1A1B03035600).

Conflicts of Interest: The authors declare no conflict of interest.

References

1. Wichard, T.; Charrier, B.; Mineur, F.; Bothwell, J.H.; De Clerck, O.; Coates, J.C. The green seaweed *Ulva*: A model system to study morphogenesis. *Front. Plant Sci.* **2015**, *6*, 72. [CrossRef]
2. Liu, X.; Wang, Z.; Zhang, X. A review of the green tides in the Yellow Sea, China. *Mar. Environ. Res.* **2016**, *119*, 189–196. [CrossRef] [PubMed]
3. Sanz-Pintos, N.; Pérez-Jiménez, J.; Buschmann, A.H.; Vergara-Salinas, J.R.; Pérez-Correa, J.R.; Saura-Calixto, F. Macromolecular antioxidants and dietary fiber in edible seaweeds. *J. Food Sci.* **2017**, *82*, 289–295. [CrossRef] [PubMed]
4. Lahaye, M.; Robic, A. Structure and functional properties of ulvan, a polysaccharide from green seaweeds. *Biomacromolecules* **2007**, *8*, 1765–1774. [CrossRef] [PubMed]
5. Tian, H.; Yin, X.; Zeng, Q.; Zhu, L.; Chen, J. Isolation, structure, and surfactant properties of polysaccharides from *Ulva lactuca* L. from South China Sea. *Int. J. Biol. Macromol.* **2015**, *79*, 577–582. [CrossRef]
6. Tabarsa, M.; Lee, S.-J.; You, S. Structural analysis of immunostimulating sulfated polysaccharides from *Ulva pertusa*. *Carbohydr. Res.* **2012**, *361*, 141–147. [PubMed]
7. Qi, H.; Sheng, J. The antihyperlipidemic mechanism of high sulfate content ulvan in rats. *Mar. Drugs* **2015**, *13*, 3407–3421. [CrossRef]
8. Yu-Qing, T.; Mahmood, K.; Shehzadi, R.; Ashraf, M.F. *Ulva lactuca* and its polysaccharides: Food and biomedical aspects. *J. Biol. Agric. Healthc.* **2016**, *6*, 140–151.
9. Athukorala, Y.; Kim, K.-N.; Jeon, Y.-J. Antiproliferative and antioxidant properties of an enzymatic hydrolysate from brown alga, *Ecklonia cava*. *Food Chem. Toxicol.* **2006**, *44*, 1065–1074. [CrossRef]
10. Yaich, H.; Garna, H.; Besbes, S.; Barthélemy, J.-P.; Paquot, M.; Blecker, C.; Attia, H. Impact of extraction procedures on the chemical, rheological and textural properties of ulvan from *Ulva lactuca* of Tunisia coast. *Food Hydrocoll.* **2014**, *40*, 53–63. [CrossRef]
11. Tsubaki, S.; Oono, K.; Hiraoka, M.; Onda, A.; Mitani, T. Microwave-assisted hydrothermal extraction of sulfated polysaccharides from *Ulva* spp. and *Monostroma latissimum*. *Food Chem.* **2016**, *210*, 311–316. [CrossRef]
12. Coste, O.; Malta, E.-J.; López, J.C.; Fernández-Díaz, C. Production of sulfated oligosaccharides from the seaweed *Ulva* sp. using a new ulvan-degrading enzymatic bacterial crude extract. *Algal Res.* **2015**, *10*, 224–231. [CrossRef]
13. Chan, C.-H.; Yusoff, R.; Ngoh, G.-C.; Kung, F.W.-L. Microwave-assisted extractions of active ingredients from plants. *J. Chromatogr. A* **2011**, *1218*, 6213–6225. [CrossRef] [PubMed]
14. Delazar, A.; Nahar, L.; Hamedeyazdan, S.; Sarker, S.D. Microwave-assisted extraction in natural products isolation. In *Natural Products Isolation*; Springer: Berlin, Germany, 2012; pp. 89–115.
15. Prajapati, V.D.; Maheriya, P.M.; Jani, G.K.; Solanki, H.K. Carrageenan: A natural seaweed polysaccharide and its applications. *Carbohydr. Polym.* **2014**, *105*, 97–112. [CrossRef] [PubMed]
16. Fleita, D.; El-Sayed, M.; Rifaat, D. Evaluation of the antioxidant activity of enzymatically-hydrolyzed sulfated polysaccharides extracted from red algae; *Pterocladia capillacea*. *LWT-Food Sci. Technol.* **2015**, *63*, 1236–1244. [CrossRef]
17. DuBois, M.; Gilles, K.A.; Hamilton, J.K.; Rebers, P.t.; Smith, F. Colorimetric method for determination of sugars and related substances. *Anal. Chem.* **1956**, *28*, 350–356. [CrossRef]

18. Bondet, V.; Brand-Williams, W.; Berset, C. Kinetics and mechanisms of antioxidant activity using the DPPH. free radical method. *LWT-Food Sci. Technol.* **1997**, *30*, 609–615. [CrossRef]
19. Hromadkova, Z.; Ebringerova, A.; Valachovič, P. Ultrasound-assisted extraction of water-soluble polysaccharides from the roots of valerian (*Valeriana officinalis* L.). *Ultrason. Sonochem.* **2002**, *9*, 37–44. [CrossRef]
20. Dahmoune, F.; Boulekbache, L.; Moussi, K.; Aoun, O.; Spigno, G.; Madani, K. Valorization of *Citrus limon* residues for the recovery of antioxidants: Evaluation and optimization of microwave and ultrasound application to solvent extraction. *Ind. Crop.Prod.* **2013**, *50*, 77–87. [CrossRef]
21. Mosmann, T. Rapid colorimetric assay for cellular growth and survival: Application to proliferation and cytotoxicity assays. *J. Immunol. Methods* **1983**, *65*, 55–63. [CrossRef]
22. Jung, C.H.; Jun, C.-Y.; Lee, S.; Park, C.-H.; Cho, K.; Ko, S.-G. *Rhus verniciflua* stokes extract: Radical scavenging activities and protective effects on H2O2-induced cytotoxicity in macrophage RAW 264.7 cell lines. *Biol. Pharm. Bull.* **2006**, *29*, 1603–1607. [CrossRef]
23. Yang, S.H.; Le, B.; Androutsopoulos, V.P.; Tsukamoto, C.; Shin, T.-S.; Tsatsakis, A.M.; Chung, G. Anti-inflammatory effects of soyasapogenol I-αa via downregulation of the MAPK signaling pathway in LPS-induced RAW 264.7 macrophages. *Food Chem. Toxicol.* **2018**, *113*, 211–217. [CrossRef] [PubMed]
24. Baş, D.; Boyacı, I.H. Modeling and optimization I: Usability of response surface methodology. *J. Food Eng.* **2007**, *78*, 836–845. [CrossRef]
25. Samavati, V. Polysaccharide extraction from *Abelmoschus esculentus*: Optimization by response surface methodology. *Carbohydr. Polym.* **2013**, *95*, 588–597. [CrossRef]
26. Maran, J.P.; Manikandan, S.; Thirugnanasambandham, K.; Nivetha, C.V.; Dinesh, R. Box–Behnken design based statistical modeling for ultrasound-assisted extraction of corn silk polysaccharide. *Carbohydr. Polym.* **2013**, *92*, 604–611. [CrossRef]
27. Qi, H.; Zhao, T.; Zhang, Q.; Li, Z.; Zhao, Z.; Xing, R. Antioxidant activity of different molecular weight sulfated polysaccharides from *Ulva pertusa* Kjellm (Chlorophyta). *J. Appl. Phycol.* **2005**, *17*, 527–534. [CrossRef]
28. Radzki, W.; Ziaja-Sołtys, M.; Nowak, J.; Rzymowska, J.; Topolska, J.; Sławińska, A.; Michalak-Majewska, M.; Zalewska-Korona, M.; Kuczmow, A. Effect of processing on the content and biological activity of polysaccharides from *Pleurotus ostreatus* mushroom. *LWT-Food Sci. Technol.* **2016**, *66*, 27–33. [CrossRef]
29. Teo, C.C.; Tan, S.N.; Yong, J.W.H.; Hew, C.S.; Ong, E.S. Evaluation of the extraction efficiency of thermally labile bioactive compounds in *Gastrodia elata* Blume by pressurized hot water extraction and microwave-assisted extraction. *J. Chromatogr. A* **2008**, *1182*, 34–40. [CrossRef]
30. Wu, L.; Hu, M.; Li, Z.; Song, Y.; Yu, C.; Zhang, H.; Yu, A.; Ma, Q.; Wang, Z. Dynamic microwave-assisted extraction combined with continuous-flow microextraction for determination of pesticides in vegetables. *Food Chem.* **2016**, *192*, 596–602. [CrossRef]
31. Li, W.; Cui, S.W.; Kakuda, Y. Extraction, fractionation, structural and physical characterization of wheat β-D-glucans. *Carbohydr. Polym.* **2006**, *63*, 408–416. [CrossRef]
32. Zhang, H.; Cai, X.T.; Tian, Q.H.; Xiao, L.X.; Zeng, Z.; Cai, X.T.; Yan, J.Z.; Li, Q.Y. Microwave-assisted degradation of polysaccharide from *Polygonatum sibiricum* and antioxidant activity. *J. Food Sci.* **2019**, *84*, 754–761. [CrossRef] [PubMed]
33. Xu, J.; Hou, H.; Hu, J.; Liu, B. Optimized microwave extraction, characterization and antioxidant capacity of biological polysaccharides from *Eucommia ulmoides* Oliver leaf. *Sci. Rep.* **2018**, *56*, 995–1007. [CrossRef]
34. Xu, Y.; Cai, F.; Yu, Z.; Zhang, L.; Li, X.; Yang, Y.; Liu, G. Optimisation of pressurised water extraction of polysaccharides from blackcurrant and its antioxidant activity. *Food Chem.* **2016**, *194*, 650–658. [CrossRef]
35. Felkai-Haddache, L.; Dahmoune, F.; Remini, H.; Lefsih, K.; Mouni, L.; Madani, K. Microwave optimization of mucilage extraction from *Opuntia ficus* indica Cladodes. *Int. J. Biol. Macromol.* **2016**, *84*, 24–30. [CrossRef]
36. Yang, W.; Wang, Y.; Li, X.; Yu, P. Purification and structural characterization of Chinese yam polysaccharide and its activities. *Carbohydr. Polym.* **2015**, *117*, 1021–1027. [CrossRef]
37. Jia, X.; Dong, L.; Yang, Y.; Yuan, S.; Zhang, Z.; Yuan, M. Preliminary structural characterization and antioxidant activities of polysaccharides extracted from Hawk tea (*Litsea coreana* var. *lanuginosa*). *Carbohydr. Polym.* **2013**, *95*, 195–199. [CrossRef]
38. Wang, J.; Zhang, Q.; Zhang, Z.; Li, Z. Antioxidant activity of sulfated polysaccharide fractions extracted from *Laminaria japonica*. *Int. J. Biol. Macromol.* **2008**, *42*, 127–132. [CrossRef]

39. Zhang, Z.; Wang, F.; Wang, X.; Liu, X.; Hou, Y.; Zhang, Q. Extraction of the polysaccharides from five algae and their potential antioxidant activity *in vitro*. *Carbohydr. Polym.* **2010**, *82*, 118–121. [CrossRef]
40. Rahimi, F.; Tabarsa, M.; Rezaei, M. Ulvan from green algae *Ulva intestinalis*: Optimization of ultrasound-assisted extraction and antioxidant activity. *J. Appl. Phycol.* **2016**, *28*, 2979–2990. [CrossRef]
41. Wang, J.; Hu, S.; Nie, S.; Yu, Q.; Xie, M. Reviews on mechanisms of in vitro antioxidant activity of polysaccharides. *Oxid. Med. Cell. Longev.* **2016**, *2016*, 5692852. [CrossRef]
42. Wu, H.; Zhu, J.; Diao, W.; Wang, C. Ultrasound-assisted enzymatic extraction and antioxidant activity of polysaccharides from pumpkin (*Cucurbita moschata*). *Carbohydr. Polym.* **2014**, *113*, 314–324. [CrossRef]
43. Lo, T.C.-T.; Chang, C.A.; Chiu, K.-H.; Tsay, P.-K.; Jen, J.-F. Correlation evaluation of antioxidant properties on the monosaccharide components and glycosyl linkages of polysaccharide with different measuring methods. *Carbohydr. Polym.* **2011**, *86*, 320–327. [CrossRef]
44. Chun, K.; Alam, M.; Son, H.-U.; Lee, S.-H. Effect of novel compound LX519290, a derivative of L-allo threonine, on antioxidant potential in vitro and in vivo. *Int. J. Mol. Sci.* **2016**, *17*, 1451. [CrossRef] [PubMed]
45. Ma, X.-T.; Sun, X.-Y.; Yu, K.; Gui, B.-S.; Gui, Q.; Ouyang, J.-M. Effect of content of sulfate groups in seaweed polysaccharides on antioxidant activity and repair effect of subcellular organelles in injured HK-2 cells. *Oxid. Med. Cell. Longev.* **2017**, *2017*, 2542950. [CrossRef] [PubMed]
46. Yan, Y.; Ren, Y.; Li, X.; Zhang, X.; Guo, H.; Han, Y.; Hu, J. A polysaccharide from green tea (*Camellia sinensis* L.) protects human retinal endothelial cells against hydrogen peroxide-induced oxidative injury and apoptosis. *Int. J. Biol. Macromol.* **2018**, *115*, 600–607. [CrossRef] [PubMed]
47. Presa, F.; Marques, M.; Viana, R.; Nobre, L.; Costa, L.; Rocha, H. The protective role of sulfated polysaccharides from green seaweed *Udotea flabellum* in cells exposed to oxidative damage. *Mar. Drugs* **2018**, *16*, 135. [CrossRef]

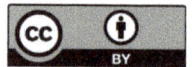

© 2019 by the authors. Licensee MDPI, Basel, Switzerland. This article is an open access article distributed under the terms and conditions of the Creative Commons Attribution (CC BY) license (http://creativecommons.org/licenses/by/4.0/).

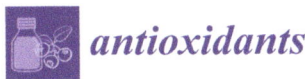

Article

Carotenoid Production by *Dunaliella salina* under Red Light

Yanan Xu and Patricia J. Harvey *

Faculty of Engineering and Science, University of Greenwich, Central Avenue, Chatham Maritime, Kent ME4 4TB, UK; y.xu@greenwich.ac.uk
* Correspondence: p.j.harvey@greenwich.ac.uk; Tel.: +44-20-8331-9972

Received: 18 April 2019; Accepted: 5 May 2019; Published: 7 May 2019

Abstract: The halotolerant photoautotrophic marine microalga *Dunaliella salina* is one of the richest sources of natural carotenoids. Here we investigated the effects of high intensity blue, red and white light from light emitting diodes (LED) on the production of carotenoids by strains of *D. salina* under nutrient sufficiency and strict temperature control favouring growth. Growth in high intensity red light was associated with carotenoid accumulation and a high rate of oxygen uptake. On transfer to blue light, a massive drop in carotenoid content was recorded along with very high rates of photo-oxidation. In high intensity blue light, growth was maintained at the same rate as in red or white light, but without carotenoid accumulation; transfer to red light stimulated a small increase in carotenoid content. The data support chlorophyll absorption of red light photons to reduce plastoquinone in photosystem II, coupled to phytoene desaturation by plastoquinol:oxygen oxidoreductase, with oxygen as electron acceptor. Partitioning of electrons between photosynthesis and carotenoid biosynthesis would depend on both red photon flux intensity and phytoene synthase upregulation by the red light photoreceptor, phytochrome. Red light control of carotenoid biosynthesis and accumulation reduces the rate of formation of reactive oxygen species (ROS) as well as increases the pool size of anti-oxidant.

Keywords: *Dunaliella salina*; microalgae; red LED; blue LED; growth; carotenoids; plastoquinol:oxygen oxidoreductase; photosynthesis

---

1. Introduction

Carotenoids are orange, yellow or red pigments which are synthesized by all photosynthetic organisms for light-harvesting and for photo-protection, and for stabilising the pigment–protein light-harvesting complexes and photosynthetic reaction centres in the thylakoid membrane. They may also be accumulated by some non-photosynthetic archaea, bacteria, fungi and animals for pigmentation [1–3]. Carotenoids are also the precursors of a range apocarotenoids of biological and commercial importance, such as the phytohormone abscisic acid, the visual and signalling molecules retinal and retinoic acid, and the aromatic or volatile beta-ionone [4]. Increasingly sought after as natural colorants, there is accumulating evidence that carotenoids protect humans against ageing and diseases that are caused by harmful free radicals and may also reduce the risks of cataract, macular degeneration, neurodegeneration and some cancers [5,6]. They have also been implicated as the actives for treating diseases associated with retinoids [4].

In most plants and algae containing chlorophyll a (λ_{max} ~680 nm) and b (λ_{max} ~660 nm), photons with a wavelength of 660–680 nm yield the highest quantum efficiencies. However the solar spectrum at the surface of the Earth is at its maximum intensity in the blue and green regions of the visible spectrum (400–550 nm), which is where carotenoids have strong absorption. In photosynthetic organisms in the light, carotenoids drive photosynthesis by transferring absorbed excitation energy to chlorophylls, which have poor absorption in this range. Carotenoids are also able to protect photosynthetic organisms from the harmful effects of excess exposure to light by permitting triplet–triplet energy transfer from chlorophyll to carotenoid and by quenching reactive oxygen species (ROS) [2].

Dunaliella salina, a halotolerant chlorophyte, is one of the richest sources of natural carotenoids and, similar to various members of the Chlorophyceae, accumulates a high content (up to 10% of the dry biomass) of carotenoids under conditions that are sub-optimal for growth i.e., high light intensity, sub-optimal temperatures, nutrient limitation and high salt concentrations. In *D. salina*, the major accumulated carotenoid is β-carotene, which is stored in globules of lipid and proline-rich, carotene globule protein in the inter-thylakoid spaces of the chloroplast (βC-plastoglobuli) [7–10]. The pathway for β-carotene synthesis and accumulation in *D. salina* has been partly mapped out [11,12], but the physiological role and signals triggering its accumulation are not well established. In other members of the Chlorophyceae, such as *Haematococcus pluvialis* and *Chlorella zofingiensis*, high levels of oxygen-rich, secondary ketocarotenoids, astaxanthin and canthaxanthin, also accumulate under high light stress or nutrient stress, often in lipid bodies located outside the chloroplast in the cytoplasm. Accumulation of these may also be accompanied by cell encystment. Lemoine and Schoefs [13] proposed that these carotenoids accumulate as a metabolic means of lowering ROS levels by lowering cellular oxygen concentration, as well as serving as a convenient way to store energy and carbon for further synthesis under less stressful conditions [13,14]. Chemically generated ROS will trigger astaxanthin accumulation [15] and recently Sharma et al. [16] showed that a small dose (up to 50 mJ cm^2) of short wavelength ultraviolet C (UV-C) light (100–280 nm) in cultures of either *D. salina* or *H. pluvialis* massively increased carotenoids accumulation as well as detached the flagellae to increase cell settling, 24 h after exposure: UV-light exposure is typically accompanied by ROS formation.

However in *D. salina* there may be additional mechanisms leading to carotene accumulation. Jahnke [17] for example found that whilst supplements to visible radiation of long wavelength ultraviolet A (UV-A) radiation (320–400 nm) specifically increased carotenoid levels and the ratio of carotenoids to chlorophylls in the closely related *D. bardawil*, neither blue light nor medium wavelength ultraviolet B (UV-B) light (290–320 nm) supplements were similarly effective. In blue light, Loeblich [8] found that green cells of *D. salina* with a low carotenoid to chlorophyll ratio had a relatively depressed photosynthetic activity, which was even more exaggerated in red cells with a high carotenoid to chlorophyll ratio. They proposed that blue light, which was absorbed by the accumulated β-carotene, was not available for photosynthetic oxygen evolution. Amotz et al. [18] on the other hand found a marked photo-inhibition for both red and green cells under high intensity red light, which is absorbed by chlorophylls, but red cells, when transferred to high intensity blue light were seemingly photoprotected. Since the accumulated carotenoids were physically distant from chlorophylls located in thylakoid membranes, Amotz et al. [18] proposed that in high intensity red light, the carotenoids were unable to provide photoprotection against chlorophyll-generated ROS or quench chlorophyll excited states, supporting the argument that carotene globules may function as a screen against high irradiation in blue light to protect photosynthetic reaction centres in *D. salina*. Fu et al. [19] examined the effects of different light intensities of red LED light on carotenoid production in *D. salina*, and showed that the major carotenoids changed in parallel to the chlorophyll b content and that both carotenoids and chlorophyll b decreased with increasing red light intensity and increased with nitrogen starvation.

Light-emitting diodes (LEDs) can be applied to adjust the biochemical composition of the biomass produced by microalgae via single wavelengths at different light intensities [20–23] and recently Han et al. [20] successfully used a low light intensity blue-red LED wavelength-shifting system to increase carotenoid productivity in *D. salina*. In this paper we explore the effects of red, blue and white LEDs on the growth and content of carotenoids and chlorophyll in four different *D. salina* strains under nutrient-sufficient conditions using a temperature-controlled photobioreactor (PBR) favouring growth. We show that in this system, cultivation using red LED was particularly effective in supporting a high rate of carotenoid productivity. We suggest that in strains of *Dunaliella salina*, accumulating carotenoids may be synthesised principally as a mechanism for maintaining cellular homeostasis under conditions which might otherwise lead to over-reduction of electron transport chains, formation ROS and of a hyperoxidant state and ultimately lead to cell death.

2. Materials and Methods

2.1. Strains and Cultivation

Strains *D. salina rubeus* CCAP 19/41 and *D. salina salina* PLY DF17 were isolated from a salt pan in Eilat, Israel. *D. salina* CCAP 19/40 was isolated from a salt pond in Monzon, Spain. Strain UTEX 2538 (*D. salina bardawil*) was purchased from the Culture Collection of Algae and Protozoa (CCAP), Scotland, UK.

Algae were cultured in 500 mL Modified Johnsons Medium [24] containing 1.5 M NaCl and 10 mM $NaHCO_3$ in Erlenmeyer flasks (Fisher Scientific, UK) in an ALGEM Environmental Modelling Labscale Photobioreactor (Algenuity, Bedfordshire, UK) at 25 °C. The cultures were shaken for 10 min at 100 rpm every hour before taking samples to monitor cell growth. Cells were grown under 12/12 light/dark (L/D) with 200 µmol photons $m^{-2} s^{-1}$ supplied by white LED light to exponential growth phase and then dark-adapted for 36 h. After dark adaption, cultures were exposed continuously to blue, red or white LED light at light intensities of 200, 500, or 1000 µmol photons $m^{-2} s^{-1}$. Cultures acclimated to white, red or blue LED light for 24 h were used to monitor the changes in cellular carotenoids after further growth for 24 h in white, red or blue LED light. Cell density of the cultures was determined by counting the cell number of cultures using a haemocytometer after fixing with 2% formalin.

2.2. Pigment Analysis

The composition of pigments was analysed by High-Performance Liquid Chromatography with Diode-Array Detection (HPLC-DAD) (Agilent Technologies 1200 series, Agilent, Santa Clara, United States), using a YMC30 250 × 4.9 mm I.D S-5µ HPLC column (YMC, Europe GmbH) at 25 °C with an isocratic solvent system of 80% methanol: 20% methyl tert-butyl ether (MTBE) and flow rate of 1 mL min^{-1} at a pressure of 78 bar. Carotenoid standards of β-carotene, α-carotene, lutein, zeaxanthin and phytoene were obtained from Sigma-Aldrich Inc. (Merck KGaA, Darmstadt, Germany) and dissolved in methanol or acetone to generate standard curves and DAD scans analysed at wavelengths of 280 nm (phytoene), 355 nm (phytofluene), 450 nm (β-carotene, α-carotene, lutein and zeaxanthin), and 663 nm (chlorophylls). Pigments were extracted from the biomass of 15 mL samples of culture. Samples were harvested by centrifugation at 3000× g for 10 min and pigments extracted after sonication for 20 s with 10 mL MTBE–MeOH (20:80). Samples were clarified at the centrifuge then filtered (0.45 µm filter) into amber HPLC vials before analysis.

Total carotenoids and total chlorophyll in the cultures were measured using a Jenway 6715 UV/Vis spectrophotometer (Cole-Parmer, Staffordshire, UK). Pigments were extracted from the harvested algal biomass of 1 mL culture using 1 mL of 80% (v/v) acetone, then clarified at 10,000× g for 10 min. The content of total carotenoids was calculated from absorbance values at 480 nm according to Strickland & Parsons [25]. Chlorophyll a, b and total chlorophyll content was measured at 664 nm and 647 nm according to Porra et al. [26].

2.3. Oxygen Evolution and Dark Respiration

Samples of cultures exposed to white, red or blue LED light were collected and the rates of O_2 evolution and dark respiration were measured as described by Brindley at al. [27] at 25 °C using a Clark-type electrode (Chlorolab 2, Hansatech Instruments Ltd, Norfolk, UK). O_2 evolution/uptake was induced by white, red, or blue LED light supplied by the manufacturer at a light intensity of 1000 µmol $m^{-2} s^{-1}$. After an initial period of 30 min of dark adaption of 1.5 mL of each culture, the rate of O_2 evolution/uptake was measured for 20 min followed by dark respiration for 20 min. The average rate of photosynthesis was determined from the linear rate of oxygen evolution during 5–15 min of the light period. Dark respiration was determined by following the same procedure, except that the rate was

3. Results

3.1. Cell Growth and Carotenoids Production in Acclimated Cultures

Figure 1a shows that in high intensity blue, white or red LED light, the growth rate recorded as cell density for *D. salina* CCAP 19/41 was the same. There was no significant difference in cell size (data not shown). However the contents of total carotenoids and total chlorophyll depended on the relative proportions of blue or red light supplied. The initial phase of growth in all high intensity light conditions, apart from blue, caused an initial sharp drop in chlorophyll content; the drop was greatest in high intensity red LED light but decreased depending on the relative proportions of red: blue light supplied. On the other hand, cultures maintained in red LED accumulated carotenoids at the highest rate; in blue, the content declined depending again on the relative proportions of red and blue light supplied (Figure 1b,c). The carotenoids/chlorophyll ratio is often used to evaluate carotenogenesis in *D. salina*. As shown in Figure 1d, the ratio increased rapidly with the increasing proportion of red light supplied but remained the same for blue light.

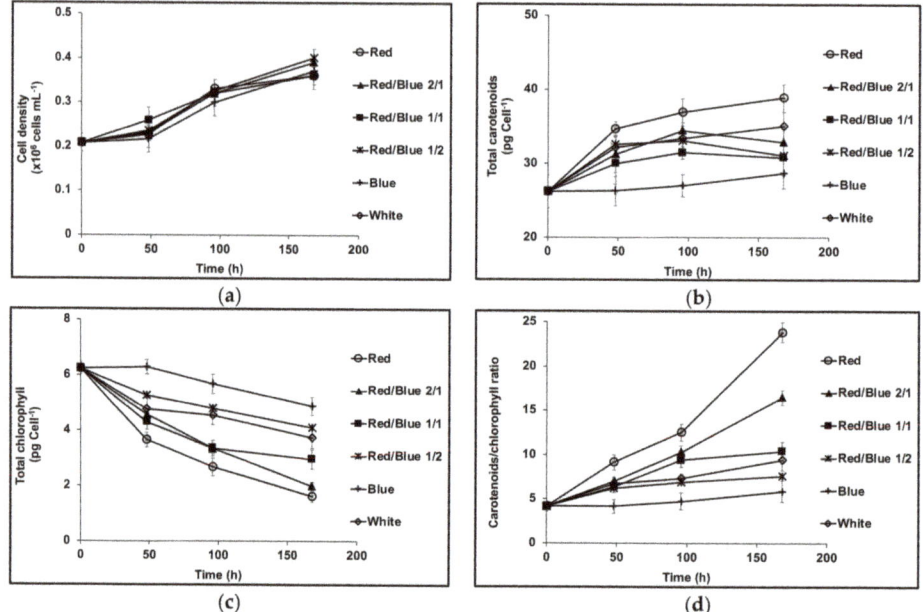

Figure 1. (a) Cell growth; (b) Cellular content of total carotenoids; (c) cellular content of total chlorophyll; (d) Carotenoids/Chlorophyll ratio in *D. salina* CCAP 19/41 grown under different ratios of red and blue light (Red/Blue 1/0, 2/1, 1/1, 1/2, 0/1) or white light with a total light intensity of 1000 µmol photons $m^{-2} s^{-1}$ after dark-acclimation. Each culture condition was set up at least in triplicate.

Different *Dunaliella* strains responded differently to cultivation in high intensity blue or white LED (see Figure 2). All showed a decline in chlorophyll content in white LED compared to cultivation in high intensity blue but only strain CCAP 19/41 showed a significant increase in carotenoid content in white compared to blue light.

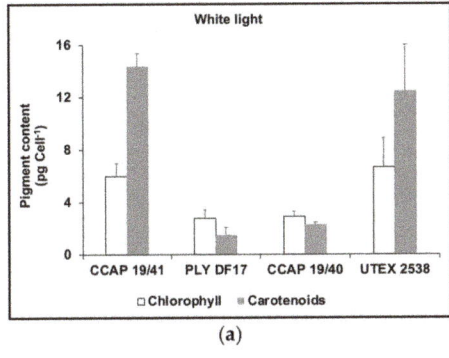
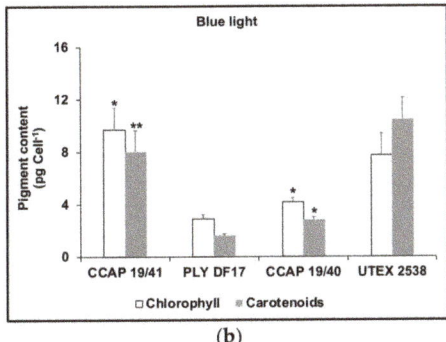

Figure 2. Cellular content of total carotenoids and of total chlorophyll for different *D. salina* strains cultivated each to the mid log phase under either white (**a**) or blue (**b**) light with a total light intensity of 1000 µmol photons m^{-2} s^{-1} after dark-acclimation. Each culture condition was set up at least in triplicate. Results were analysed by one way ANOVA comparing blue light to white light, **: $0.001 < p \leq 0.01$; *: $0.01 < p \leq 0.05$.

Carotenoids in *D. salina* CCAP 19/41 cultures exposed to different light conditions: white, red or blue LED light at 1000 µmol photons m^{-2} s^{-1}, a mixture of white and red (1:1) or a mixture of white and blue (1:1) with a total intensity of 1000 µmol photons m^{-2} s^{-1} for 48 h were extracted and the major carotenoids were identified and quantified by HPLC. Cultures exposed to continuous red LED light had the highest contents of all the identified carotenoids, while cultures maintained under blue LED light showed the lowest content. The difference was mainly due to variation in β-carotene content between treatments: there was no significant difference in relative content of all other carotenoids (Figure 3).

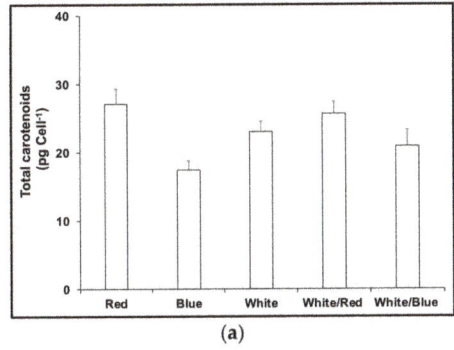
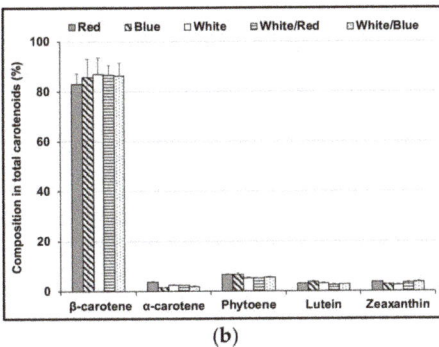

Figure 3. (**a**) Cellular content of total carotenoids; (**b**) Relative composition of major carotenoids characterised by HPLC in total carotenoids in *D. salina* CCAP19/41 cells exposed to continuous LED of different wavelength distribution (red, blue, white, white/red 1:1, and white/blue 1:1) for 48 h. The total light intensity for all conditions was the same at 1000 µmol photons m^{-2} s^{-1}. Results were analysed by one way ANOVA.

The total carotenoids and total chlorophyll contents after 48 h exposure to red or blue LED at different light intensities are shown in Figure 4. Carotenoids accumulated with increasing blue LED intensity between 200 µmol m^{-2} s^{-1} and 1000 µmol m^{-2} s^{-1}. In red LED light, cultures contained high amounts of carotenoids even under low light intensity and the content increased with increasing red LED intensity up to 500 µmol m^{-2} s^{-1}. With further increase in light intensity to 1000 µmol m^{-2} s^{-1}, carotenoids declined slightly (<10% of the value recorded at 500 µmol m^{-2} s^{-1}), but chlorophylls declined 34%. The carotenoids/chlorophyll ratio increased with the increase of light intensity both red and blue LED light, however, under red LED light a much higher carotenoids/chlorophyll ratio was recorded than under blue. Cellular content of β-carotene and phytoene showed a similar trend to that of total carotenoids, except that the highest β-carotene content under red light was achieved at 500 µmol m^{-2} s^{-1}, while the highest phytoene content under red light was achieved at 1000 µmol m^{-2} s^{-1}.

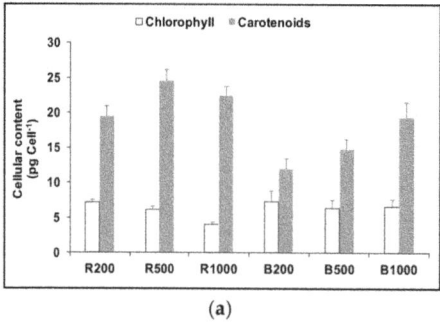 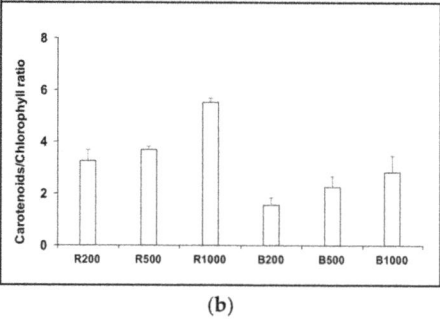

(a) (b)

Figure 4. Cellular content of total carotenoids and total chlorophyll (a) and carotenoids/chlorophyll ratio (b) in *D. salina* CCAP19/41 grown under continuous red (R200; R500; R1000) or blue (B200; B500; B1000) LED light at three different light intensities of 200, 500 and 1000 µmol m^{-2} s^{-1} for 48 h. Each culture condition was set up at least in triplicate.

A phytoene desaturase inhibitor norflurazon known to cause accumulation of phytoene was used to treat *D. salina* cultures maintained under red, blue or white LED light. Figure 5 shows that under these conditions the cellular content of phytoene increased, as expected, but cultures maintained under red LED accumulated a significantly higher amount of phytoene compared to cultures maintained under white or blue light.

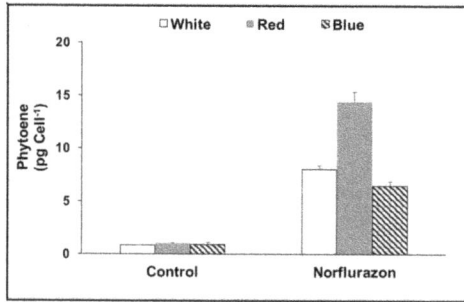

Figure 5. Cellular content of phytoene in cultures treated with no inhibitors (control) or with 5 µM norflurazon. Cultures were maintained under red, blue and white LED light at 200 µmol m^{-2} s^{-1} for 48 h.

3.2. Acclimation and Carotenoids Production in Response to Wavelength Switching

Dark-adapted cultures of *D. salina* CCAP19/41 were cultivated in red, white or blue LED light for 24 h (T0), and then cultivated for a further 24 h in red, blue, or a mixture of red and blue LED light (1:1), or the dark. Blue-acclimated cells produced slightly more carotenoids (14% greater content) when transferred to red LED but chlorophyll content declined from that at the start of the experiment to an amount only 62% of that in continuous blue (Figure 6a). On the other hand the chlorophyll content increased when red-acclimated cells were exposed to blue light, but the total carotenoids content declined sharply, approximately in proportion to the amount of blue LED supplied (see Figure 6b). Red LED cultures maintained for a further 24 h in red LED accumulated 24.5 ± 1.3 pg carotenoid cell^{-1}, but after 24 h in blue LED instead of red, the carotenoid content was 50% lower (11.4 ± 0.4 pg carotenoid cell^{-1}) and less than if they had been transferred to the dark (12.3 ± 0.5 pg carotenoid cell^{-1}).

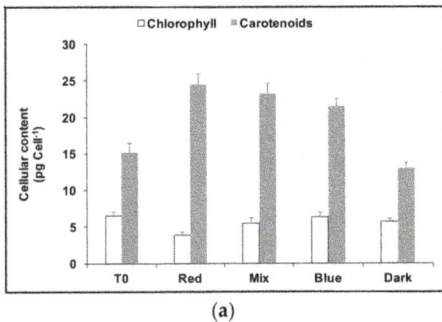
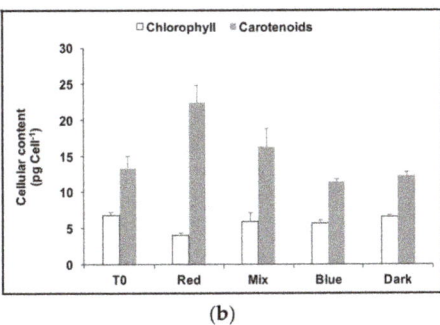

Figure 6. Cellular content of total carotenoids and chlorophyll under continuous blue (**a**) or red (**b**) LED light at 1000 µmol m^{-2} s^{-1} for 24 h followed by 24 h growth under either red light, a mix of 1:1 red and blue light, blue light at the same light intensity of 1000 µmol m^{-2} s^{-1} or dark. Each culture condition was set up at least in triplicate. T0: time point after growth for 24h only, in either blue (**a**) or red (**b**) light at 1000 µmol m^{-2} s^{-1}.

Dark-adapted cultures were cultivated in red, blue or white light at 1000 µmol m^{-2} s^{-1} for 48 h before measuring the rates of oxygen evolution/uptake over a 20 min period with illumination supplied once more by white, red or blue LED lights at 1000 µmol m^{-2} s^{-1} (Figure 7a). Dark respiration was also recorded (Figure 7b). The rate profiles of oxygen uptake/evolution are shown in Figure 8. Red LED supported net oxygen evolution (55 ± 15 nmol O$_2$ h^{-1} µg chlorophyll^{-1}) but on transfer to blue light in the Clark-type electrode, photo-oxidation massively exceeded the rate of oxygen evolution and oxygen was consumed at an exponentially increasing rate (Figure 7a; 222 ± 32 nmol O$_2$ h^{-1} µg chlorophyll^{-1}). Significantly cultures grown in red LED also supported the highest rate of dark respiration (320 ± 17 nmol O$_2$ h^{-1} µg chlorophyll^{-1}, ~2.6-fold greater than that for cultures maintained in either blue or white LED light), but this also declined when cultures were transferred to blue light in the Clark-type electrode. By contrast, cultures maintained in blue LED supported ~3-fold higher rate of net oxygen evolution (141 nmol O$_2$ h^{-1} µg chlorophyll^{-1}) in the Clark-type electrode in blue light, compared to those in maintained in red LED. On transfer of blue light cultures to red light in the Clark-type electrode, the rate of oxygen evolution doubled to 280 nmol O$_2$ h^{-1} µg chlorophyll^{-1} (Figure 7b), and was maintained at a linear rate during the period of measurement. The rate of dark respiration also increased slightly from 123 ± 2.7 nmol O$_2$ h^{-1} µg chlorophyll^{-1} to 175 ± 5.0 nmol O$_2$ h^{-1} µg chlorophyll^{-1}.

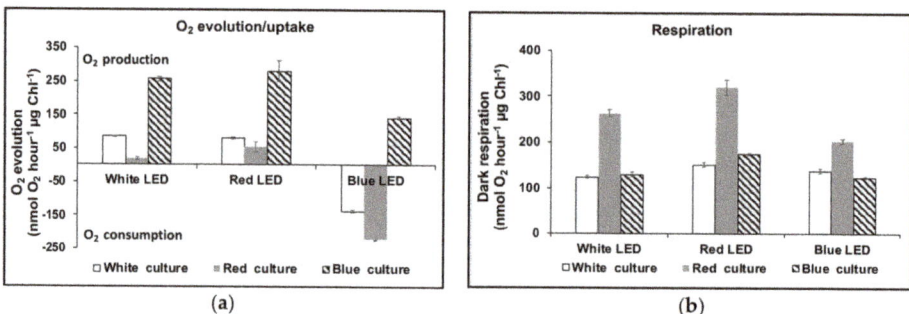

Figure 7. Oxygen evolution/uptake by *D. salina* cultures in different white, red or blue LED light sources (**a**) and in the dark (**b**). Cultures were grown under continuous red, blue or white light at 1000 µmol m^{-2} s^{-1} for 48 h before measurement.

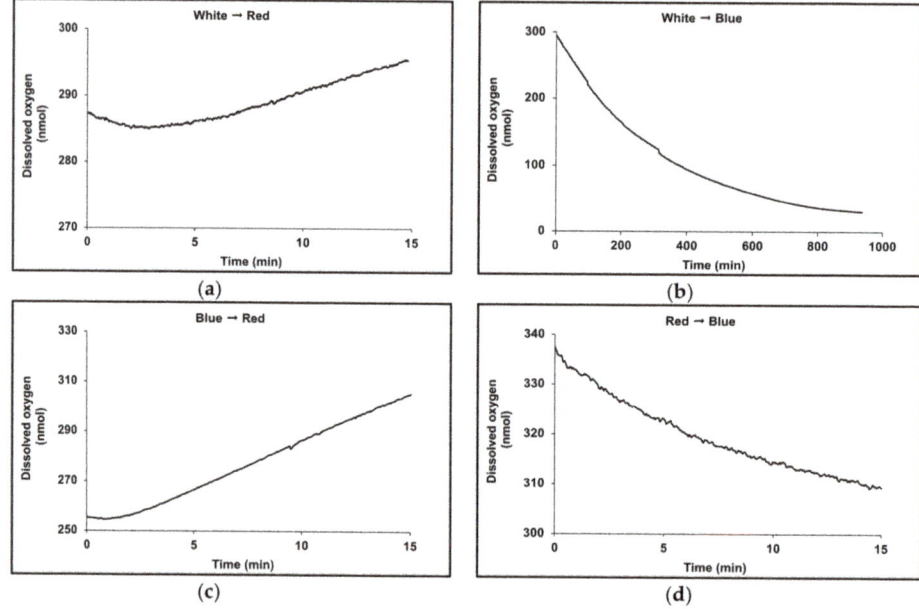

Figure 8. Rate profiles for oxygen uptake/evolution measured with different wavelengths of LED lights measured using a Clark-type electrode for 1.5 mL cultures of *D. salina* CCAP19/41 maintained at 25 °C. (**a**) Red light acclimated cultures measured under blue light. (**b**) Blue light acclimated cultures measured under red light; (**c**) White light acclimated cultures measured under red light; (**d**) White light acclimated cultures measured under blue light.

4. Discussion

LEDs with different wavelengths have been increasingly used to study the wavelength effects on the growth and productivity of photoautotrophic microalgae, and much effort is being invested to understand the most energy-efficient way to incorporate their use for large-scale algal cultivation [20–23,28,29]. In the present work we explored the effects of using red, white, blue and mixtures of red and blue LEDs at different intensities to evaluate the basis for carotenoid accumulation in strains of *Dunaliella salina*.

The emission spectrum of the red LED used in the present work (625–680 nm) emits photons with the exact range required by molecules of chlorophyll a and chlorophyll b to initiate photosynthesis [30]. In *D. salina*, action spectra of O_2 evolution rates show maximum photosynthetic activity within the red absorption bands of the chlorophylls [8]. Photosystems I and II (PSI, PSII), which both contain chlorophyll a, work together in a series of more than 40 steps that proceed with the efficiency of nearly 100% to transfer electrons from water to nicotinamide adenine dinucleotide phosphate in its oxidised form ($NADP^+$) [2]. Consequently the wavelength range of the red LED should be the most efficient emission required for photosynthesis in this alga and deliver the highest specific growth rate. However this also depends on the rate at which the absorbed light energy from any given applied photon flux density is converted to chemical energy: with increasing photon flux density, photosynthesis eventually achieves a light-saturated maximum rate that is limited by the rate of carbon fixation in the Calvin cycle. *Spirulina platensis* for example exhibited the highest specific growth rate using high intensity red LED [28]. *C. reinhardtii* however, showed unstable growth in high intensity orange-red and deep red LED, which ceased completely after a few days and was accompanied by cell agglomeration [22]: agglomeration is typical of oxidant stress and formation of a hyperoxidant state [31].

In the present work, we found that in high intensity red light in conditions of nutrient sufficiency, *D. salina* strains maintained a growth rate at least equal to that in white light or blue LED light, seemingly in contrast with the work of others [8,18,19]. However we also found that some but not all strains accumulated carotenoids rapidly, within 48 h of exposure. Carotenoids are known antioxidants that are synthesized by many microalgae as part of the battery of photoprotective mechanisms necessary to prevent photo-inhibition caused by photo-oxidation of photosynthetic reaction centres [2,32,33]. Photo-oxidation may occur in photon flux density levels that result in absorption of more light than is required to saturate photosynthesis. At the molecular level, when a photon is absorbed by a chlorophyll molecule, it enters a short-lived singlet excited state ($^1Chl^*$): the longer the excitation of $^1Chl^*$ lasts, which increases under saturating light conditions, the greater the chance that the molecule will enter the triplet excited state ($^3Chl^*$) via intersystem crossing. $^3Chl^*$ has a longer excitation lifetime and can transfer energy to the ground state of O_2 to form singlet oxygen, $^1O_2$, predominantly at the reaction centre of PSII and, to a lesser extent, in the light-harvesting complexes. Photo-oxidative damage occurs to the photosynthetic apparatus when species such as $^1O_2$ react with fatty acids form lipid peroxides, setting up a chain of oxygen activation events that may eventually lead to a hyperoxidant state and cell death. Carotenoids may protect the photosystems by reacting with lipid peroxidation products to terminate these chain reactions; by scavenging $^1O_2$ and dissipating the energy as heat; by reacting with $^3Chl^*$ to prevent formation of $^1O_2$ or by dissipation of excess excitation energy through the xanthophyll cycle. It is tempting therefore to suppose that the differences observed by different workers simply reflects differences in carotenoids content between different strains, but this does not explain what triggered the differences in carotenoids content.

In the *D. salina* strain CCAP 19/41, accumulation of carotenoids was accompanied by the highest rate of O_2 consumption and a low rate of net O_2 evolution, which might imply $^1O_2$ formation and ROS accumulation. In the non-photosynthetic, astaxanthin-accumulating yeast, *Phaffia rhodozyma*, artificially generated $^1O_2$ was proposed to degraded astaxanthin to relieve feedback inhibition of carotenoid biosynthesis and also to induce carotenoid synthesis by gene activation [34]. However these authors also found that carotenoid biosynthesis was linked to O_2 consumption by a cyanide-insensitive alternative oxidase, serving to consume oxygen without chemiosmotic synthesis of adenosine triphosphate (ATP). In *C. reinhardtii*, a specific thylakoid-associated, terminal plastoquinol:oxygen oxidoreductase has been identified with homology to the mitochondrial alternative oxidase [35]. The smaller rate of oxygen uptake compared to mitochondrial respiration suggested a function in directly coupling oxygen uptake and the exergonic reaction of plastoquinol oxidation with plastoquinone reduction by a phytoene/phytoene desaturase couple, to permit endergonic carotene desaturation without ATP involvement [35]. In *D. bardawil*, a decrease in oxygen consumption rate coupled to phytoene accumulation caused by norflurazon inhibition of phytoene desaturase also suggests a connection between direct desaturation of phytoene and chloroplastic oxygen dissipation [36].

In the present work, high intensity red light in conditions of nutrient sufficiency maintained growth at the same rate as in blue or white light, and red light also led to carotenoid accumulation albeit to different extents in different strains. These data support involvement of a plastoquinol:oxygen oxidoreductase as originally proposed for *C. reinhardtii* [35], but controlled by red photon flux intensity (see Scheme 1). In this scheme, chlorophyll absorption of red light photons is coupled to plastoquinone reduction in photosystem II, and oxygen reduction is coupled to phytoene desaturation by plastoquinol:oxygen oxidoreductase leading to carotenoid accumulation. Partitioning of electrons between photosynthesis and carotenoid biosynthesis would depend on both red photon flux intensity as well as upregulation of phytoene synthase. The observed increase in O_2 consumption coupled to accumulation of carotenoids via the carotenoid biosynthetic pathway would reduce the tendency for $^1O_2$ formation under high photon flux and maintain cytosolic redox potential.

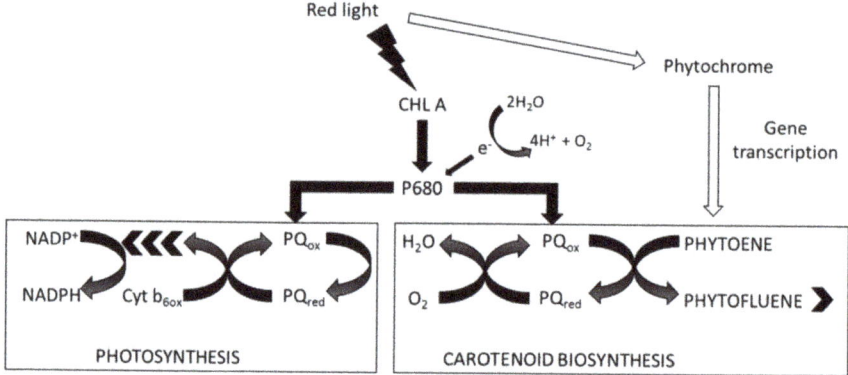

Scheme 1. Partitioning electron flux between photosynthesis and carotenoid biosynthesis. Red photon flux intensity controls the partitioning of electrons either for carotenoid biosynthesis or for photosynthesis, via energy absorption by chlorophyll and the plastoquinone (PQ) pool. Red photon flux density also controls phytochrome regulation of phytoene synthase. CHL A: chlorophyll a; P680: chlorophyll a, primary electron donor of Photosystem II; PQ_{ox}: plastoquinone, oxidised form; PQ_{red}: plastoquinone, reduced form; Cyt b_{6ox}: cytochrome b6f complex, oxidised form; $NADP^+$: NADP oxidised form; NADPH: NADP reduced form.

The coupling of reduction of the plastoquinone pool to carotenoid synthesis driven by chlorophyll absorption of red light may involve the red light photoreceptor phytochrome. Photosynthetic organisms are known to perceive red light signals via phytochrome. The synthesis of phytoene by phytoene synthase is under phytochrome regulation [37–39] and is upregulated by both red and far-red light [37]. Red light also lowers the concentration of the transcription factor PIF1, a repressor of carotenoid biosynthesis [40]. In those strains which do not accumulate carotenoids, alternative mechanisms may serve to consume energy e.g., via NAD(P)H reduction of dihydroxyacetone phosphate to form glycerol [41].

In support of this model, transfer from high intensity red light to blue with higher energy content caused a massive drop in the accumulated carotenoid content, very high rates of photo-oxidation and low respiratory rates. Carotenoids in both the accumulated pool and in the light harvesting antenna, but not chlorophyll, absorb photons in the range 400–550 nm, exactly overlapping the emission spectrum of the blue LED (440–500 nm). Failure of chlorophyll molecules to use the absorbed energy to reduce the plastoquinone pool would be expected to reduce the rate of electron flux through the plastoquinol:oxygen oxidoreductase as well as uncouple carotenoid synthesis and consequently increase cellular O_2 concentration. This would lead in turn to increased ROS formation by reaction of O_2 with reduced electron transport chains, initiating further oxygen radical chain reactions, and carotenoid oxidation. Furthermore, in continuous high intensity blue LED, growth was maintained without carotenoid accumulation, but transfer to high intensity red LED light stimulated a small increase in carotenoid content, once again putting red light absorption by chlorophylls and transfer of absorbed energy to the plastoquinone pool at the centre of carotenoid biosynthesis. Transfer from blue to red light in the Clark-type electrode would cause absorption of more light than was required to saturate photosynthesis; if upregulation of the carotenoid biosynthetic pathway via phytochrome perception was required before coupling with O_2 uptake via the plastoquinol:oxygen oxidoreductase, this would result in initial increase in the rate of photoinhibition and O_2 uptake in the Clark-type electrode, and consequent loss in chlorophyll content, as was observed.

β-carotene accumulation in βC-plastoglobuli has parallels with that for astaxanthin accumulation, serving both as a carbon sink and end-product of an alternative oxygen-consuming biosynthetic pathway that on the one hand, controls over-reduction of photosynthetic (and respiratory) electron transport chains at the same time as removes oxygen from the plastid to limit formation of ROS. It is also able to quench any ROS that form. In blue light it may serve as a screen to absorb excess irradiation [7,18] but clearly offers photoprotection in red light as well. These functions are seen as distinct from its role as an accessory pigment in light-harvesting antennae systems.

Recently Davidi et al. [10] showed that the formation of cytoplasmic triacylglyceride (TAG) under N deprivation preceded that of βC-plastoglobuli, reaching a maximum after 48h of N deprivation and then decreasing. They suggested that βC-plastoglobuli are made in part from hydrolysis of chloroplast membrane lipids and in part by a continual transfer of TAG or of fatty acids derived from cytoplasmic lipid droplets. TAG synthesis represents a pathway for restricting over-reduction of electron transport chains [42] and its recruitment in formation of βC-plastoglobuli is entirely consistent with steps to dissipate excessive energy absorbed by chlorophyll in high intensity red light.

Overall, cultivation with red light may hold potential to enhance carotenoids production in carotenoid-accumulating strains of *D. salina*. Red light treatment has also been reported as an effective way to accelerate ripening of tomato fruit and increase the content of carotenoids [43]. Compared to other commonly used approaches to induce carotenogenesis, such as high light stress, high salt stress and addition of hydrogen peroxide or sodium hypochlorite, the use of red light provides a clean, convenient and economic alternative to promote carotenoids production from *D. salina* in a short time.

5. Conclusions

This study shows that under conditions of nutrient sufficiency, high intensity red light enhanced the production of carotenoids, mostly β-carotene, by upregulating the entire biosynthetic pathway of carotenoids, and that accumulation of carotenoids was accompanied by the highest rate of O_2 consumption and a low rate of net O_2 evolution. The data support a model of flexible co-operation between photosynthesis and carotenoid production via the plastoquinone pool. Chlorophyll absorption of red light photons and plastoquinone reduction in photosystem II is coupled to oxygen reduction and phytoene desaturation by plastoquinol:oxygen oxidoreductase. Partitioning of electrons between photosynthesis and carotenoid biosynthesis depends on photon flux intensity as well as upregulation of phytoene synthase by the red light photoreceptor phytochrome. Red light control of carotenoid biosynthesis and accumulation reduces the rate of formation of ROS as well as increases the pool size of anti-oxidant.

Red light may have industrial value as an energy-efficient light source for carotenoid production by *D. salina*.

Author Contributions: Conceptualization, Y.X., P.J.H.; methodology, Y.X.; formal analysis, Y.X., P.J.H.; data curation, Y.X.; writing—original draft preparation, Y.X., P.J.H; writing—review and editing, Y.X., P.J.H.; supervision, P.J.H.; project management, P.J.H.

Funding: This research received funding from EU KBBE.2013.3.2-02 programme (D-Factory: 368 613870) and from the Interreg 2 Seas programme 2014-2020 co-funded by the European Regional Development Fund under subsidy contract No ValgOrize 2S05017.

Conflicts of Interest: The authors declare no conflict of interest.

References

1. Tanaka, Y.; Sasaki, N.; Ohmiya, A. Biosynthesis of plant pigments: Anthocyanins, betalains and carotenoids. *Plant J.* **2008**, *54*, 733–749. [CrossRef] [PubMed]
2. Hashimoto, H.; Sugai, Y.; Uragami, C.; Gardiner, A.T.; Cogdell, R.J. Natural and artificial light-harvesting systems utilizing the functions of carotenoids. *J. Photochem. Photobiol. C Photochem. Rev.* **2015**, *25*, 46–70. [CrossRef]
3. Rodriguez-Concepcion, M.; Avalos, J.; Bonet, M.L.; Boronat, A.; Gomez-Gomez, L.; Hornero-Mendez, D.; Limon, M.C.; Meléndez-Martínez, A.J.; Olmedilla-Alonso, B.; Palou, A.; et al. A global perspective on carotenoids: Metabolism, biotechnology, and benefits for nutrition and health. *Prog. Lipid Res.* **2018**, *70*, 62–93. [CrossRef] [PubMed]
4. Auldridge, M.E.; McCarty, D.R.; Klee, H.J. Plant carotenoid cleavage oxygenases and their apocarotenoid products. *Curr. Opin. Plant Biol.* **2006**, *9*, 315–321. [CrossRef]
5. Zhang, J.; Sun, Z.; Sun, P.; Chen, T.; Chen, F. Microalgal carotenoids: Beneficial effects and potential in human health. *Food Funct.* **2014**, *5*, 413–425. [CrossRef] [PubMed]
6. Gong, M.; Bassi, A. Carotenoids from microalgae: A review of recent developments. *Biotechnol. Adv.* **2016**, *34*, 1396–1412. [CrossRef]
7. Ben-Amotz, A.; Katz, A.; Avron, M. Accumulation of β-Carotene in Halotolerant Algae: Purification and Characterization of β-Carotene-Rich Globules from *Dunaliella bardawil* (Chlorophyceae). *J. Phycol.* **1982**, *18*, 529–537. [CrossRef]
8. Loeblich, L.A. Photosynthesis and pigments influenced by light intensity and salinity in the halophile *Dunaliella salina* (Chlorophyta). *J. Mar. Biol. Assoc. UK* **1982**, *62*, 493–508. [CrossRef]
9. Lamers, P.P.; Janssen, M.; De Vos, R.C.H.; Bino, R.J.; Wijffels, R.H. Exploring and exploiting carotenoid accumulation in *Dunaliella salina* for cell-factory applications. *Trends Biotechnol.* **2008**, *26*, 631–638. [CrossRef]
10. Davidi, L.; Shimoni, E.; Khozin-Goldberg, I.; Zamir, A.; Pick, U. Origin of β-carotene-rich plastoglobuli in *Dunaliella bardawil*. *Plant Physiol.* **2014**, *164*, 2139–2156. [CrossRef]
11. Lers, A.; Biener, Y.; Zamir, A. Photoinduction of massive beta-carotene accumulation by the alga *Dunaliella bardawil*: Kinetics and dependence on gene activation. *Plant Physiol.* **1990**, *93*, 389–395. [CrossRef]
12. Jin, E.; Polle, J. Carotenoid biosynthesis in *Dunaliella* (Chlorophyta). In *The Alga Dunaliella Biodiversity, Physiology, Genomics and Biotechnology*, 1st ed.; Ben-Amotz, A., Polle, E.W., Subba Rao, D.V., Eds.; CRC Press: Enfield, NH, USA, 2009; pp. 147–171.
13. Lemoine, Y.; Schoefs, B. Secondary ketocarotenoid astaxanthin biosynthesis in algae: A multifunctional response to stress. *Photosynth. Res.* **2010**, *106*, 155–177. [CrossRef]
14. Takaichi, S. Carotenoids in algae: Distributions, biosyntheses and functions. *Mar. Drugs* **2011**, *9*, 1101–1118. [CrossRef]
15. Ip, P.F.; Chen, F. Employment of reactive oxygen species to enhance astaxanthin formation in *Chlorella zofingiensis* in heterotrophic culture. *Process Biochem.* **2005**, *40*, 3491–3496. [CrossRef]
16. Sharma, K.K.; Ahmed, F.; Schenk, P.M.; Li, Y. UV-C mediated rapid carotenoid induction and settling performance of *Dunaliella salina* and *Haematococcus pluvialis*. *Biotechnol. Bioeng.* **2015**, *112*, 106–114. [CrossRef]
17. Jahnke, L.S. Massive carotenoid accumulation in *Dunaliella bardawil* induced by ultraviolet-A radiation. *J. Photochem. Photobiol. B Biol.* **1999**, *48*, 68–74. [CrossRef]
18. Ben-Amotz, A.; Shaish, A.; Avron, M. Mode of action of the massively accumulated β-carotene of *Dunaliella bardawil* in protecting the alga against damage by excess irradiation. *Plant Physiol.* **1989**, *91*, 1040–1043. [CrossRef] [PubMed]
19. Fu, W.; Guðmundsson, Ó.; Paglia, G.; Herjólfsson, G.; Andrésson, Ó.S.; Palsson, B.Ø.; Brynjólfsson, S. Enhancement of carotenoid biosynthesis in the green microalga *Dunaliella salina* with light-emitting diodes and adaptive laboratory evolution. *Appl. Microbiol. Biotechnol.* **2013**, *97*, 2395–2403. [CrossRef] [PubMed]

20. Han, S.I.; Kim, S.; Lee, C.; Choi, Y.E. Blue-Red LED wavelength shifting strategy for enhancing beta-carotene production from halotolerant microalga, *Dunaliella salina*. *J. Microbiol.* **2018**, *57*, 101–106. [CrossRef]
21. Schulze, P.S.C.; Barreira, L.A.; Pereira, H.G.C.; Perales, J.A.; Varela, J.C.S. Light emitting diodes (LEDs) applied to microalgal production. *Trends Biotechnol.* **2014**, *32*, 422–430. [CrossRef] [PubMed]
22. de Mooij, T.; de Vries, G.; Latsos, C.; Wijffels, R.H.; Janssen, M. Impact of light color on photobioreactor productivity. *Algal Res.* **2016**, *15*, 32–42. [CrossRef]
23. Nwoba, E.G.; Parlevliet, D.A.; Laird, D.W.; Alameh, K.; Moheimani, N.R. Light management technologies for increasing algal photobioreactor efficiency. *Algal Res.* **2019**, *39*, 101433. [CrossRef]
24. Borowitzka, M.A. Algal growth media and sources of cultures. In *Microalgal Biotecnology*; Borowitzka, M.A., Borowitzka, L.J., Eds.; 1988; pp. 456–465.
25. Strickland, J.; Parsons, T.R. *A Practical Handbook of Seawater Analysis*, 2nd ed.; Fisheries Research Board of Canada: Ottawa, Canada, 1972; pp. 185–190.
26. Porra, R.J.; Thompson, W.A.; Kriedemann, P.E. Determination of accurate extinction coefficients and simultaneous equations for assaying chlorophylls a and b extracted with four different solvents: Verification of the concentration of chlorophyll standards by atomic absorption spectroscopy. *Biochim. Biophys. Acta Bioenerg.* **1989**, *975*, 384–394. [CrossRef]
27. Brindley, C.; Acién, F.G.; Sevilla, J.M.F. The oxygen evolution methodology affects photosynthetic rate measurements of microalgae in well-defined light regimes. *Biotechnol. Bioeng.* **2010**, *106*, 228–237. [CrossRef] [PubMed]
28. Wang, C.Y.; Fu, C.C.; Liu, Y.C. Effects of using light-emitting diodes on the cultivation of *Spirulina platensis*. *Biochem. Eng. J.* **2007**, *37*, 21–25. [CrossRef]
29. Gordon, J.M.; Polle, J.E.W. Ultrahigh bioproductivity from algae. *Appl. Microbiol. Biotechnol.* **2007**, *76*, 969–975. [CrossRef]
30. Milne, B.F.; Toker, Y.; Rubio, A.; Nielsen, S.B. Unraveling the intrinsic color of chlorophyll. *Angew. Chem. Int. Ed. Engl.* **2015**, *54*, 2170–2173. [CrossRef]
31. Hansberg, W.; Aguirre, J. Hyperoxidant states cause microbial cell differentiation by cell isolation from dioxygen. *J. Theor. Biol.* **1990**, *142*, 201–221. [CrossRef]
32. Erickson, E.; Wakao, S.; Niyogi, K.K. Light stress and photoprotection in *Chlamydomonas reinhardtii*. *Plant J.* **2015**, *82*, 449–465. [CrossRef]
33. Yokthongwattana, K.; Jin, E.; Melis, A. Chloroplast acclimation, photodamage and repair reactions of Photosystem-II in the model green alga, *Dunaliella salina*. In *The Alga Dunaliella Biodiversity, Physiology, Genomics and Biotechnology*, 1st ed.; Ben-Amotz, A., Polle, E.W., Subba Rao, D.V., Eds.; CRC Press: Enfield, NH, USA, 2009; pp. 273–299.
34. Schroeder, W.A.; Johnson, E.A. Singlet oxygen and peroxyl radicals regulate carotenoid biosynthesis in *Phaffia rhodozyma*. *J. Biol. Chem.* **1995**, *270*, 18374–18379. [CrossRef] [PubMed]
35. Bennoun, P. Chlororespiration and the process of carotenoid biosynthesis. *Biochim. Biophys. Acta Bioenerg.* **2001**, *1506*, 133–142. [CrossRef]
36. Salguero, A.; de la Morena, B.; Vigara, J.; Vega, J.M.; Vilchez, C.; León, R. Carotenoids as protective response against oxidative damage in *Dunaliella bardawil*. *Biomol. Eng.* **2003**, *20*, 249–253. [CrossRef]
37. Bonk, M.; Batschauer, A. Light-dependent regulation of carotenoid biosynthesis occurs at the level of phytoene synthase expression and is mediated by phytochrome in *Sinapis alba* and *Arabidopsis thaliana* seedlings. *Plant J.* **1997**, *12*, 625–634.
38. Welsch, R.; Beyer, P.; Hugueney, P.; Kleinig, H.; von Lintig, J. Regulation and activation of phytoene synthase, a key enzyme in carotenoid biosynthesis, during photomorphogenesis. *Planta* **2000**, *211*, 846–854. [CrossRef]
39. Welsch, R.; Wüst, F.; Bär, C.; Al-Babili, S.; Beyer, P. A Third Phytoene Synthase Is Devoted to Abiotic Stress-Induced Abscisic Acid Formation in Rice and Defines Functional Diversification of Phytoene Synthase Genes. *Plant Physiol.* **2008**, *147*, 367–380. [CrossRef]
40. Llorente, B.; Martinez-Garcia, J.F.; Stange, C.; Rodriguez-Concepcion, M. Illuminating colors: Regulation of carotenoid biosynthesis and accumulation by light. *Curr. Opin. Plant Biol.* **2017**, *37*, 49–55. [CrossRef]
41. Xu, Y.; Ibrahim, I.M.; Wosu, C.I.; Ben-Amotz, A.; Harvey, P.J. Potential of New Isolates of Dunaliella Salina for Natural β-Carotene Production. *Biology* **2018**, *7*, 14. [CrossRef]

42. Johnson, X.; Alric, J. Central carbon metabolism and electron transport in *Chlamydomonas reinhardtii*: Metabolic constraints for carbon partitioning between oil and starch. *Eukaryot. Cell* **2013**, *12*, 776–793. [CrossRef]
43. Panjai, L.; Noga, G.; Fiebig, A.; Hunsche, M. Effects of continuous red light and short daily UV exposure during postharvest on carotenoid concentration and antioxidant capacity in stored tomatoes. *Sci. Hort.* **2017**, *226*, 97–103. [CrossRef]

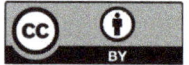

© 2019 by the authors. Licensee MDPI, Basel, Switzerland. This article is an open access article distributed under the terms and conditions of the Creative Commons Attribution (CC BY) license (http://creativecommons.org/licenses/by/4.0/).

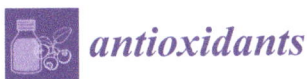

Article

The Long-Term Algae Extract (*Chlorella and Fucus sp*) and Aminosulphurate Supplementation Modulate SOD-1 Activity and Decrease Heavy Metals (Hg^{++}, Sn) Levels in Patients with Long-Term Dental Titanium Implants and Amalgam Fillings Restorations

José Joaquín Merino [1,*], José María Parmigiani-Izquierdo [1], Adolfo Toledano Gasca [2] and María Eugenia Cabaña-Muñoz [1]

[1] Clínica CIROM, Centro de Implantología and Rehabilitación Oral Multidisciplinaria, 30001 Murcia, Spain; jmparmi@clinicacirom.com (J.M.P.-I.); mecjj@clinicacirom.com (M.E.C.-M.)
[2] Department of Neuroanatomy, Instituto Cajal (CSIC), 28002 Madrid, Spain; atoledano@cajal.csic.es
* Correspondence: josem2005@yahoo.es

Received: 16 February 2019; Accepted: 9 April 2019; Published: 16 April 2019

Abstract: The toxicity of heavy metals such as Hg^{++} is a serious risk for human health. We evaluated whether 90 days of nutritional supplementation (d90, $n = 16$) with *Chlorella vulgaris* (CV) and *Fucus sp* extracts in conjunction with aminosulphurate (nutraceuticals) supplementation could detox heavy metal levels in patients with long-term titanium dental implants (average: three, average: 12 years in mouth) and/or amalgam fillings (average: four, average: 15 years) compared to baseline levels (d0: before any supplementation, $n = 16$) and untreated controls (without dental materials) of similar age (control, $n = 21$). In this study, we compared levels of several heavy metals/oligoelements in these patients after 90 days ($n = 16$) of nutritional supplementation with CV and aminozuphrates extract with their own baseline levels (d0, $n = 16$) and untreated controls ($n = 21$); 16 patients averaging 44 age years old with long-term dental amalgams and titanium implants for at least 10 years (average: 12 years) were recruited, as well as 21 non-supplemented controls (without dental materials) of similar age. The following heavy metals were quantified in hair samples as index of chronic heavy metal exposure before and after 90 days supplementation using inductively coupled plasma-mass spectrometry (ICP-MS) and expressed as µg/g of hair (Al, Hg^{++}, Ba, Ag, Sb, As, Be, Bi, Cd, Pb, Pt, Tl, Th, U, Ni, Sn, and Ti). We also measured several oligoelements (Ca^{++}, Mg^{++}, Na^+, K^+, Cu^{++}, Zn^{++}, Mn^{++}, Cr, V, Mo, B, I, P, Se, Sr, P, Co, Fe^{++}, Ge, Rb, and Zr). The algae and nutraceutical supplementation during 90 consecutive days decreased Hg^{++}, Ag, Sn, and Pb at 90 days as compared to baseline levels. The mercury levels at 90 days decreased as compared with the untreated controls. The supplementation contributed to reducing heavy metal levels. There were increased lithium (Li) and germanium (Ge) levels after supplementation in patients with long-term dental titanium implants and amalgams. They also (d90) increased manganesum (Mn^{++}), phosphorum (P), and iron (Fe^{++}) levels as compared with their own basal levels (d0) and the untreated controls. Finally, decreased SuperOxide Dismutase-1 (SOD-1) activity (saliva) was observed after 90 days of supplementation as compared with basal levels (before any supplementation, d0), suggesting antioxidant effects. Conversely, we detected increased SOD-1 activity after 90 days as compared with untreated controls. This SOD-1 regulation could induce antioxidant effects in these patients. The long-term treatment with algae extract and aminosulphurates for 90 consecutive days decreased certain heavy metal levels (Hg^{++}, Ag, Sn, Pb, and U) as compared with basal levels. However, Hg^{++} and Sn reductions were observed after 90 days as compared with untreated controls (without dental materials). The dental amalgam restoration using activated nasal filters in conjunction with long-term nutritional supplementation enhanced heavy metals removal. Finally, the long-term supplementation with these algae and aminoazuphrates was safe and non-toxic in patients. These supplements prevented certain deficits in oligoelements without affecting their Na$^+$/K$^+$ ratios after long-term nutraceutical supplementation.

Keywords: algae; Chlorella; Fucus; detoxification; environmental pollution; antioxidants; heavy metals; selenium; SOD-1; neurotoxicology; aminoazuphrates; clinical medicine; nutrition; neuropathology

1. Introduction

Humans are exposed to pollutants, xenobiotics, and heavy metals that can be accumulated in the body when detox mechanisms are defective. Heavy metals can affect metallothionein and glutathione levels (its reduced form labeled herein as GSH) as well as SuperOxide Dismutase-1 (SOD-1) enzymatic activity [1–4]. Selenium (Se) is a crucial element for heavy metal removal by conjugation with GSH [2]. These xenobiotics can provoke hypertension and other clinical alterations in patients [5,6]. Mercury may cause neurodevelopmental disorders as autism spectrum disorders. Dental amalgams contain 50% of mercury (Hg), 41% of silver (Ag), Tin (Sn: 5–8%), Zn^{++}, and Cu^{++} as minority oligoelements; titanium dental implants contain Ti-6Al-4V alloy [7]. Levels of heavy metals/oligoelements can be measured by inductively coupled plasma-mass spectrometry (ICP-MS) [8] in human samples such as urine, plasma, or hair [9,10]. The toxicity of heavy metals (e.g., mercury, cadmium) depends on the route, the concentration [11], and the exposure time and mixtures of heavy metals [12]. The function of oligoelements in odontology is still little studied (to review its functions, consult reference number [13]).

The increasing concern of health problems associated with environmental pollutants is a serious one in humans because aluminum (Al) [14], lead (Pb), mercury (Hg^{++}), cadmium (Cd), arsenic (As), nickel (Ni), copper (Cu^{++}), iron (Fe^{++}), chromium (Cr), and cobalt (Co) could provoke health problems in the case of heavy metal accumulation [14–16], which could be reduced by microalgae [17]. The occupational exposure to Cd and Hg^{++} are associated with antropometric activities, cremation, plastics, glass, and metal alloys. These heavy metals are also present in electrode material, nickel-cadmium batteries, water, and cigarette smoke [18,19].

Detoxification is the ability to remove drugs, mutagens, and other harmful agents from the body. The detoxification takes place in the intestinal tract, the liver, and the kidneys by microbiota able to chelate several heavy metals [20,21]. For instance, increased blood lead, mercury, and zinc levels were associated with Sarcopenia in the elderly population [6]. In addition, increased hair mercury levels (but not urinary levels) were correlated with the elevated title for the Lupus Eritematose marker in women (nuclear antigen: ANA) [10]. Several metabolic pathways in food-derived compounds are involved in detoxification [21]. Thus, clinical protocols able to prevent heavy metal accumulation are necessary in patients in conjunction with long-term nutritional supplementation. Antioxidants contribute to chelating reactive oxygen species (ROS) by removing heavy metals; thus, the screening of new antioxidants from plants is important from a clinical view point.

Some microalgae can remove heavy metals from wastewater. *Chlorella vulgaris* (CV) is a unicellular marine algae rich in chlorophyll (1–4%) that contains 55–67% protein, 9–18% dietary fiber, minerals, vitamins, and several oligoelements [17,22]. The CV algae are considered to be highly resistant to heavy metals and are widely used as a food supplement in Japan [17,23]. The *Chlorella sorokiniana* can promote antioxidant responses under zinc tolerance by increasing antioxidant enzymatic activities and increasing flavonoids, polyphenols, tocopherols, glutathione, and ascorbate (ASC) levels [24]. The CV extract can also excrete dioxin [25] and remove Cd levels by inducing metallotionein-like proteins. The biosorption of Pb^{2+} and Cd^{2+} have been described on a fixed bed column with immobilized Chlorella algae biomass [26]. *Chlorella prototothecoides* algae promote heavy metal detoxification in chlordecone poisoned-treated rats by reducing the half-life of the toxin from 40 to 19 days. In addition, the *Fucus spiralis* is a marine brown alga (spiral wrack) that contains phlorotannins (antioxidant) [22].

The phytochelatins are short produced peptides from plants, algae, and fungi in response to heavy metal exposure, which detoxificate heavy metals by its high cysteine-content. *Fucus versiculosus* also may chelate Zn^{++} [22,27]. Phytochelatins are a natural source of novel angiotensin-I converting enzyme (ACE) inhibitors [28].

Our hypothesis is that the use of nasal filters (active carbon) in conjunction with long-term algae extract (*Chlorella and Fucus sp*) and aminosulphurates supplementation for 90 consecutive days contributes to the removal of heavy metals (Hg^{++}, Ag, Sn, Pb) in patients with long-term dental titanium implants and amalgam fillings restorations.

2. Aim

We evaluated whether dietary chronic supplementation with CV and aminoazuphrates during 90 consecutive days could contribute to detoxificating heavy metals and/or prevent certain oligoelement deficits in patients with long-term dental titanium implants and amalgam fillings restorations. Therefore, the study was conducted to investigate whether long-term dietary CV contributed to the prevention of heavy metal accumulation after 90 days of supplementation (d90) in patients with long-term dental titanium implants and amalgam fillings restorations as compared with their own baseline levels (before any nutritional supplementation: d0) as well as untreated controls (without dental materials).

3. Materials and Methods

3.1. Patients

All selected patients were 49–68 years old (average: 58.5 years). The percentage of smokers was 7%, and their sociocultural states were medium-high levels (higher school education: 70%). Similar untreated (non-supplemented) control patients were included in this study. Their average age was similar to the rest of the patients. These untreated controls did not receive nutritional supplementation with the formulations. They did not have dental materials in their mouths ($n = 21$ controls).

The average number of dental amalgam fillings was 4, and there were 3 dental titanium implant alloys on average. All selected patients had a dental filling at least 10 years in their mouths (average: 15 years) and long-term titanium dental alloys for at least 10 years as well (average: 12 years). We selected 16 patients who had at least two or more long-term dental amalgams.

The number of enrolled patients suitable according to inclusion criteria was 21 untreated controls as well as 16 patients.

They received nutritional algae extracts (*Chlorella/Fucus sp*) and aminoazuphrates supplementation during 90 consecutive days (d90). Their heavy metal/oligoelement levels were compared at day 90 (d90, $n = 16$) with their basal levels (d0: before any supplementation, baseline, $n = 16$) as well as untreated controls (without dental materials in mouth, $n = 21$). These controls did not receive supplementation.

Their dental amalgams fillings were progressively replaced by composites (bisphenol A free) every 20 days following a clinical safe protocol by using active carbon filters ([@]InspiraHealth, Barcelona, Spain) and nutritional supplementation [29]. There are four quadrants in the mouth, and these amalgams were progressively replaced by each quadrant (each session within 20 days). Thus, some patients still had dental fillings during the 90 consecutive days of supplementation before their complete removal. The patients took supplements by oral intake (formulations) from the beginning (day 0, baseline levels) until the end of supplementation (d90: 90 consecutive days). We also compared levels of heavy metals/oligoelements after 90 days of supplementation with untreated controls (control, $n = 21$) and baseline levels (day zero, d0: before any supplementation). The nutritional supplementation took place during the time of dental amalgam restoration by composites. It is noteworthy that all dental materials were progressively replaced by composites at the time of collecting hair samples (90 days of supplementation). The fish consumption was 1–2 times per week in all recruited patients, including the controls. The basal heavy metals/oligoelements levels were taken at the initial visit to the dental clinic (CIROM: Centro de Implantología y Rehabilitación Oral Multidisciplinaría, https://clinicacirom.com/) before taking any nutritional supplementation, which were termed d0 (day 0) patients in the present study.

All supplemented patients received nutritional treatment by oral intake during 90 consecutive days with the following formulations: GREEN-FLOR (2-0-2; 4 capsules/day: *Chlorella and Fucus* algae extract), ERGYTAURINE (1-0-1; 2 capsule/day), and ERGYLIXIR formulations (Laboratorios Nutergia) during 90 consecutive days [from the initial day that patients visited the dental clinic (day 0) until the end of nutritional supplementation (d90: day 90)]. Controls without dental materials did not receive these treatments.

All ICP-MS heavy metal or oligoelements data were evaluated as percentiles (median, 25% and 75%) for non-parametric data (Kruskal-Wallis) and expressed as µg/g of hair in all cases (except vadanium). The ANOVA (analysis of variance) evaluated differences for vanadium levels, which were expressed as mean values ± standard error media (S.E.M). S.E.M was the variance divided by root square, and n was the size simple. The size sample was $n = 16$ patients at d90 and d0 and $n = 21$ untreated controls; the following heavy metals and oligoelements, respectively, were quantified by ICP-MS in the hair samples (Al, Hg^{++}, Ba, Sn, Ag, Sb, As, Be, Bi, Cd, Pb, Pt, Tl, Th, U, Ni, Sn, Ti); (Ca^{++}, Mg^{++}, Na^+, K^+, Cu^{++}, Zn^{++}, Mn^{++}, Cr, V, Mo, B, I, P, Se, Sr, P, Co, Fe, Ge, Rb, Zr).

These heavy metal/oligoelements were compared after 90 days of nutritional supplementation (d90) with their own basal levels (d0: before any supplementation) as well as untreated controls without dental materials (control, $n = 21$, non-supplemented). These untreated controls did not receive supplements and they did not carry dental materials. Saliva samples were taken at these study times for SOD-1 determination.

The limitation of the present study was the size sample (pilot study) and the absence of a placebo group. However, we included untreated controls (without dental materials and non-supplemented). This placebo group in patients with long-term dental implants and amalgam fillings could be not ethically justifiable since it is not possible to keep dental amalgam fillings, which release mercury in patients [9]. The implementation of this protocol in the Caucasian population (Spaniards) was the other limitation.

A dentist assessed 152 interviews or call phones to select potentially eligible patients. There were 35 patients who declined to participate and 30 patients who did not meet the inclusion criteria. We also excluded patients with fish consumption higher than 2 times by week. We did not enroll patients with periodontal disease or metabolic alterations. Thus, we selected 40 patients, and 37 participated in the end, which comprised the untreated controls ($n = 21$) and the baseline patients [before taking supplements (d0, $n = 16$) and after 90 days of nutritional supplementation (d90, $n = 16$), see study groups in Figure 1]. All statistical analyses were evaluated in 37 patients and 53 hair samples for each heavy/metal oligoelement determination here.

3.2. Inclusion Criteria

This study followed the Declaration of Helsinki (1974, updated 2000), and it was approved by the Institutional Review Board from CIROM (Murcia, #2016/014). All subjects were properly instructed by signing the appropriate consent paperwork. In addition, all efforts were made to protect patient privacy and anonymity. The CIROM Center was approved and certified by AENOR Spain (Spain; CIROM CERTIFICATE for dentist services, CD-2014-001 number; ER-0569/2014 following UNE-EN ISO 9001: 2008 as well as UNE 179001-2001 Directive from Spain). We selected 16 patients who had at least two or more long-term dental amalgams. They had long-term dental amalgam fillings for at least 10 years in their mouths (average: 15 years) and long-term titanium dental implants for at least 10 years (average: 12 years). The fish consumption was 1-2 times per week in all recruited patients. The average number of dental amalgam fillings was 4, and the average number of dental titanium implant alloys was 3.

Controls were selected after clinical examination. They did not have dental materials in their mouths, nor did they show signs of periodontal diseases. We excluded patients who had fish consumption higher than 2 times by week.

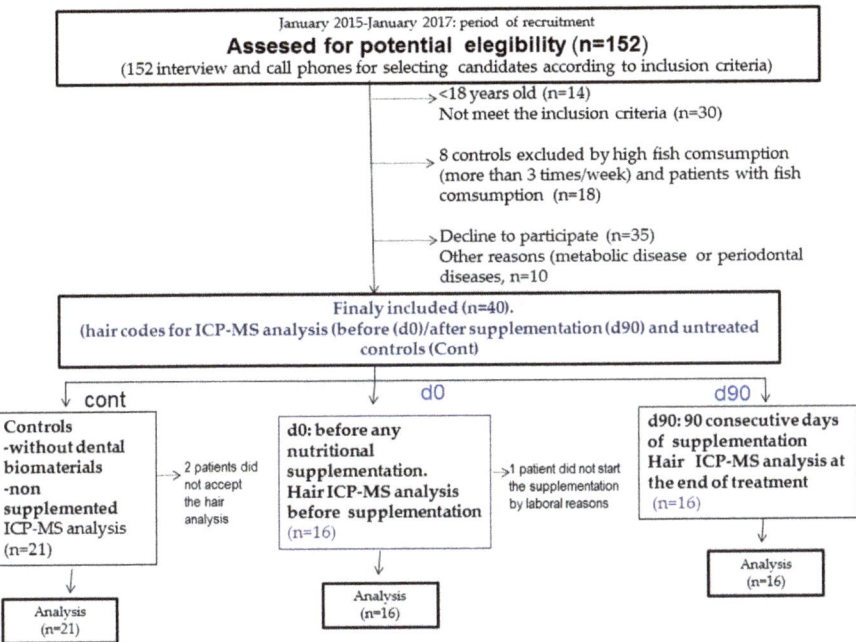

Figure 1. Study groups.

3.3. Exclusion Criteria

Physically handicapped patients who had metabolic diseases [diabetes, metabolic syndrome, liver/kidney disease, systemic inflammation, lupus/autoimmune disease, thyroid disease, adrenal disease, or neuropsychiatry disorders Diagnostic and Statistical manual of Mental disorders (4th Edition, DSM IV)] [30], were excluded in the present study. Patients taking regular medication or stimulants, anticonvulsants, atypical antipsychotic drugs, or those who had history of liver/kidney disease or DMSA (dimercaptosuccinic acid) prescribed (or chelators) patients were also excluded. Particularly, hypertensive patients and those who had periodontal disease tattoos or were taking nutritional supplements were excluded in the present study. Finally, patients who had orthodontic devices were not included here. The correct diagnostic of periodontal disease was based on several parameters, such as visual exploration (palpation), presence of dental calculus, radiographic evaluation, dental mobility, and oclusal exploration (pathological eroding facets). Periodontal disease was also a cause of exclusion, which was identified by following several criteria by an expert dentist, such as a deep dental probe higher than 3 mm, loss of bone (radiography), possible bleeding, and dental mobility [31].

3.4. Composition of Nutritional Supplementation (Algae and Other Bioactive Phytomolecules)

All patients took the following nutritional supplementation during 90 consecutive days (oral intake): GREEN-FLOR (2-0-2), ERGYTAURINE (1-0-1), and ERGYLIXIR formulation (Nutergia, 1 bottle/month) following the patterns of their antioxidants properties (see Table 1). The controls of the intakes were registered by dentists every 20 days, and we administered the following dosages according our previous clinical experience.

Table 1. Composition (nutraceuticals) of formulations.

GREEN-FLOR (Formulation-1)	
Nutritional supplementation during 90 consecutive days (4 capsules/day 2-0-2)	dosage (mg/day)
Chlorella: 80 mg/capsule	320 mg/day
Spirulina: 80 mg/capsule	320 mg/day
Kelp of Pacific: 60 mg/capsule	240 mg/day
Fucus: 30 mg/capsule	120 mg/day
Cardille: 25 mg/capsule	100 mg/day
Pectine of apple: 60 mg/capsule	240 mg/day
Acerole (rich in vitamin C): 50 mg/capsule	200 mg/day
Fructooligosacarides: 280 mg	1120 mg/day
Scolymus hispanicus: 60 mg/capsule	240 mg/day
ERGYTAURINE (Formulation-2)	
Treatment: 90 consecutive days (2 capsules/day; 1-0-1)	dosage (mg or µg/day)
Selenium (Se): 25 µg/capsule	50 µg/day
Vitamin B6: 0.8 µg/capsule	1.6 µg/day
Folic Acid (B-9): 100 µg/capsule	200 µg/day
Zinc (Zn++): 3.5 mg/capsule	50 µg/day
Taurine: 120 mg/capsule	240 mg/day
Extract of *Raphanus niger L.* 15 mg/capsule	30 mg/day
ERGYLIXIR (Formulation-3)	
Extracts from:	dosage: mg/month
Cynara scolymus (artichoe)	1440 mg
Raphanus niger	900 mg
Taraxacum officinale	400 mg
Arctium lappa	320 mg
Vaccinium macrocarpo	228 mg
Solidago virgaurea	200 mg
Rosmarinus officinalis	640 mg
Sambucus niger (elderberry: antocianines)	200 mg
Sodium Moligdate	50 µg
Selenium	50 µg

3.5. Inductible Coupled Mass Spectromery Analysis (ICP-MS)

In the weight of the dental amalgam fillings, mercury (Hg) was 50%, and silver (Ag) was 41%, Sn was approximately 5–8%, and Cu^{++} and Zn^{++} levels were in the minority. Hair samples close to the scalp were taken from all subjects (0.25 g from the occipital area) to measure a plethora of heavy metals/oligoelements by ICP-MS (Doctor's Data, USA). Doctor's Data is a pioneer laboratory specializing in the toxicology of heavy metals with over 35 years of experience, and they provide analytical tests for healthcare practitioners. ICP-MS values for heavy metals were expressed in µg/g of hair.

3.6. Super Oxide Dismutase-1 (SOD-1 Activity)

The saliva SOD-1 activity was measured following a modified protocol by [9] Cabaña-Muñoz et al., 2015. Briefly, the buffer assay contained 0.1 mM EDTA (Ethylenediaminetetraacetic acid), 50 mM sodium carbonate, and 96 mM of nitro blue tetrazolium (NBT). Then, 470 µL of the above mixture was added to 100 µL of saliva, and the auto-oxidation of hydroxylamine was observed by adding 0.05 mL of hydroxylamine hydrochloride (pH 6.0). Finally, SOD-1 activity was measured by the change in optical density at 560 nm for 2 min at 30/60 s intervals and normalized as optical density (D.O) by protein [9].

3.7. Statistical Analysis

All data were analyzed by SPSS software (v17.0) (U.C.M: Universidad Complutense, Madrid, Spain) and Sigma Plot (v11.0, U.C.M, Madrid, Spain). Mean 25%, 75%, and median values (µg/g of hair) were estimated for heavy metals/oligoelements in the hair samples. Non-parametric tests were applied in cases without homogeneity of variance (Mann Whitney/Kruskal Wallis). The Bonferroni tests were applied for multiple comparisons when there was homogeneity of variance (e.g., vanadium, V). All results were expressed as percentiles 25%, 75%, and median (µg/g of hair) according to Kruskal Wallis values (H value) and Mann Whitney (MW) and Dunn's post hoc test in the case of non-parametric data between (d0: $n = 16$, d90: $n = 16$) and controls (control: $n = 21$). The Levene test identified whether or not there was homogeneity of variance depending on its significance. Correlations between variables were performed by Spearman's rank correlation. Differences were considered statistically significant if $p < 0.05$ and highly significant when $p < 0.01$.

4. Results

4.1. SOD-1 Activation Reflects Antioxidants Responses in Patients after Long-Term Supplementation with Algae Extract and Aminoazuphrates Compared with Untreated Controls

There was a statistically significant effect for SOD-1 activity in the Kruskal Wallis analysis (H = 45.1, $p \leq 0.001$) for SOD-1 activity (saliva). The parametric Dunn's non-analysis revealed decreased SOD-1 activity after 90 days of supplementation (d90) compared to their basal levels (d0: before any supplementation, $p < 0.05$); Conversely, increased activity SOD-1 activity was detected before any supplementation as compared with untreated controls (without dental materials, $p < 0.05$, Table 2).

Table 2. Regulation of SuperOxide Dismutase-1 (SOD-1) by long-term algae and aminosulphurate supplementation and SOD-1 activity.

Group	Median	25%	75%
SOD-1 activity (control)	100	100	100
SOD-1 activity (d0)	143.5	139.500 *	149
SOD-1 activity (d90)	121	119.000 *,#	125
SOD-1 Activity	**Difference of Ranks**	**Q**	**$p < 0.05$?**
Control vs. d0 (before treatment)	34.000	6.7	Yes
d0 vs. d90 (after 90 days)	16.000	2.920	Yes
d90 vs. Cont: controls	18.500	3.600	Yes

* $p < 0.05$ vs. control, # $p < 0.05$ d90 vs. d0; control: controls without dental materials and non-supplemented ($n = 21$); d0: patients with long-term titanium implants and dental amalgam fillings restorations before any nutritional supplementation (d0, $n = 16$); d90: patients with long-term titanium implants and dental amalgam fillings restorations after 90 days of supplementation (d90, $n = 16$).

4.2. Reduced Mercury (Hg^{++}) and Silver (Ag) Levels after 90 Days of Nutritional Supplementation (d90) as Compared with Their Baseline Levels (d0) as ell as Untreated Controls (Without Dental Materials and non Supplemented, cont)

We compared levels of heavy metals (Hg^{++}, Ag, Sn) as well as titanium alloys (Ti-6Al-4V) in patients with long-term dental titanium implants and amalgams fillings after 90 days of nutritional supplementation as compared with their own basal levels (before any supplementation, d0) as well with non-supplemented controls (without dental materials, controls). The Kruskal Wallis and Mann Whitney post hoc analyses revealed mercury (Hg^{++}) and tin (Sn) reductions after 90 days of supplementation as compared with their own basal levels (d0) without reaching a significant effect in Zn^{++}, Co, Ni, or Cu^{++} levels (Table 3).

Finally, Ag levels decreased after 90 days as compared to their basal levels (d0, before any supplementation) without reaching a significant effect as compared to untreated the controls.

The aluminium (Al) levels decreased after 90 days of supplementation (d90) as compared with untreated controls ($p < 0.05$); increased d90 vanadium (V) levels were observed as compared with basal levels (d0, $p < 0.05$). There were no effects in Ti or Co levels by treatment ($p > 0.05$, non-supplemented, Table 3).

Table 3. Heavy metals/oligoelements of dental materials.

Heavy Metals from Dental Amalgams				
Hg++	**Median**	**25%**	**75%**	**H**
Control	1.6	1.25	2.3	$H = 13.85, p < 0.001$.
d0	1.9	1.9	3.7 *	MW (* $p < 0.005$).
d90	1.15	0.34	2.1 *,#	MW (# d90 vs. d0, $p = 0.049$); * $p < 0.05$ d90 vs. Cont
Ag	**Median**	**25%**	**75%**	**H**
Control	0.03	0.02	0.06	$H = 9.3, p = 0.01$.
d0	0.1	0.03	0.155 #	MW (* $p = 0.005$ d0 vs. control). (# d90 vs. d0, $p = 0.031$)
d90	0.055	0.025	0.075	
Sn	**Median**	**25%**	**75%**	**H**
Control	0.045	0.02	0.095	$H = 6.27, p = 0.43$.
d0	0.11	0.04	0.20 *	MW (* d0 vs. Cont, $p = 0.023$).
d90	0.03	0.02	0.105 #	MW (# d90 vs. d0, $p = 0.047$).
Zn++	**Median**	**25%**	**75%**	**H**
Control	195	180	230	$H = 5, p = 0.078$
d0	245	208	275 *	MW (* $p < 0.05$ d0 vs. control).
d90	210	180	242	
Cu++	**Median**	**25%**	**75%**	**H**
Control	13.5	10.5	35.5	$H = 1.01, p = 0.6$, n.s
d0	15	11	31	
d90	13.5	10	19.5	
Materials from Dental Titanium Alloys (Cr, Ni, Co)				
Al	**Median**	**25%**	**75%**	**H**
Control	2.9	2.05	5.6	$H = 4.6, p = 0.1$, n.s.
d0	3	1.6	4.6	
d90	1.6	1.5	2.4 *	MW (* d90 vs. control, $p = 0.029$).
Cr	**Median**	**25%**	**75%**	**H**
Control	0.35	0.31	0.39	$H=9.64, p = 0.008$
d0	0.35	0.35	0.39	
d90	0.41	0.36	0.45 *,#	MW or Dunn's.* $p < 0.05$ vs. cont, # $p < 0.05$ d90 vs. d0
Co	**Median**	**25%**	**75%**	**H**
Control	0.004	0.004	0.010	$H = 4.97, p = 0.083$, n.s.
d0	0.017	0.04	0.035 *	MW * $p < 0.05$ d0 vs. control.
d90	0.06	0.035	0.012	

Table 3. Cont.

Ni	Median	25%	75%	H
Control	0.055	0.04	0.10	$H = 3.07, p = 0.21$, n.s.
d0	0.09	0.08	0.16 *	MW (* $p < 0.05$, d0 vs. Cont).
d90	0.11	0.04	0.16	
V	Media	S.E.M		F
Control	0.04	0.003		$F (2.50) = 2.73, p = 0.07$, n.s.
d0	0.031	0.004 *		Bonferroni ($p = 0.043$, alpha (α) = 0.05, beta (β) = 0.42). * $p < 0.05$ vs. control
d90	0.041	0.0035 #		(# $p < 0.05$, d90 vs. d0)
	* $p < 0.05$ vs. Cont		# $p < 0.05$ d90 vs. d0	n.s: non significant effect ($p > 0.05$, n.s).

Percentiles analysis for heavy metals/oligoelement levels in Kruskal-Wallis (H) between patients with long-term titanium implant and dental fillings after 90 days of supplementation (d90, $n = 16$) as compared with their own basal levels (d0: before any supplementation, $n = 16$) and untreated (non-supplemented) controls without dental materials (control, $n = 21$). All heavy metals and oligoelements were expressed as µg/g of hair. H is the Krukal-Wallis analysis and F is ANOVA data. MW = Mann Whitney, S.E.M = standard error media; Control: controls without dental materials and non-supplemented ($n = 21$); d0: patients with long-term titanium implants and dental amalgam fillings restorations before any supplementation (d0, $n = 16$); d90: patients with long-term titanium implants and amalgams after 90 days of supplementation ($n = 16$); n.s: not significant effect, $p > 0.05$. * $p < 0.05$ vs. Control; # $p < 0.05$ d90 vs. d0.

4.3. Levels of Oligoelements Involved in Metabolic Functions (Se, Mn^{++}, Li, Mg^{++}, Ge, S, P, I, Ca^{2+}, Sr, Na^+, K^+)

Patients with long-term titanium implants and amalgam fillings increased germanium (Ge), manganesum (Mn^{++}), chromium (Cr), vanadium (V), phosphorum (P), and lithium levels (Li) after 90 days of supplementation (day 90) as compared with untreated controls (control, $n = 21$). In addition, after 90 days (d90, $n = 16$), their selenium (Se) levels decreased in comparison to their basal levels (d0, $n = 16$, $p < 0.05$, µg/g of hair); however, they were higher than the control values (Table 4, $p < 0.05$). These supplements could promote antihypertensive effects by rising certain oligoelements. Finally, there were no effects in other oligoelements (Ca^{2+}, Mg^{2+}, I, Sr, B, Rb) or for Be, Bi, Tl, To (data not shown, $p > 0.05$, n.s).

Table 4. Percentiles for oligoelements involved in metabolic functions in patients with long-term titanium implant and dental fillings after 90 days of supplementation (d90, $n = 16$) and their basal levels (d0: before any supplementation, $n = 16$) and non-supplemented controls (control: without dental materials and non-supplemented, $n = 21$). All heavy oligoelements were expressed as µg g/g of hair.

Se	Median	25%	75%	H
Control	0.66	0.59	0.73	$H = 10.91, p = 0.004$.
d0	0.6	0.47	0.67 *	MW (* d0 vs. control, $p = 0.05$).
d90	0.55	0.48	0.62 * #	MW (# d90 vs. d0, $p = 0.039$; * $p < 0.05$ vs. cont).
Mo	Median	25%	75%	H
Control	0.034	0.0140	0.0032	$H = 14.5, p < 0.001$.
d0	0.022	0.0079	0.023 *	MW or Dunn's (* $p < 0.05$ d0 vs. control).
d90	0.020	0.0084	0.150 *	MW or Dunn's: * $p < 0.05$ d90 vs. control
Mn^{++}	Median	25%	75%	H
Control	0.075	0.06	0.10	$H = 5.42, p = 0.066$, n.s.
d0	0.085	0.04	0.11	
d90	0.115	0.07	0.18 * #	MW (* d90 vs. control, $p = 0.05$); MW (d90 vs. d0, $p < 0.05$; * $p < 0.05$ vs. cont)

Table 4. *Cont.*

Li	Median	25%	75%	H
Control	0.008	0.006	0.012	H = 1.45, $p < 0.001$.
d0	0.005	0.0045	0.0075 *	MW (* d0 vs. control, $p = 0.03$).
d90	0.023	0.010	0.010 * #	MW (* d90 vs. control, $p < 0.05$); MW (# d90 vs. d0, $p = 0.05$).
Ge	**Median**	**25%**	**75%**	**H**
Control	0.031	0.024	0.033	H = 13.1, $p = 0.01$.
d0	0.024	0.021	0.032	MW (* d0 vs. control, $p = 0.1$, n.s).
d90	0.023	0.032	0.035 #	MW or Dunn's (# $p < 0.05$ d90 vs. d0).
S	**Median**	**25%**	**75%**	**H**
Control	47700	47200	49250	H = 3.97, $p = 0.13$, n.s.
d0	46900	46350	47600 *	MW (* d0 vs. control, $p < 0.05$).
d90	46850	45600	49950	
P	**Median**	**25%**	**75%**	**H**
Control	185	155	197	H = 8.88, $p = 0.012$.
d0	153	134	160 *	MW (* d0 vs. control, $p < 0.05$).
d90	170	154	179 #	MW (# d90 vs. d0, $p = 0.004$).
I	**Median**	**25%**	**75%**	**H**
Control	0.58	0.37	2.05	H=3.67, $p = 0.15$, n.s
d0	0.39	0.29	0.5	
d90	0.47	0.31	0.77	
Ca^{++}	**Median**	**25%**	**75%**	**H**
Control	488	285	705	H = 1.37, $p = 0.5$, n.s
d0	785	410	1262	
d90	676	380	1060	
Sr	**Median**	**25%**	**75%**	**H**
Control	2.7	0.93	6.55	H = 4.41, $p = 0.11$, n.s
d0	7	2.97	11.7	d0 vs. control, $p = 0.064$, n.s.
d90	11.81	1.9	17.75	d90 vs. control, $p = 0.099$, n.s
B	**Median**	**25%**	**75%**	**H**
Control	0.5	0.41	0.87	H = 1.5, $p = 0.46$, n.s.
d0	0.63	0.56	1.1	
d90	0.71	0.52	0.8	
Na$^+$	**Median**	**25%**	**75%**	**H**
Control	35	14.5	73.25	H = 6, $p = 0.05$.
d0	62.5	52	140 *	MW or Dunn's (* d0 vs. control, $p = 0.046$).
d90	48	33	75	d90 vs. control, $p = 0.1$, n.s.
K$^+$	**Median**	**25%**	**75%**	**H**
Control	13.5	4	31.5	H = 1.3, $p = 0.52$, n.s
d0	5.5	3.5	44	
d90	8.5	3	15	
Mg^{++}	**Median**	**25%**	**75%**	**H**
Control	50	32.5	94	H = 3.63, $p = 0.16$, n.s.
d0	99	43.5	184.5	
d90	137	57	345	MW (d90 vs. control, $p = 0.088$, n.s).
Rb	**Median**	**25%**	**75%**	**H**
Control	0.015	0.0045	0.031	H = 2.72, $p = 0.25$, n.s.
d0	0.014	0.0040	0.019	
d90	0.011	0.0030	0.013	

Table 4. Cont.

Fe^{++}	Median	25%	75%	H
Control	6.7	6.2	7.7	H = 3.7, p = 0.15, n.s.
d0	6.6	6.4	7.4	
d90	7.7	6.5	8.4 #	MW (d90 vs. d0, # p = 0.022).
	* p < 0.05 vs. control		# p < 0.05 d90 vs. d0	

* $p < 0.05$ vs. control; # $p < 0.05$ d90 vs. d0; controls (without dental materials and non-supplement; control, $n = 21$); d0: patients with long-term titanium implants and dental amalgam fillings restorations before any supplementation (d0, $n = 16$); d90: patients with long-term titanium implants and dental amalgams after 90 days of supplementation (d90, $n = 16$); (n.s: not significant effect, $p > 0.05$; * $p < 0.05$ vs. Control; # $p < 0.05$ d90 vs. d0).

4.4. Metals of Environmental Exposure

The algae extract and aminoazuphrates supplements decreased lead (Pb) levels after 90 days of supplementation (day 90) as compared with baseline levels (d0: before any supplementation); the aluminium (Al) levels were reduced after 90 days in comparison to untreated controls (see Table 5).

There was a lack of effect in several heavy metals (As, Ti, Pt, Sb, Tl, To, Cd, Be, Bi, Zr, $p > 0.05$, n.s) and oligoelements by treatment (Zn^{++}, Cu^{++}, Ca^{++}, Sr, B, I, K$^+$, Mg^{++}, Rb) after 90 days of supplementation as compared with their baseline (d0) and control levels.

Table 5. Decreased lead (Pb) levels after 90 days of supplementation as compared with baseline levels.

Ba	Median	25%	75%	H
Control	0.17	0.1	0.33	H = 7.73, p = 0.021.
d0	0.54	0.25	0.84 *	MW (* d0 vs. control, p = 0.05).
d90	0.28	0.2	0.36	MW (d90 vs. control, p = 0.11, n.s).
Pb	**Median**	**25%**	**75%**	**H**
Control	0.11	0.07	0.3	H = 3.41, p = 0.18, n.s.
d0	0.14	0.09	0.21	
d90	0.085	0.05	0.14 #	MW (# d90 vs. d0, p = 0.047).
Cd	**Median**	**25%**	**75%**	**H**
Control	0.009	0.009	0.010	H = 4.73, p = 0.094, n.s.
d0	0.009	0.009	0.009	
d90	0.009	0.009	0.009	MW (d90 vs. control, p = 0.08, n.s).
Sb	**Median**	**25%**	**75%**	**H**
Control	0.01	0.01	0.018	H = 3.5, p = 0.16, n.s.
d0	0.01	0.01	0.01	
d90	0.01	0.01	0.01	
As	**Median**	**25%**	**75%**	**H**
Control	0.038	0.01	0.018	H = 0.9, p = 0.62, n.s.
d0	0.028	0.022	0.042	
d90	0.028	0.023	0.052	
	* p < 0.05 vs. Cont		# p < 0.05 d90 vs. d0	

These tables show percentile values (median, 25%, and 75%) in Kruskal Wallis analysis for several heavy metals/oligoelements (Hg^{++}, Ag, Sn, Zn^{++}, Cu^{++}, Al, Cr, V, Co, and Ni), metabolic oligoelements (Se, Mo, Mn^{++}, Li, Ge, S, P, I, Ca^{++}, Sr, B, Na$^+$, K$^+$, Mg^{++}, Rb, B, and Fe^{++}), and metals of environmental exposure in Table 6 (Ba, As, Pt, Sb, Tl, To, Cd, Be, Bi, Zr, Pb, Cd, As, and U). The ANOVA data for V are shown by mean values ± S.E.M [the root square divided by n; n was the size sample; $n = 16$ (d90), $n = 16$ (d0), $n = 21$ controls]. Post hoc differences were evaluated by the Mann Whitney or Dunn's method; Control: controls without dental materials and non-supplemented ($n = 21$); d0: patients with long-term titanium implants and dental amalgam fillings restorations (d0, $n = 16$); d90: patients with long-term titanium implants and dental amalgams after 90 days of supplementation ($n = 16$); n.s: not significant effect, $p > 0.05$). * $p < 0.05$ vs. Control; # $p < 0.05$ d90 vs. d0).

4.5. Effects on Selenium (Se) Ratios and Heavy Metals after 90 Days of Nutritional Supplementation

For example, we found decreased Se/Hg^{++}, and increased Se/Al, and Mo/Hg^{++} ratios after 90 days of supplementation (d90) compared to their respective basal levels (before any treatment, d0, $p < 0.05$); However, these Se/Hg^{++}, Se/Ag, and Mo/Hg^{++}, and Na^+/K^+ ratios decreased before any treatment (d0) as compared with non-supplemented patients (controls, $p < 0.05$, Table 6).

Table 6. Effects on Se/Hg^{++}, Se/Ag, Se/Al, Se/Pb, Mo/Hg^{++}, $Na+/K+$ before/after nutritional supplementation and untreated controls.

Se/Hg^{++} Ratio	Median	25%	75%	H
Control	2.21	1.6	3.2	$H = 31.42, p < 0.001$.
d0	0.23	0.17	0.31 *	MW (* d0 vs. control, $p < 0.001$).
d90	0.28	0.24	0.56 * #	MW (# d90 vs. d0, $p = 0.05$. * $p < 0.05$ vs. cont.
Se/Ag ratio	**Median**	**25%**	**75%**	**H**
Control	22.3	12.26	37.7	$H = 6.25, p = 0.044$
d0	7.16	4.12	20.5	MW (* d0 vs. control, $p = 0.04$).
d90	11	6.8	18.2 *	MW (* d90 vs. control, $p = 0.032$).
Se/Al ratio	**Median**	**25%**	**75%**	**H**
cont	0.26	0.1	0.39	$H = 3.76, p = 0.15$, n.s.
d0	0.14	0.07	0.29	
d90	0.34	0.19	0.36 #	MW (# d90 vs. d0, $p = 0.05$).
Se/Pb	**Median**	**25%**	**75%**	**H**
Control	4.57	1,79	9.1	$H = 1.12, p = 0.57$, n.s
d0	3.81	2.2	6.9	
d90	5.72	3.76	8.24	
Mo/Hg^{++}	**Median**	**25%**	**75%**	**H**
Control	0.018	0.011	0.03	$H = 13.51, p = 0.001$
d0	0.0089	0.0067	0.011 *	MW or Dunn's, * d0 vs. Cont, $p = 0.001$
d90	0.026	0.011	0.112 * #	MW or Dunn's, # d90 vs. d0, $p < 0.001$, * $p < 0.05$ vs. control
Na^+/K^+	**Median**	**25%**	**75%**	**H**
Control	3.57	4.46	0.94	$H = 2.59, p = 0.2$, n.s.
d0	7.74	16.3	0.82 *	MW (* $p < 0.05$, d0 vs. control).
d90	8	13.6	0.79	MW (d90 vs. control, $p = 0.065$, n.s).
* $p < 0.05$ vs. control		# $p < 0.05$ d90 vs. d0		

Control: controls without dental materials and non-supplemented ($n = 21$); d0: patients with long-term titanium implants and dental amalgam fillings restorations (d0, $n = 16$); d90: patients with long-term titanium implants and dental amalgams after 90 days of supplementation ($n = 16$). n.s: not significant effect, $p > 0.05$; * $p < 0.05$ vs. Control; # $p < 0.05$ d90 vs. d0.

4.6. Correlations between Selenium (Se) and Heavy Metals Ratios after 90 Days of Nutritional Supplementation

The r Spearman correlations between selenium and heavy metal ratios are shown in Table S1. For example, there was a strong correlation between the Se/Hg^{++} (d90) ratio and Se levels after 90 days of supplementation [Se (d90), $r = -0.76, p = 0.004$] as well as with Mo/Hg^{++} (d90) ratio after 90 days (d90, $r = 0.6, p = 0.02$). Two outlier values were excluded for statistical analysis herein (Table S1, see Supplementary Materials). Table S2 showed other correlations between heavy metals and oligoelements (see Supplementary Materials).

5. Discussion

This section discusses the effects of dental amalgam restoration in mercury reduction in patients with long-term titanium implants and dental amalgam restorations using carbon active (nasal filters) and long-term algae and aminoazuphrates supplementation.

The exposure derived from amalgam fillings exceeds that from food, air, or beverages. Chronic nutritional supplementation contributes to preventing mercury release peaks caused by dental amalgam restoration (replacement by biocompatible materials like Bisphenol A free composites). A study of 12 patients demonstrated that the long-term presence of dental amalgam (at least five years) did not result in any remarkable changes in mercury or tin levels in the pulp tissue after comparing 12 restored amalgams and 12 non-restored patients. However, elevated blood mercury levels were observed even five years after the placement of the restoration [32]. These data suggest that mercury release is important even after complete dental amalgam restoration with composites, because five years after its restoration, mercury is still present in the blood [32]. Bergerow et al. reported that within 12 months after removing dental amalgam fillings (restoration by composites), patients showed substantially lower urinary mercury levels [33]. In the present study, the period of supplementation was shorter (three months: 90 days), which minimized mercury release by using carbon active (nasal filters) during dental restorations [29]. The synergic algae and aminoazuphrates treatment contributed to activating the detoxification because the mercury reached peaks shortly at 24 h after replacement with composites until 3–7 days later [34].

5.1. Detoxification of Heavy Metals in Patients with Long-Term Amalgam Fillings and Titanium Dental Implants

We determined that chronic nutritional *Chlorella* and *Fucus* algae extract supplementation in conjunction with aminosulphurates lowered certain heavy metal levels in patients with long-term titanium implants and dental amalgams restoration using activated carbon active nasal filter as well as the nutraceuticals. Preclinical findings suggest a role of *Chlorella vulgaris* as a heavy chelator in preventing toxicity of certain xenobiotics and accelerating dioxin excretion in rats [25,35]. The mercury and tin reduction after 90 days in patients agreed with enhanced heavy metal removal by *Chlorella sp* [36–38]. However, the exact mechanism by which chronic algae consumption removes heavy metals has not been tested yet in humans. Our aim is to develop a clinical and practical protocol to chelate heavy metals with a mixture of bioactive nutraceuticals such as algae extracts and aminosulphurates that could act independently of signaling pathways involved in detoxification.

Supplementation with *Chlorella sp* promoted detoxification of heterocyclic amines (carcinogenic chemical) in six young Korean adults [39]. This randomized, double blind, placebo-controlled crossover study was performed in six female supplemented-patients; the nutritional period of three months in our study was longer than in the Korean study. Our findings also reflected enhanced removal of certain heavy metals, including lead (a metal of environmental exposure). Our patients' Hg^{++}, Sn, and Pb accumulations were strongly reduced after 90 days of consecutive nutritional supplementation as compared with basal levels (before any supplementation). Interestingly, mercury and Sn levels reductions were observed after 90 days as compared with untreated controls (without dental materials and non-supplemented).

5.2. SOD-1 Activity in Patients with Long-Term Dental Titanium Implants and Amalgams Restorations

Although it was not possible to elucidate the exact nutraceutical involved in SOD-1 activation here, we must consider that SOD-1 activation decreased after 90 days as compared with their basal levels (d0, before any supplementation). Conversely, higher SOD-1 activity was observed after long-term supplementation (day 90) compared with untreated controls; this suggests algae and aminoazuphates treatment may activate SOD-1. In addition, increased Mn^{++} levels could suggest enhanced antioxidant responses after 90 days of supplementation. In fact, Ala16Val MnSOD-2 polymorphism has been described in cells exposed to methylmercury [40]. We have previously observed higher SOD-1 activation in women with long-term dental amalgams only (without titanium dental alloys) as compared with controls (without dental materials) [9]. Our clinical findings were in consonance with the detoxification induced by Ag nanoparticles through inducing SOD, peroxidase, catalase, and glutamine synthetase enzymatic activities [41,42]. The silver (Ag) reduction after 90 days of supplementation as compared with the patients' baseline levels (before any supplementation) agreed with the enhanced removal of heavy metals. However, silver levels after 90 days did not differ with controls.

Heavy metals detox requires (i) a healthy gut microbiome state [20], (ii) the induced-activation of endogenous hepatic I-II-enzyme, which can be activated by phytonaturals in these formulations [43], and (iii) the chelation and excretion of these heavy metals [44]. Steps (i) and (ii) are activated by natural products from these formulations. The ERGYLIXIR formulation contains synergic depurative bioactive compounds from extracts such as *Cinara scolymus* (artichoke) [45], *Raphanus niger* [46], *Taraxacum officinale* [47], *Arctium lappa* (dandelion root) [48], *Vaccinium macrocarpo* [49], *Solidago virgaurea* (quercitin, afzelin) [50], *Rosmarinus officinallis* [51], *Scolymus hispanicus* [52], and *Sambucus nigra* (elderberry with antocianines) [53]. In addition, sulfur-rich extracts such as garlic acid (*Allium sativa* in the ERGYTAURINE formulation) may enhance heavy metal removal by inducing antioxidant activities [54–56]. Apple pectin [56] and acerole (very rich in vitamin C) also contribute to heavy metals removal [57]. In addition, *Sambucus nigra* (elderberry) contains antocyanines that supply 87% of the daily vitamin C levels necessary for humans [57]. Vitamins B6, B-9, and B-12, as well as Se, Zn^{++}, and Mg^{++} (ERGYTAURINE formulation) [58] are necessary for certain enzymatic activities.

5.3. Possible Role of Selenium (Se) in Detox after Long-Term Chlorella CV Supplementation in Patients

Because Se levels decreased after 90 days of supplementation, we cannot exclude the possibility that selenomercurials reflect the Se-heavy metal complex formation in order to prevent mercury toxicity (or other metals) in patients with long-term dental amalgams and titanium alloys. As the Na^+/K^+ ratio did not differ after 90 days as compared with their basal levels (before any supplementation), we can confirm that chronic algae and aminoazuphrates supplementation are safe and non-toxic for humans. The increased Se/Hg^{++} ratios suggest enhanced detoxification after 90 days compared to their basal levels (before any supplementation) as well as untreated controls. Surprisingly, a toxic effect has been demonstrated in autistic children who had elevated hair selenium levels [59]. These lower Se levels observed in conjunction with the lack of effect on the Na^+/K^+ and Se/Pb ratios could prevent mercury accumulation at 90 consecutive days of supplementation. In fact, antagonistic interaction between selenomethionine enantiomers and methylmercury toxicity was described with *Chlorella sorokiniana* [60]. Mercury loss with *Chlorella vulgaris* is largely influenced by amino acids, cysteine being the most effective in promoting the detoxification of mercury $(Hg^{2+})^-$ in *Chlorella sp* exposed to this metal [61]. The amino acid taurine (ERGYTAURINE formulation) is derived from cysteine [62] and also contributes to heavy metal detoxification. In fact, increased oxidative stress and low systemic taurine levels were demonstrated in patients with long-term dental amalgam fillings and/or titanium alloys [63]. This indirect evidence agreed with a study in which selenocystine ($SeCys_2$) reduced MeHg cytotoxicity in Hepatic $HepG_2$ cells by inducing MeHg-glutathione (GSH) and also formed MeHg-cysteine (Cys) complex in vitro [64]. These indirect findings suggest that selenium contributed to detoxification in the present clinical study. Uchikawa et al. (2011) described the enhanced removal of tissue methylmercury in (BP) *Parachlorella beijerinckii*-fed mice; this continuous BP intake (10%) accelerated MeHg excretion and subsequently decreased tissue mercury accumulation by inducing the GSH metabolism [65].

Other metals such as Pb, Cd, and U that are associated with occupational exposure were significantly decreased after three consecutive months of supplementation compared with their basal levels (before any supplementation) without affecting the untreated controls (without dental materials). The biosorption of Pb^{2+} and Cd^{2+} was detected using a fixed bed column analysis with immobilized Chlorella algae biomass [66]. Pb levels decreased after 90 days of supplementation, agreeing with the 56% Pb reduction at four days of algae *Chlorella sp* supplementation, 69% at eight days, and

77% at 12 days of treatment [26]. Although U levels were within the normal detection range in our patients, their decrease after 90 days of supplementation was crucial. As selenium-enriched spirulina formulation reduces the development radiation that is *pneumonitis*-induced [67], the lower U levels after chronic algae supplementation are important from a clinical view point. In addition, a glutathione-dependent detoxification pathway has been described in *Chlorella algae* exposed to U [68–70].

5.4. The Nutritional Supplementation after 90 Days Prevented Certain Oligoelements Deficit in Patients with Long-Term Titanium Implants and Dental Amalgam Restorations

These polyphenols from Azorean brown algae (*Fucus spiralis* or *Fucus vesiculosus* in GREEN-FLOR formulation) may enhance heavy metal removal in patients with long-term dental fillings and titanium alloys. In fact, the marine algae *Ulva lactuca* and *Fucus vesiculosus* can sequester Cd and Cu^{++} [70], which explained the induced-detoxification here. The phlorotannins have potential impact on public health, particularly in hypertensive patients [71,72]. The in situ determination of trace elements in fucoids by field-portable-X-ray fluorescence (FP-XRF) provides a rapid monitoring environmental contamination [73]. Increased mercury levels can provoke hypertension, and Se may exhibit a protective effect against cardiovascular disease [6]. Long-term nutritional supplementation could increase germanium (Ge) levels in patients with long-term dental amalgam fillings and titanium implants, seemingly by reflecting antihypertensive effects. However, a direct causal relationship between antihypertensive effects and Cr and Ge elevations was not conclusive in the present study. The Sn-Se correlation observed in conjunction with Ge, Li, Cr, P and I elevations after 90 days of supplementation could be explained by the high oligoelement content (10–15%) in the supplement, resulting from its marine origin [74]. The detoxification of Hg^{++} and Cd levels here agreed with the enhanced Hg^{++}, Cd^{++}, and Pb removal by *Fucus* from contaminated salt waters exposed to heavy metals for seven days [74]. The *Fucus sp* algae is also traditionally used to prevent obesity or gastrointestinal diseases. As *Fucus vesiculosus* extracts reduced the blood glucose peak in mice fed with a normal diet [75], the possibility that chromium Cr and Ge elevation could contribute to these antihypertensive effects should not be excluded here. These oligoelements also increased after 90 days of supplementation as compared with untreated controls. The increased Li levels suggest a better regulation of gut microbiota after treatment with these formulations, since the host serotonine biosynthesis is regulated by intestinal microbiota [76]. In fact, the strong r Spearman correlation together with the Se/Li ratio and Li correlation suggest a better state of gut microbiota in treated patients at 90 days of supplementation as compared with their basal and control levels. Finally, the augmented phosphorous (P) levels described here may have been a consequence of chronic spirulina supplementation (GREEN-FLOR). Since undernourished children receiving *Spirulina platensis* plus Misola extract treatment have a better hematocrite that those taking Misola alone [77], the chronic algae-supplementation could prevent iron deficit. These synergic supplementations contribute to heavy metal removal in these patients. Moreover, increased systemic malondialdehyde levels and lower Mo/Co and Mo/Fe^{2+} ratios have been described in patients with long-term dental titanium implants and dental amalgams [74]. Further studies should evaluate detoxification pathways by which long-term supplementation *Chlorella* or *Fucus vesiculosus* treatment contribute to the removal of heavy metals in patients with long-term dental amalgam fillings and titanium implants. The absence of placebo, the non-RCT (randomised controlled trials), the size sample (pilot study), as well as the Caucasian population (Spaniards) are limitations in this study.

6. Conclusions

The aminosulphurates and *Chlorella and Fucus sp* algae supplementation enhanced detoxification of heavy metals by reducing Hg^{++}, Ag, Sn, and Pb levels in patients with long-term dental amalgam filling and titanium implants. The chronic nutritional supplementation with algae extract reduced Hg^{++} and Sn levels in patients with long-term titanium implants and dental amalgam restorations as compared with untreated controls (without dental materials). In addition, increased Mn^{++}, Li, Ge, Cr and lower U levels, and decreased Se levels were observed after 90 days of supplementation as compared to their basal levels (before any supplementation). These findings suggest that these nutraceuticals promote beneficial effects in patients. The safety of long-term algae and aminoazuphrates supplementation were confirmed by the lack of effect in Ka^+/K^+ and Se/Pb ratios after 90 days compared to their basal levels (before any supplementation) and untreated controls. The SOD-1 activity could explain antioxidant and enhanced detoxification of certain heavy metals by nutritional supplementation in the present study.

Supplementary Materials: The following are available online at http://www.mdpi.com/2076-3921/8/4/101/s1, Table S1: correlations between Se, Mo and heavy metal ratios, Table S2: correlations between heavy metals and oligoelements (r Spearman).

Author Contributions: J.J.M., M.E.C.-M.: writing the manuscript; M.E.C.-M., J.M.P.-I.: performed the samples collection and clinical data; J.J.M., J.M.P.-I., A.T.G., M.E.C.-M.: statistical analysis and experimental design; J.J.M., J.M.P.-I., A.T.G., M.E.C.-M. planned and supervised and the final revision.

Funding: Funds # 20151602 from CIROM (Murcia, Spain), Article processing charge (APC) supported by Nutergia Laboratories (San Sebastian).

Acknowledgments: We thank Laboratorios Nutergia (Basque Country) the support of this research project to Jose Joaquin Merino. We also thank InspiraHealth® (Barcelona) for the supplying of nasal filters. GREEN-FLOR (Nutergia), ERGYLIXIR (Nutergia), ERGYTAURINE (Nutergia) were supplied by Nutergia Laboratories. We also thank all enrolled patients from CIROM (Murcia, Spain) in the present study. The principal researcher of this project Jose Joaquin Merino thanks the support of Nutergia laboratories and CIROM Clinic (Murcia, Spain). IP Research project: "Detoxification of heavy metals by long-term algae and aminoazuphrate supplementation in patients with long-term dental amalgam fillings and titanium implants to Jose Joaquin Merino.

Conflicts of Interest: The authors declare no conflict of interest.

References

1. Dierickx, P.J. In vitro interaction of organic mercury compounds with soluble glutathione s-transferases from rat liver. *Pharmacol. Res. Commun.* **1985**, *17*, 489–500. [CrossRef]
2. Valko, M.; Leibfritz, D.; Moncol, J.; Cronin, M.T.; Mazúr, M.; Telser, J. Free radicals and antioxidants in normal physiological functions and human disease. *Int. J. Biochem. Cell Biol.* **2007**, *39*, 44–84. [CrossRef] [PubMed]
3. Farina, M.; Aschner, M.; Rocha, J.B.T. Oxidative stress in MeHg induced neurotoxicity. *Toxicol. Appl. Pharmacol.* **2011**, *256*, 405–417. [CrossRef] [PubMed]
4. Belyaeva, E.A.; Sokolova, T.V.; Emelyanova, L.V.; Zakharova, I.O. Mitochondrial Electron Transport Chain in Heavy Metal-Induced Neurotoxicity: Effects of Cadmium, Mercury, and Copper. *Sci. J.* **2012**, *2012*, 1–14. [CrossRef] [PubMed]
5. Hu, X.F.; Eccles, K.M.; Chan, H.M. High selenium exposure lowers the odds ratios for hypertension, stroke, and myocardial infarction associated with mercury exposure among Inuit in Canada. *Environ. Int.* **2017**, *102*, 200–206. [CrossRef] [PubMed]
6. Yoo, J., II; Ha, Y.-C.; Lee, Y.-K.; Koo, K.-H. High levels of heavy metals increases the prevalence of sarcopenia in the Ederly population. *J. Bone Metab.* **2016**, *23*, 101–109. [CrossRef] [PubMed]
7. Joska, L.; Fojt, J.; Cvrcek, L.; Březina, V. Properties of titanium-alloyed DLC layers for medical applications. *Biomatter* **2014**, *4*, e29505. [CrossRef] [PubMed]
8. Puchyr, R.F.; Bass, D.A.; Gajewski, R.; Calvin, M.; Marquardt, W.; Urek, K.; Druyan, M.E.; Quig, D. Preparation of hair for measurement of elements by inductively coupled plasma-mass spectrometry (ICP-MS). *Biol. Elem. Res.* **1998**, *62*, 167–182. [CrossRef] [PubMed]
9. Cabaña-Muñoz, M.E.; Parmigiani-Izquierdo, J.M.; Bravo-González, L.A.; Kyung, H.M.; Merino, J.J. Increased Zn/Glutathione Levels and Higher Superoxide Dismutase-1 Activity as Biomarkers of Oxidative Stress in Women with Long-Term Dental Amalgam Fillings: Correlation between Mercury/Aluminium Levels (in Hair) and Antioxidant Systems in Plasma. *PLoS ONE* **2015**, *10*, e0126339. [CrossRef]
10. Somers, E.C.; Ganser, M.A.; Warren, J.S.; Basu, N.; Wang, L.; Zick, S.M.; Park, S.K. Mercury Exposure and Antinuclear Antibodies among Females of Reproductive Age in the United States: NHANES. *Environ. Health Perspect.* **2015**, *123*, 792–798. [CrossRef]

11. López, E.; Arce, C.; Oset-Gasque, M.; Cañadas, S.; González, M. Cadmium induces reactive oxygen species generation and lipid peroxidation in cortical neurons in culture. *Free Radic. Biol. Med.* **2006**, *40*, 940–951. [CrossRef] [PubMed]
12. Cobbina, S.J.; Chen, Y.; Zhou, Z.; Wu, X.; Zhao, T.; Zhang, Z.; Feng, W.; Wang, W.; Li, Q.; Wu, X.; et al. Toxicity assessment due to sub-chronic exposure to individual and mixtures of four toxic heavy metals. *J. Hazard. Mater.* **2015**, *294*, 109–120. [CrossRef]
13. Soetan, K.O.; Olaiya, C.O.; Otewole, O.E. The importance of mineral elements for humans, domestic animals and plants. A review. *Afr. J. Food Sci.* **2010**, *4*, 200–222.
14. Fattoretti, P.; Bertoni-Freddari, C.; Balietti, M.; Giorgetti, B.; Solazzi, M.; Zatta, P.; Bertoni-Freddari, C. Chronic Aluminum Administration to Old Rats Results in Increased Levels of Brain Metal Ions and Enlarged Hippocampal Mossy Fibers. *Ann. N. Y. Acad. Sci.* **2004**, *1019*, 44–47. [CrossRef]
15. Vig, E.K.; Hu, H. Lead toxicity in older adults. *J. Am. Geriatr. Soc.* **2000**, *48*, 1501–1506. [CrossRef] [PubMed]
16. Jaishankar, M.; Tseten, T.; Anbalagan, N.; Mathew, B.B.; Beeregowda, K.N. Toxicity, mechanism and health effects of some heavy metals. *Interdiscip. Toxicol.* **2014**, *7*, 60–72. [CrossRef]
17. Travieso, L.; Cañizares, R.O.; Borja, R.; Benitez, F.; Domínguez, A.R.; Dupeyrón, R.; Valiente, V. Heavy metals removal by microalgae. *Bull. Environ. Contam. Toxicol.* **1999**, *62*, 144–151. [CrossRef]
18. Waisberg, M.; Joseph, P.; Hale, B.; Beyersmann, D. Molecular and cellular mechanisms of cadmium carcinogenesis. *Toxicology* **2003**, *192*, 95–117. [CrossRef]
19. Pacyna, J.M.; Pacyna, E.G.; Aas, W. Changes of emissions and atmospheric deposition of mercury, lead, and cadmium. *Atmos. Environ.* **2009**, *43*, 117–127. [CrossRef]
20. Monachese, M.; Burton, J.P.; Reid, G. Bioremediation and Tolerance of Humans to Heavy Metals through Microbial Processes: A Potential Role for Probiotics? *Appl. Environ. Microbiol.* **2012**, *78*, 6397–6404. [CrossRef] [PubMed]
21. Hodges, R.E.; Minich, D.M. Modulation of Metabolic Detoxification Pathways Using Foods and Food-Derived Components: A Scientific Review with Clinical Application. *J. Nutr. Metab.* **2015**, *2015*, 1–23. [CrossRef] [PubMed]
22. Jervis, L.; Rees-Naesborg, R.; Brown, M. Biochemical responses of the marine macroalgae *Ulva lactuca* and *Fucus vesiculosus* to cadmium and copper-from sequestration to oxidative stress. *Biochem. Soc. Trans.* **1997**, *25*, 63. [CrossRef]
23. Ben-Bassat, D.; Mayer, A.M. Volatilization of mercury by algae. *Pshysiol. Plant.* **1975**, *33*, 128–132. [CrossRef]
24. Hamed, S.M.; Zinta, G.; Klöck, G.; Asard, H.; Selim, S.; AbdelGawad, H. Zinc-induced differential oxidative stress and antioxidant responses in *Chlorella sorokiniana* and *Scenedesmus acuminatus*. *Ecotoxicol. Environ. Saf.* **2017**, *140*, 256–263. [CrossRef] [PubMed]
25. Kim, Y.H.; Hwang, Y.K.; Lee, Y.W.; Yun, J.Y.; Hwang, J.M.; Yoo, J.D. Effect of Chlorella diet supplementation on blood and urine cadmium levels in cadmium poisoned rats. *J. Biomed. Lab. Sci.* **2003**, *9*, 133–137.
26. Cantu, V.; Garza-González, M.T.; de la Rosa, J.R.; Loredo-Medrano, J.A. Biosorption of Pb2+ and Cd2+ in a fixed bed column with immobilised *Chorella* sp. biomass. *J. Nutr.* **1999**, *129*, 1731–1736.
27. Castro, L.; Blázquez, M.L.; González, F.; Muñoz, J.A.; Ballester, A. Biosorption of Zn (II) from industrial effluents using sugar beet pulp and *F. vesiculosus*: From laboratory tests to a pilot approach. *Sci. Total Environ.* **2017**, *598*, 856–866. [CrossRef] [PubMed]
28. Isuru, W.; Se-Kwon, K. Angiotensin-I-Converting Enzyme (ACE) Inhibitors from Marine Resources: Prospects in the Pharmaceutical Industry. *Mar. Drugs* **2010**, *8*, 1080–1093. [CrossRef]
29. APA. American Psychiatric Association. *Diagnostic and Statistical Manual of Mental Disorders: DSM-IV-TR*; American Psychiatric Association: Washington, DC, USA, 2006.
30. Cabaña-Muñoz, M.E.; Parmigiani-Izquierdo, J.M.; Merino, J.J. Safe renoval of dental amalgams by using nasal filtres and phytoteraphy. *IJSR Int. J. Sci. Res.* **2015**, *4*, 2391–2395.
31. Salvi, G.E.; Lindhe, J.; Lang, N.P. Examination of patients with periodontal disease. In *Clinical Periodontology and Implants Dentistry*, 5th ed.; Lindh, J., Lan, N.P., Karring, T., Eds.; Wiley: Oxford, UK, 2008; pp. 573–586.
32. Saghiri, M.A.; Banava, S.; Sabzian, M.A.; Gutmann, J.L.; Asatourian, A.; Ramezani, G.H.; García-Godoy, F.; Sheibani, N. Correlation between long-term in vivo amalgam restorations and the presence of heavy elements in the dental pulp. *J. Elem. Med. Biol.* **2014**, *28*, 200–204. [CrossRef]
33. Begerow, J.; Zander, D.; Freier, I.; Dunemann, L. Long-term mercury excretion in urine after removal of amalgam fillings. *Int. Arch. Occup. Environ. Health* **1994**, *66*, 209–212. [CrossRef] [PubMed]

34. Kremers, L.; Halbach, S.; Willruth, H.; Mehl, A.; Welzl, G.; Wack, F.-X.; Greim, H.; Wack, F.; Hickel, R. Effect of rubber dam on mercury exposure during amalgam removal. *Eur. J. Oral Sci.* **1999**, *107*, 202–207. [CrossRef] [PubMed]
35. Morita, K.; Matsueda, T.; Iida, T.; Hasegawa, T. Chlorella Accelerates Dioxin Excretion in Rats. *J. Nutr.* **1999**, *129*, 1731–1736. [CrossRef] [PubMed]
36. Mahltig, B.; Soltmann, U.; Haase, H. Modification of algae with zinc, copper and silver ions for usage as natural composite for antibacterial applications. *Mater. Sci. Eng. C* **2013**, *33*, 979–983. [CrossRef] [PubMed]
37. Rai, U.N.; Singh, N.K.; Upadhyay, A.K.; Verma, S. Chromate tolerance and accumulation in *Chlorella vulgaris*. A role of antioxidant enzymes and biochemical changes in detoxification of metals. *Bioresour. Technol.* **2013**, *136*, 604–609. [CrossRef] [PubMed]
38. Jiang, Y.; Purchase, D.; Jones, H.; Garelick, H. Effects of arsenate (As5+) on growth and production of glutathione (GSH) and phytochelatins (PCS) in *Chlorella vulgaris*. *Int. J. Phytoremediation* **2011**, *13*, 834–844. [CrossRef]
39. Lee, I.; Tran, M.; Evans-Nguyen, T.; Stickle, D.; Kim, S.; Han, J.; Park, J.Y.; Yang, M. Detoxification of chlorella supplement on heterocyclic amines in Korean young adults. *Environ. Toxicol. Pharmacol.* **2015**, *39*, 441–446. [CrossRef]
40. Algaerve, T.D.; Barbisan, F.; Ribeiro, E.E.; Duarte, M.M.; Manica-Cattani, M.F.; Mostardeiro, C.P.; Lenz, A.F.; da Cruz, I.B. In vitro effects of Ala16Val manganese superoxide dismutase gene polymorphism on human white blood cells exposed to methylmercury. *Genet. Mol. Res.* **2014**, *12*, 5133–5144. [CrossRef]
41. Mohseniazar, M.; Barin, M.; Zarredar, H.; Alizadeh, S.; Shanehbandi, D. Potential of Microalgae and Lactobacilli in Biosynthesis of Silver Nanoparticles. *Bioimpacts* **2011**, *1*, 149–152.
42. Qian, H.; Zhu, K.; Lu, H.; Lavoie, M.; Chen, S.; Zhou, Z.; Deng, Z.; Chen, J.; Fu, Z. Contrasting silver nanoparticle toxicity and detoxification strategies in *Microcystis aeruginosa* and *Chlorella vulgaris*: New insights from proteomic and physiological analyses. *Sci. Total Environ.* **2016**, *572*, 1213–1221. [CrossRef]
43. Hinson, J.A.; Forkert, P.G. Phase II enzymes and bioactivation. *Can. J. Physiol. Pharmacol.* **1995**, *73*, 1407–1413. [CrossRef]
44. Ben-Bassat, D.; Mayer, A.M. Reduction of mercury chloride by Chlorella: Evidence for a reducing agent. *Physiol. Plant.* **1977**, *40*, 157–162. [CrossRef]
45. Walker, A.F.; Middleton, R.W.; Petrowicz, O. Artichoke leaf extract reduces symptoms of irritable bowel síndrome in a post-marketing surveillance study. *Phytother. Res.* **2001**, *15*, 58–61. [CrossRef]
46. N'jai, A.U.; Kemp, M.Q.; Metzger, B.T.; Hanlon, P.R.; Robbins, M.; Czuyprynski, C.; Barnes, D.M. Spanish Black Radish (*Raphanus sativus L. var niger*) diet enhances clearance of DMBA and diminishes toxic effects on bone marrow progenitor cells. *Nutr. Cancer* **2012**, *64*, 1038–1048. [CrossRef]
47. Wei, S.; Wang, S.; Zhou, Q.; Zhan, J.; Ma, L.; Wu, Z.; Sun, T.; Prasad, M.N. Potential of *Tarazacum mongolium* hand-mazz for accelerating phytoextration of cadmium in combination with eco-friendly amendments. *J. Hazard. Mater.* **2010**, *15*, 480–484. [CrossRef]
48. Chan, Y.S.; Cheng, L.N.; Wu, J.H.; Chan, E.; Kwan, Y.W.; Lee, S.M.Y.; Leung, G.P.H.; Yu, P.H.; Chan, S.W. A review of the pharmacological effects of *Arctium lappa* (burbock). *Inflammapharmacology* **2010**, *19*, 245–254. [CrossRef]
49. Yan, X.; Murphy, B.T.; Hammond, G.B.; Vinson, J.A.; Neto, C.C. Antioxidant Activities and Antitumor Screening of Extracts from Cranberry Fruit (*Vaccinium macrocarpon*). *J. Agric. Chem.* **2002**, *50*, 5844–5849. [CrossRef]
50. Wang, Z.; Kim, J.H.; Jang, Y.S.; Lee, J.Y.; Lim, S.S. Anti-obesity effect of *Solidago virgaurea* vs. Gigantea extract through regulation of adipogenesis and lipogenesis pathways in high-fat diet-induced obese mic (C57BL/6N). *Food Nutr. Res.* **2017**, *13*, 1273479. [CrossRef]
51. Lara, M.S.; Gutierrez, J.I.; Timón, M.; Andrés, A.I. Evaluation of two natural extracts (*Rosmarinus officinalis* L. and *Melissa officinalis* L). as antioxidants in cooked pork patties packed in MPA. *Meat Sci.* **2011**, *88*, 481–488. [CrossRef] [PubMed]
52. Kirimer, N.; Tunalier, Z.; Başer, K.C.; Cingi, I. Antispasmodic and Spasmogenic Effects of *Scolymus hispanicus* and Taraxasteryl Acetate on Isolated Ileum Preparation. *Planta Med.* **1997**, *63*, 556–558. [CrossRef] [PubMed]
53. Viapiana, A.; Wesolowski, M. The phenolic contents and antioxidant activities of infussions of *Sambucus nigra* L. *Plant Foods Hum. Nutr.* **2017**, *72*, 82–87. [CrossRef] [PubMed]

54. Lawal, A.O.; Lawal, A.F.; Ologundudu, A.; Adeniran, O.Y.; Omonkhua, A.; Obi, F. Antioxidant effects of heated garlic juice on cadmium-induced liver damage in rats as compared to ascorbic acid. *J. Toxicol. Sci.* **2011**, *36*, 549–557. [CrossRef]
55. Yun, H.M.; Ban, J.O.; Park, K.R.; Lee, C.K.; Jeong, H.S.; Han, S.B.; Hong, J.T. Potential terapeutic effects of functional active compounts from garlic. *Pharmacol. Ther.* **2013**, *142*, 183–195. [CrossRef]
56. Khotimchenko, M.; Serguschenko, I.; Khotimchenko, Y. Lead Absorption and Excretion in Rats Given Insoluble Salts of Pectin and Alginate. *Int. J. Toxicol.* **2006**, *25*, 195–203. [CrossRef] [PubMed]
57. Sato, Y.; Uchida, E.; Aoki, H.; Hanamura, T.; Nagamine, K.; Kato, H.; Koizumi, T.; Ishigami, A. Acerola (*Malpica emarginarta* DC) juice intake supress UVB-induced skin pigmentation in SMP30/GNL knockout hairless mice. *PLoS ONE* **2017**, *23*, e0170438.
58. Dean, C. *The Magnesium Miracle*; Ballantine books: New York, NY, USA, 2007.
59. El-Ansary, A.; Bjorklund, G.; Tinkow, A.A.; Skalny, A.V. Relationship between selenium, lead, and mercury in red blood cells of Saudi austistic children. *Metab. Brain Dis.* **2017**, *32*, 1073–1080. [CrossRef] [PubMed]
60. Moreno, F.; García-Barrera, T.; Gómez-Jacinto, V.; Gómez-Ariza, J.L.; Garbayo-Nores, I.; Vilchez-Lobato, C. Antagonistic interaction of selenomethionine enantiomers on methylmercury toxicity in the microalgae *Chlorella sorokiniana*. *Metallomics* **2014**, *6*, 347. [CrossRef] [PubMed]
61. Mohapatra, D.K.; Mohanty, L.; Mohanty, R.C.; Mohapatra, P.K. Biotoxicity of mercury to *Chlorella vulgaris* as influenced by amino acids. *Acta Biol. Hung.* **1997**, *48*, 497–504.
62. Ripps, H.; Shen, W. Review: Taurine: A "very essential" amino acid. *Mol. Vis.* **2012**, *18*, 2673–2686. [PubMed]
63. Cabaña-Muñoz, M.E.; Parmigiani-Izquierdo, J.M.; Camacho-Alonso, F.; Merino, J.J. Increased Systemic Malondialdehyde Levels and Decreased Mo/Co, Co/Fe^{2+} Ratios in Patients with Long-Term Dental Titanium Implants and Amalgams. *J. Clin. Med.* **2019**, *8*, 86. [CrossRef]
64. Shi, C.; Zhou, X.; Zhang, J.; Wang, J.; Xie, H.; Wu, Z. Alpha lipoic acid protects against the cytotoxicity and oxidative stress induced by cadmum in HepG2 cells through regeneration of glutathione by glutathione reductase via Nrf-2/ARE signaling pathway. *Environ. Toxicol. Pharmacol.* **2016**, *45*, 274–281. [CrossRef] [PubMed]
65. Uchikawa, T.; Kumamoto, Y.; Maruyama, I.; Kumamoto, S.; Ando, Y.; Yasutake, A. The enhanced elimination of tissue methylmercury in *Parachlorella beijerinckii*-fed mice. *J. Toxicol. Sci.* **2011**, *36*, 121–126. [CrossRef] [PubMed]
66. Kumar, R.M.; Frankilin, J.; Raj, S.P. Accumulation of heavy metals (Cu, Cr, Pb and Cd) in freshwater micro algae (*Chlorella* sp.). *J. Environ. Sci. Eng.* **2013**, *55*, 371–376.
67. Bai, Y.; Wang, D.; Cui, X.; Yang, Z.; Zhu, M.; Zhang, Z.; Xia, G.; Gong, Y. Preventive effects of selenium-enriched spiruline (SESP) on radiation pneumonitis. *J. Environ. Pathol. Toxicol. Oncol.* **1998**, *17*, 159–163. [PubMed]
68. Evseeva, T.I.; Maĭstrenko, T.A.; Geras'kin, S.A. An assessment of relative contribution of DNA reparation and glutathione-dependent pathway of detoxification in response of Chlorella algae to uranium. *Radiats Biol. Radioecol.* **2013**, *53*, 236–245.
69. Horikoshi, T.; Nakajima, A.; Sakaguchi, T. Update of uranium by various cell fractions of *Chlorella vulgaris*. *Radioisotopes* **1979**, *28*, 485–488. [CrossRef] [PubMed]
70. Simmons, D.B.D.; Hayward, A.R.; Hutchinson, T.C.; Emery, R.J.N. Identification and quantification of glutathione and phytochelatins from *Chlorella vulgaris* by RP-HPLC ESI-MS/MS and oxygen-free extraction. *Anal. Bioanal. Chem.* **2009**, *395*, 809–817. [CrossRef] [PubMed]
71. Paiva, L.; Lima, E.; Neto, A.I.; Baptista, J. Angiotensin I-converting enzyme (ACE) inhibitory activity of *Fucus spiralis* macroalgae and influence of the extracts storage temperature—A short report. *J. Pharm. Biomed. Anal.* **2016**, *131*, 503–507. [CrossRef]
72. Lopes, G.; Andrade, P.B.; Valentão, P.; McPhee, D.J. Phlorotannins: Towards New Pharmacological Interventions for Diabetes Mellitus Type 2. *Molecules* **2016**, *22*, 56. [CrossRef]
73. Turner, A.; Poon, H.; Taylor, A.; Brown, M.T. In situ determination of trace elements in *Fucus sp* by field-portabel-XRF. *Sci. Total Environ.* **2017**, *593–594*, 227–235. [CrossRef] [PubMed]
74. Henriques, B.; Lopes, C.B.; Figueira, P.; Rocha, L.S.; Duarte, A.C.; Vale, C.; Pardal, M.A.; Pereira, E. Bioaccumulation of Hg, Cd and Pb by *Fucus vesiculosus* in single and multi-metal contamination scenarios and its effect on growth rate. *Chemosphere* **2017**, *171*, 208–222. [CrossRef] [PubMed]

75. Gabbia, D.; Dall'Acqua, S.; Di Gangi, I.M.; Bogialli, S.; Caputi, V.; Albertoni, L.; Marsilio, I.; Paccagnella, N.; Carrara, M.; Giron, M.C.; et al. The Phytocomplex from *Fucus vesiculosus* and *Ascophyllum nodosum* Controls Postprandial Plasma Glucose Levels: An In Vitro and In Vivo Study in a Mouse Model of NASH. *Mar. Drugs* **2017**, *15*, 41. [CrossRef] [PubMed]
76. Yano, J.M.; Yu, K.; Donaldson, G.P.; Shastri, G.G.; Ann, P.; Ma, L.; Nagler, C.R.; Ismagilov, R.F.; Mazmanian, S.K.; Hsiao, E.Y. Indigenous Bacteria from the Gut Microbiota Regulate Host Serotonin Biosynthesis. *Cell* **2015**, *163*, 258. [CrossRef]
77. Simpore, J.; Kabore, F.; Zongo, F.; Dansou, D.; Bere, A.; Pignatelli, S.; Biondi, D.M.; Ruberto, G.; Musumeci, S. Nutrition rehabilitation of undernourished children utilizing Spiruline and Misola. *Nutr. J.* **2006**, *5*, 3. [CrossRef]

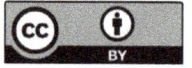

© 2019 by the authors. Licensee MDPI, Basel, Switzerland. This article is an open access article distributed under the terms and conditions of the Creative Commons Attribution (CC BY) license (http://creativecommons.org/licenses/by/4.0/).

MDPI
St. Alban-Anlage 66
4052 Basel
Switzerland
Tel. +41 61 683 77 34
Fax +41 61 302 89 18
www.mdpi.com

Antioxidants Editorial Office
E-mail: antioxidants@mdpi.com
www.mdpi.com/journal/antioxidants

www.ingramcontent.com/pod-product-compliance
Lightning Source LLC
LaVergne TN
LVHW070711100526
838202LV00013B/1072